DEAF PEOPLE

Evolving Perspectives from Psychology, Education, and Sociology

JEAN F. ANDREWS

Lamar University

IRENE W. LEIGH

Gallaudet University

MARY T. WEINER

Gallaudet University

Boston ■ New York ■ San Francisco
Mexico City ■ Montreal ■ Toronto ■ London ■ Madrid ■ Munich ■ Paris
Hong Kong ■ Singapore ■ Tokyo ■ Cape Town ■ Sydney

Executive Editor and Publisher: *Stephen D. Dragin*
Series Editorial Assistant: *Barbara Strickland*
Manufacturing Buyer: *Andrew Turso*
Marketing Manager: *Tara Whorf*
Production Coordinator: *Pat Torelli Publishing Services*
Editorial-Production Service: *TKM Productions*
Electronic Composition: *TKM Productions*

For related titles and support materials, visit our online catalog at www.ablongman.com.

Between the time Website information is gathered and then published, it is not unusual
for some sites to have closed. Also, the transcription of URLs can result in unintended
typographical errors. The publisher would appreciate notification where these occur so
that they may be corrected in subsequent editions.

Library of Congress Cataloging-in-Publication Data

Andrews, Jean F.
    Deaf people : evolving perspectives from psychology, education, and sociology/
    Jean F. Andrews, Irene W. Leigh, Mary T. Weiner
        p. cm.
    Includes bibliographical references and indexes.
    ISBN 0-205-33813-5
        1. Deaf. 2. Deaf--Psychology. 3. Deafness--Psychological aspects. 4. Deaf--Means of
communication. 5. Deaf--Education. I. Leigh, Irene W. II. Weiner, Mary T. III. Title.

HV2380.A63 2004
362.4'2--dc21

                                2003043723

Printed in the United States of America

10 9 8 7 6 5 4 3 2 1   07 06 05 04 03

CONTENTS

Preface   xi

Acknowledgments   xvii

CHAPTER ONE

**Historical Perspectives of Deaf People and Psychology:
1950 to the Present   1**
by McCay Vernon, Ph.D.

CHAPTER OBJECTIVES   2

PSYCHOLOGY AND DEAF PEOPLE   2

THE LAST HALF CENTURY   3
Court Decisions and Legislation in the 1970s, 1980s, and 1990s   4

PSYCHOLOGISTS AND EDUCATIONAL POLICY   6

PROFESSIONAL TRAINING   7

PROFESSIONAL ASSOCIATIONS   7

PSYCHIATRY AND MENTAL HEALTH   8

DEAF CULTURE   10

CONCLUSION   13

SUGGESTED READINGS   13

CHAPTER TWO

The Deaf Community: A Diverse Entity   15

CHAPTER OBJECTIVES   16

DEAF PEOPLE   16

DEMOGRAPHICS   17

LABELS OF DIFFERENT PERSPECTIVES   18

TWO MODELS   20
The Medical/Disability Model   20
The Sociolinguistic/Cultural Model   22

iii

BELIEF SYSTEMS   23

DEAF CULTURE: THE ANTHROPOLOGY VIEW   25

VALUES AND CUSTOMS   26

MEMBERSHIP   27
Deaf of Deaf Parents   27
Deaf of Hearing Parents   27
Hearing Members in Deaf Families   27
Hard-of-Hearing Children of Deaf or Hearing Parents   28
Deaf Adoptive and Foster Children   28
Late-Deafened Persons   29
Deaf-Blind Persons   29
Ethnic Differences   30

TRANSMISSION OF DEAF CULTURE   30
Deaf Studies Programs   33

DEAF COMMUNITIES   33

CONCLUSION   34

SUGGESTED READINGS   35

CHAPTER THREE

Where Does It All Begin?   37

CHAPTER OBJECTIVES   38

ETIOLOGY: THE CAUSES OF HEARING LOSS   38
The Significance of Etiology   38
Major Nongenetic Causes of Deafness   39
Genetic Causes of Deafness   43
Genetic Transmission of Deafness   44
Major Genetic Syndromes Involving Deafness   48
Genetic Counseling   50

THE DIAGNOSIS OF DEAFNESS   52
Hearing Screening   52
The Diagnostic Phase   53
Deaf Parents   56
The Aftermath of Diagnosis and Psychological Considerations   56

CONCLUSION   58

SUGGESTED READINGS   59

APPENDIX: THE BASICS OF AUDIOLOGY   60

CHAPTER FOUR

Language, Cognition, and the Mind   67

CHAPTER OBJECTIVES   68

EARLY GESTURAL ROOTS   68

ASL AND ENGLISH STRUCTURE: A COMPARISON   70

LANGUAGE PATHS   75

THE CRITICAL PERIOD   78

THE BRAIN AND THE ENVIRONMENT   79

BILINGUALISM, INTELLIGENCE, AND THINKING   81

LEARNING HOW TO THINK, REMEMBER, AND LEARN   82

TRANSFER OF COGNITIVE ABILITIES TO ACADEMIC LEARNING   83

CONCLUSION   87

SUGGESTED READINGS   87

CHAPTER FIVE

From Communication to Language to Literacy   89

CHAPTER OBJECTIVES   90

FIRST CONVERSATIONS   90

THE READING PROCESS   92
  Recognizing Words   93
  Reading, Writing, and Spelling Development   96
  Reading Comprehension   97
  Language-Teaching Approaches and Bridges to Literacy   98
  Literacy and Content Subjects   100
  Miscue (Error) Analysis and Eye Movements   101

SOCIOCULTURAL PROCESSES   101
  Bilingualism and Reading English as a Second Language   102
  Technology in the Classroom   103
  Unique Populations with Literacy Needs Using Sign Language   106

CONCLUSION   108

SUGGESTED READINGS   108

CHAPTER SIX

Educational Aspects   109

CHAPTER OBJECTIVES   110

PLACEMENT ISSUES   110

INDIVIDUALS WITH DISABILITIES EDUCATION ACT (IDEA)   111

SCHOOL PLACEMENTS   113
Early Intervention Programs   113
Residential Schools   114
Day Schools   116
Charter Schools   116
Public School Placement Alternatives   117
Placement Changes and Consequences   124

USE OF TESTING IN EDUCATION   125

MULTICULTURAL ISSUES   126

TEACHER TRAINING ISSUES   128
Training Deaf Teachers   130
Training Minority Teachers   131

INTERNATIONAL DEAF EDUCATION   131

BILL OF RIGHTS FOR DEAF AND HARD-OF-HEARING CHILDREN   132

CONCLUSION   132

SUGGESTED READINGS   132

CHAPTER SEVEN

**Language Learning and Language Teaching Approaches:
A Sociocultural View   135**

CHAPTER OBJECTIVES   136

COMMUNICATION COMPETENCE   136

MONOLINGUAL APPROACHES   138
Issues with Monolingual Approaches   141

LANGUAGE-MIXING   144
Issues with Language-Mixing Approaches   150

BILINGUAL APPROACHES   150
Issues with Bilingual Approaches   154

CONCLUSION   155

SUGGESTED READINGS   155

CHAPTER EIGHT

Psychological Issues in Childhood   157

CHAPTER OBJECTIVES   158

THE PARENT/CHILD RELATIONSHIP   158

ATTACHMENT   159

EARLY INTERVENTION PROGRAMS   163

CHILD DEVELOPMENT AND DEAFNESS   165
  Foundations for Language Development   165
  The Role of Play in Early Cognitive Development   166
  Psychosocial Development   167
  The Role of Deaf Professionals in Psychosocial Development   173

CHILDHOOD PSYCHOPATHOLOGY   173

CHILD ABUSE AND ITS CONSEQUENCES   175

TREATMENT PROGRAMS   177

PSYCHOLOGICAL EVALUATION OF DEAF CHILDREN   177

CONCLUSION   178

SUGGESTED READINGS   179

CHAPTER NINE

Being a Deaf Adult: Viewpoints from Psychology   181

CHAPTER OBJECTIVES   182

POSITIVE PSYCHOLOGY AND POSITIVE HEALTH   182

THE DEAF ADULT: PSYCHOLOGICAL PERSPECTIVES   183

PSYCHOLOGICAL ASSESSMENT OF DEAF ADULTS   188

PSYCHOPATHOLOGY   195
  Prevalence   195
  Service Delivery   197
  Diversity   198

CONCLUSION   199

SELECTED BOOKS ABOUT DEAF PEOPLE   199

CHAPTER TEN

Being a Deaf Adult: Viewpoints from Sociology   201

CHAPTER OBJECTIVES   202

SOCIOLOGICAL PERSPECTIVES OF THE DEAF COMMUNITY   202

DEAF PRESIDENT NOW: IMPLICATIONS FOR THE DEAF COMMUNITY   203

DEAF ORGANIZATIONS   206
Specialized Organizations   208
Ethnic Deaf Groups   210
Religious Groups   210
Deaf Clubs   211
Sports   211

HEALTH CARE ISSUES   212

THE WORLD OF WORK   213

LEGAL ISSUES   216

CONCLUSION   217

SUGGESTED READINGS   218

APPENDIX: ORGANIZATIONS' WWW ADDRESSES   219

CHAPTER ELEVEN

Deaf-Hearing Relationships in Context   221

CHAPTER OBJECTIVES   222

"INTERESTING" ATTITUDES   223

THE INFLUENCE OF PERCEPTIONS   224

MEANINGS OF DISABILITY AND DEAFNESS   225

THE OTHER SIDE   226

PROFESSIONAL ATTITUDES   227

OPPRESSION   230

HEALTHY WAYS OF RELATING   231

INTERPRETER ISSUES   233

ATTITUDES WITHIN THE DEAF COMMUNITY   237

CONCLUSION   238

SUGGESTED READINGS   239

CHAPTER TWELVE
To the Future   241

ADVANCES IN MENTAL HEALTH SERVICES   242

AMERICAN SIGN LANGUAGE   244

CHANGES IN THE DEAF COMMUNITY   246

ADVANCES IN MOLECULAR GENETICS AND COCHLEAR IMPLANTATION   249

EDUCATION ISSUES   251

TECHNOLOGY   253

CONCLUSION   254

Appendix: Websites   255

References   259

Name Index   285

Subject Index   291

Daily, most of us encounter individuals who do not hear. Hearing loss is increasingly common and currently affects almost 28 million Americans, whereas profound, congenital deafness is relatively less common, occurring in 0.1 percent of the population. Yet, it is everywhere. You may have elderly family members who wear hearing aids and use amplifiers on their telephones. Or you may have a neighbor who has a noise-induced hearing loss from working in a manufacturing plant. Possibly you work at a business that employs a deaf coworker. Sitting next to you in a college classroom may be a deaf student with a sign language interpreter. Possibly you have seen a deaf actress in a movie or in a commercial or seen a sign language interpreter next to a political candidate. Some of you have friends with deaf family members. You may be deaf or hard of hearing yourself. Such encounters—ranging from superficial to significant—raise many questions.

What causes hearing loss? Can it be cured with genetic engineering? Should it? Can it be fixed with a hearing aid or a cochlear implant? Just how effective are these devices? Can deaf persons lip-read? What is sign language? Should deaf children go to special schools or mainstream public schools with appropriate services? Just what are appropriate services? How do deaf children think and learn? How are deaf persons bilingual and bicultural? How do deaf children learn to read without being able to hear the words? Are there differences in personalities between deaf and hearing persons? Do deaf people consider themselves monolingual, bilingual, or trilingual? What is Deaf culture? Do deaf people consider themselves bicultural or multicultural? Do deaf communities isolate deaf people from the hearing world? What types of education levels do deaf persons achieve? What kinds of jobs do deaf people have? What kinds of visual assistive devices do deaf persons like to use? What kind of life does an elderly deaf person have—one of isolation or one of community? How do individuals who have a hearing loss combined with cognitive disabilities, learning disabilities, or vision losses cope in our society? Persons interested in hearing loss and its implications ask such questions. We address these topics in this text.

This book is about trying to understand deafness through our own experiences and years of study. Historians, philosophers, and scientists have pondered these questions for centuries. Psychologists have studied behaviors, personalities, and the nature of intelligence in those who are deaf. Linguists have analyzed how sign languages are structured. Developmental psychologists and sociolinguists have studied how deaf children acquire and learn languages. Anthropologists and sociologists have investigated Deaf culture and how deaf communities* are formed and maintained, and how they change over time. Geneticists and biologists have

*The lowercase *d* reflects the inability to hear, whereas a capital *D* is frequently used to represent a group of people who share a signed language and culture. Also see pages xiv and 16.

determined hereditary causes of deafness and have attempted to map the genes involved in hearing. Speech pathologists and audiologists have researched the impact of limited auditory input on the acquisition of speech. Cognitive scientists have studied the way deaf children think, remember, and learn. Teachers have addressed issues deaf children face. Deaf artists have painted pictures and created sculptures. Deaf writers have composed stories, poems, plays, and histories about the deaf experience.

In recent years, hearing loss has gained increased attention in the media. The personal stories of celebrities who have lost their hearing later in life, such as Hollywood actress Nanette Fabray and radio personality Rush Limbaugh, have increased our understanding of the impact of hearing loss on late-deafened individuals. There have also been newspaper stories of deaf individuals working in the towers of the World Trade Center on September 11, 2001, that have heightened our awareness of the need for special emergency evacuation procedures for deaf employees. News articles on the anthrax scare have shown that deaf postal workers in New Jersey, Washington, DC, Illinois, and Minnesota were not given full information on medical precautions nor did they have access to sign language interpreters during these national emergencies (Suggs, 2001b). Such events have helped bring public attention to the effects of hearing loss.

How do these varied insights of different disciplines, personal histories, and media stories mesh together? Although many books have been written that cover a breadth of issues concerning the development of deaf, hard-of-hearing, and deaf-blind people throughout the life span, there have been few books that have looked under the surfaces of these issues related to the deaf experience from the perspective of deaf authors. Most existing texts have been shortsighted in that they have emphasized what deaf people *cannot* do—speak normally and hear—rather than what they *can* do—grow, think, learn, create, and become contributing members of society. This book explains how being deaf affects people's lives not only from the professional perspective but also from the adult deaf persons' viewpoint.

The absence of hearing affects a person's life in profound ways, altering experiences, interpersonal relationships, and communication styles. It results in different auditory experiences and often cognitive and linguistic deprivation, not because of the deafness itself, but because an optimum visually accessible environment for language and communication is not provided. These causes and consequences are what comprise understanding the psychological, linguistic, sociological, and educational impact of hearing loss on deaf people—the subject of this book.

Although the lives of many people who are deaf do not necessarily center on access to auditory experiences, we will not ignore this issue. Hearing loss varies on a continuum from mild to profound, and a good number of individuals do benefit from auditory rehabilitation (e.g., hearing aids, cochlear implants, and other assistive devices). Nor can we ignore the medical aspects. Many of the varied etiologies of hearing loss, whether congenital or occurring after birth, also result in health problems, such as ear infections, heart malfunctions, diabetes, emotional disturbances, and cognitive and behavioral difficulties, among others. These warrant medical attention, treatment, and special services (Vernon, 1969a).

There are also an increasing number of deaf individuals, young and old, who are confronting issues of diminishing vision and hearing. The prevalence of deaf-blindness, considered a low-incidence disability, has been estimated to be about 735,000 people (Schein & Delk, 1974). Special considerations are needed, such as mobility, technology access, vocational and employment training, counseling, transportation, housing, literacy, life skills, and interpreter services.

We need to keep in mind the fact that there is much more to understanding life as a deaf person or a deaf-blind person than a focus on auditory and medical perspectives. This is where we, the two deaf authors of this book, enter the picture. We have experienced what it means to be deaf in a multitude of ways. We are the consequences of what professional advice was imparted to our hearing parents when they discovered we did not hear. We have experimented with auditory amplification. We are the products of varied educational systems, and in the process, we have explored different communication and language parameters. We have interacted with deaf individuals from different walks of life and with different ways of adapting. We are part of the deaf community and are intimately aware of Deaf culture. The information and the life experiences of people who are deaf that are presented in this book have been filtered through our eyes.

The concept of *Deaf culture* has strongly impacted the way deaf persons are viewed by hearing people, and especially by deaf people. For many, Deaf culture provides a pathway for achieving a healthy psychosocial development and adjustment to life. Deaf culture has the potential both to prevent and limit social isolation. It allows for a shared experience and a sense of commonality among deaf people that they rarely experience in the majority hearing society. Many deaf people use American Sign Language (ASL) and its contact variations (Lucas & Valli, 1992).* Not only does this permit easy communication through vision, gestures, and movement unfettered by speech that becomes tedious and difficult to produce without clear access to auditory feedback but it also strengthens the bonding within the deaf community.

The three authors—one hearing and two deaf—present perspectives on current issues, including the following topics:

- Historical perspective of Deaf people and psychology
- The deaf community—a diverse entity
- Etiologies or causes of deafness
- Cognition, language, and communication
- Communication, language, and literacy
- Educational aspects
- Bilingual and monolingual approaches to language learning
- Childhood psychological issues
- Psychological viewpoints of deaf adults
- Sociological viewpoints of deaf adults

---

* Contact signing in the Deaf community is that kind of signing that results from the contact between ASL and English and exhibits features of both languages (Lucas & Valli, 1992, p. xiv).

- Psychodynamics of interaction between deaf and hearing people
- Research implications

Each of these topics can be thought of as one of a number of pieces of colored glass which, when arranged together, form a window through which you can better understand deaf people and their experiences.

A word about terminology: In common parlance, people tend to use the word *deaf* in a narrow sense to mean persons who cannot hear at all or those who will remain mute. Many audiologists and medical professionals are also reluctant to use the word *deaf* due to misinterpretations of that word. Rarely are deaf persons mute. In fact, the term *deaf-mute* is inappropriate and offensive. It should not be used to describe a person who is deaf. Deaf people vary in their ability to use whatever level of residual hearing they have, depending on a multitude of factors. Often, audiologists and medical professionals are shortsighted in counseling parents. In their attempts to quantify the nature of hearing loss on an audiogram, they often mislead families about the functional and realistic use of residual hearing for everyday communication and learning in the classroom. This misleading is not intentional. In fact, these professionals are often unaware that the information is misleading to parents. This well-intentioned error results in an enormous emotional and psychological cost to the deaf and hard-of-hearing child. For example, a deaf child may have sufficient residual hearing to hear environmental noises or even some speech sounds, but not enough to make speech understandable. To simply put amplification on the child and expect him or her to function in a large, noisy classroom of hearing children without appropriate visual support services jeopardizes the child's academic progress, negatively affects the child's emotional adjustment, and leads to an experience that is tedious, tiring, and counterproductive. In this book, we describe educational programs that build on all the strengths the child has, with particular attention to visual assets, rather than building solely on auditory avenues. Many parents dream of deaf children hearing and speaking, but the reality is that there is much variability in a deaf child's abilities to speak and hear. Professionals would do well to remember this and communicate it to parents, rather than imply that all deaf people can talk, hear, and lip-read.

We acknowledge the pride that culturally Deaf people have when it comes to the term *deaf*. They prefer to use the term *Deaf* to represent them, even if some of them are audiologically considered to be only hard of hearing. Such Deaf people proudly identify themselves as being *culturally Deaf*. To culturally Deaf people, the terms *hearing impaired* and *hard of hearing* are offensive. Those Deaf people who consider themselves as part of that culture are identified as *Deaf* with the uppercase *D* letter; whereas those who are not affiliated with Deaf culture are viewed as being just *deaf*, with the lowercase letter *d*. This distinction is important and respected in Deaf culture, but not known by most of the general population. This uppercase *Deaf* and lowercase *deaf* terminology reflects fundamentally different ways of coping with and feeling about hearing loss.

Our intended audience is a wide range of undergraduate and graduate students, parents, and professionals interested in working with deaf and hard-of-hearing persons—such as psychologists, linguists, social workers, physicians and nurses, educators and administrators, special educators, artists, anthropologists, sociologists, and other interested persons. We hope that researchers will be stimulated by our efforts to raise and examine key issues that puzzle us all in terms of the deaf experience and its implications on how we think, socialize, learn, behave, and acquire languages, whether we hear or not.

We use the term *deaf* in a positive manner to mean a person who does not necessarily rely primarily on audition for everyday speech conversations but must also use visual means of communication in relating with the people and the environment. We use the term *hard of hearing* to mean a person who can use audition to understand speech but who can also benefit from visual forms of communication and support services. Our use of the words *deaf* and *hard of hearing* also encompasses the positive values of identity and inclusion in a vital support group—the Deaf culture and the deaf community. Most Deaf Americans would like physicians, audiologists, and speech-language pathologists to learn about their Deaf culture and to share this information with parents and other professionals. We also hope that deaf and hard-of-hearing people and their families will be interested in comparing their own personal experiences with what we present in this book.

ACKNOWLEDGMENTS

This book reflects the observations and knowledge culled from lifetimes of experience. It also reflects a collective endeavor, and we gratefully acknowledge the help of those who helped us bring this book to completion.

In the process of producing a book, precision is enhanced by those who help to ensure accuracy in content and editing. In this respect, we gratefully acknowledge McCay Vernon, Ph.D., who not only agreed to write Chapter 1 but also spent considerable time reviewing the entire manuscript and emphasizing points we needed to make. Additionally, we thank the following reviewers who provided thoughtful comments on earlier versions of this manuscript: James C. Blair, Utah State University; Brenda Cartwright, Lansing Community College; Jack Foreman, University of Tulsa; Ann E. Geers, Central Institute for the Deaf; P. Lynn Hayes, Alabama School for the Deaf; David A. Stewart, Michigan State University; and Barbara K. Strassman, The College of New Jersey. We also greatly appreciate the assistance of Kathleen Arnos, Ph.D., and John Niparko, M.D., who made sure that the information presented in Chapter 3 was genetically and medically accurate. Dr. Arnos also provided additional documentation to support the reference base for the chapter. Dr. Michael Stinson provided information on steno-based and computer-assisted note-taking systems in Chapter 5. In addition, John B. Christiansen, Ph.D., reviewed Chapter 10 from the perspective of a sociologist and provided comments that aided the revision process. Lisa Devlin, M.S., and James G. Phelan, Au.D., made sure that the information in the audiology appendix was accurately and impeccably presented. Also, we give our profound thanks to our editors, Steve Dragin and Barbara Strickland. They took considerable time to assist us with this book and bring it to fruition.

Gallaudet University graduate research assistants Thomas Zangas, Lydia Prentiss, Michael John Gournaris, Robert Baldwin, and Sarah Jerger, as well as Lamar University graduate research assistants Anna Miller and Becky Icken, ably contributed reference sources, checked the accuracy of citations, and organized the references in final form. To them, we express appreciation. We also thank Taryn M. Sykes for her photography.

We authors are all university professors. The inspiration for our work comes from our students, who challenge us to teach them using the most recent knowledge. We are also inspired by the desire to impart to all students our dedication to the training of new generations of professionals working with deaf children, youth, and adults. To these students, we give profound thanks. We know that our students, both deaf and hearing, are our future. We hope this book stimulates them to question traditional practices, look critically and thoughtfully at our varied perspectives, and add to our research base in their future work.

Even though two of us authors are deaf and one hears, each one of us knows in her own way what it means to be deaf and how deaf people live their lives in different ways. Our perceptions were not always in agreement, because we come from divergent backgrounds. But these perceptions definitely have been enlarged by our varied experiences with the deaf community and Deaf culture. Without knowing the deaf community, our lens would have had a much more narrow focus, and finding common ground would have been more arduous. We thank the deaf community for enriching us with their zest for life, their worldviews, and their confidence in their own abilities to assert themselves in the face of a world that is not always accommodating.

Jean F. Andrews is indebted to Dr. Steve Nover, director of the Center for ASL/English Bilingual Education and Research (CAEBER) at the New Mexico School for the Deaf, who led her to the bilingual literature and influenced her thinking on language learning and language teaching. She also gratefully acknowledges Mindy Bradford, Dr. Laurene Gallimore, Dr. Cindy Bailes, Dr. Victoria Everhart, and Dr. Jay Innes for the many pleasurable hours of debate and discussions about bilingualism, multiculturalism, literacy, and technology. Jean F. Andrews also thanks Dennis Vail, Ph.D., for his editorial advice. She gratefully thanks Dr. Tony Martin, Dr. Mary Ann Gentry, and Dr. Zanthia Smith, her Lamar colleagues who read chapters of the manuscript and covered some of her university duties so she could meet the book deadline.

Irene W. Leigh would like to express appreciation to Gallaudet University for awarding her the 2001–02 Schaefer Professorship, which provided her with release time from courses, thereby enabling her to complete the work for this book on schedule. She also wants to remember Elberta Pruitt, former principal of the A. G. Bell Elementary School in Chicago (which housed a day program for deaf students), who believed in her abilities and advocated for her throughout her elementary, high school, and college years during a time when professionals tended to say "Deaf people can't . . . . " Irene W. Leigh also thanks the mental health staff at the Lexington School for the Deaf/Center for the Deaf in New York City who shaped her professional perspectives early on and her colleagues at Gallaudet University who provided ongoing professional stimulation.

Mary T. Weiner extends her gratitude and appreciation to Jean F. Andrews and Irene W. Leigh for being wonderful mentors. Preliminary editing was done with the assistance of Robert Weinstock, and the credit for final editing goes to one of the mentors, Irene W. Leigh.

Last, but not least, all three of us express our love and appreciation for those on the home front who patiently endured our lengthy sessions at the computer. The support of these loved ones motivated us all throughout the hours as we struggled to find the words to convey to the readers of this book what deafness is all about.

CHAPTER ONE

HISTORICAL PERSPECTIVES OF DEAF PEOPLE AND PSYCHOLOGY

1950 to the Present

MCCAY VERNON, PH.D.

The use of history is to give value to the present hour and its duty.
—Emerson, 1870

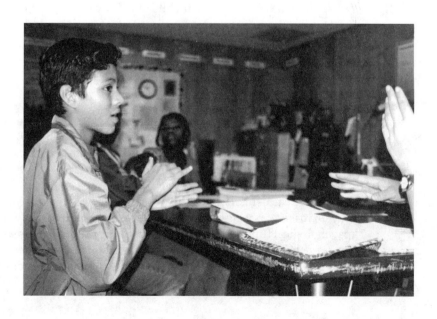

Today, as a consequence of their demand for greater equality and the presence of a more enlightened populace, deaf people are realizing more their potential in education, communications (especially with computers), theater, law, and many other areas. Within the domain of psychology and mental health, psychologists, psychiatrists, and linguists, in particular, have played an important supporting role in these changes. A sequence of events has led to our current understanding of deaf people and psychology.

CHAPTER OBJECTIVES

In this chapter, we describe the history and role of psychologists, psychiatrists, and linguists as they developed approaches that facilitated the mental health and well-being of deaf Americans from the 1950s onward. Critical court decisions are reviewed. The impact of professionals' use of sign language in counseling, in teaching, and in the training of teachers is described. Readers will learn about the way in which professionals highlighted and tied together American Sign Language (ASL) and Deaf culture as they incorporated these into the development of services with deaf individuals.

PSYCHOLOGY AND DEAF PEOPLE

Prior to the 1950s, there were fewer than 10 psychologists and no psychiatrists in the United States with full-time commitment to the mental health of deaf and hard-of-hearing people (Levine, 1977). The few available psychologists were employed in residential schools for deaf children. They essentially functioned as psychometrists, with the primary responsibility of administering IQ tests to incoming students in order to identify those with low IQs or severe behavior problems. The intention was to exclude from enrollment programs for deaf youths those with mental retardation or severe mental illnesses and to refer them to hospitals. Although the state hospitals serving individuals with mental illness or mental retardation were required by law to accept these deaf patients, they offered them no special programs nor were their staffs trained to provide deaf persons treatment or to communicate with them in sign language (Levine, 1977).

This sad state of affairs had two unfortunate consequences: First, deaf people with mental illness or mental retardation got, at best, what was essentially anti-therapeutic custodial care—care that was more for the convenience of society than for their treatment. The second consequence of this dearth of psychologists and psychiatrists was a lack of any quality research into the ways being deaf influenced psychological functioning. For example, prior to 1950, there had been only 18 studies on behavioral aspects of deafness, all done on children (Vernon & Andrews, 1990). Most of these investigations involved the use of grossly inappropriate psychological tests, many of which were verbal or based on the knowledge of English, or behavioral checklists with many items unfair to deaf youth. The results seemed to demonstrate that multiple types of pathology were present, many of which have been proven false by subsequent more valid types of testing and assessment.

In addition to the research on personality and behavioral traits present in deaf children, some 21 studies were conducted involving IQ testing (Vernon, 1967). The summary finding from these studies was that, if nonverbal performance-type tests were used, the IQs of deaf and hearing children did not significantly differ.

No formal research was done on deaf adults because the only psychologists working with deaf individuals were those employed in schools, with the exception of a few college professors, including well-known psychologists and educators of that era, such as Pintner and Paterson (Pollard, 1992–93). These psychologists were part of the first cohort of psychological researchers interested in deaf people. They wanted to see how deaf individuals would perform on IQ tests. Psychologists not only were testing deaf people but were also testing immigrants in Ellis Island. In many cases, they gave verbal IQ tests in English to both groups, thinking that was appropriate, and as a result, classified many as mentally retarded. During these years, the ultimate goal in exploring IQ tests and other psychological instruments was to evaluate their use with different populations. (For a history of the use of IQ tests with immigrants, see Gould, 1981.)

THE LAST HALF CENTURY

Starting in the 1950s, interest in deafness began to increase, partly as the outgrowth of audiological training that developed as a consequence of the impact of World War II on hearing loss. Helmer Myklebust's books, *Auditory Disorders in Children* (1954) and *The Psychology of Deafness* (1960), exemplify research done during those years. For example, he conducted studies using the Minnesota Multiphasic Personality Inventory (MMPI), a verbal-based psychological instrument, with deaf subjects. He did work on diagnosing aphasia in deaf youth and wrote on educating aphasic children. Although much of Myklebust's research has not been supported by later findings, in part because of the inappropriate use of existing instrumentation at the time, he was a psychological pioneer in the field of deafness. His work and that of his students at Northwestern University were important stages in the effort to understand the psychological impact of deafness. In particular, Myklebust was among the first to emphasize that there may be functionally different ways in which deaf children interact with the world, with implications for psychological development (Marschark, 1993). Current neuropsychological research is beginning to demonstrate this phenomenon.

Edna Levine, a contemporary of Mykelbust, was for many years a psychologist at the Lexington School for the Deaf, a prominent oral school for deaf children in New York City, and later became a professor at New York University. Levine had an excellent academic background in psychology, coupled with in-depth exposure to deafness. She, too, published a number of books and articles over a 25-year period, including *Youth in a Silent World* (1956), *Psychology of Deafness* (1960), and *The Ecology of Early Deafness* (1981). Her research monograph on the use of the Hand Test (Levine & Wagner, 1974) as a personality measure for deaf persons, a study on rubella deafened children (Levine, 1951), and her other works have stood the test of time. She was among the first to suggest that the environment was a critical factor in the development of the deaf child, and therefore its influence required critical study (Levine, 1981).

In addition to her contributions to the field of deafness through her work in psychology, Levine also was a major factor in the establishment of the National Theater of the Deaf, which enhanced the careers of deaf actors. She also authored a fictional story about a deaf child—*Lisa and Her Soundless World*, which oriented hearing children to what it meant to be deaf—and she played an influential role in determining federal policies impacting deaf children and adults.

Court Decisions and Legislation in the 1970s, 1980s, and 1990s

Two major court decisions and a series of laws enacted by Congress during the last three decades had major impacts on psychology and deafness. The court decisions were the *Pennsylvania Association for Retarded Citizens* v. *Commonwealth of Pennsylvania* (1972) and *Mills* v. *Board of Education* (1972). The legislation included the Education of All Handicapped Children Act and Section 504 of the Rehabilitation Act of 1973. The Americans with Disabilities Act (ADA) was signed into law in 1990. The ADA expanded the provisions of Section 504 into the private sector. This law also gave deaf persons greater access to public accommodation, transportation, employment, and telecommunications.

The Education for All Handicapped Children Act (Public Law 94-142) was later expanded and renamed the Individuals with Disabilities Act of 1990 (IDEA). This law brought changes to educational programming by requiring a free and appropriate public education for all children with disabilities. The IDEA mandated the development of an individualized family service plan for each child, required that children with disabilities be educated with nondisabled children to the greatest extent possible, and stated that parents have an active role in the decisions related to their children's educational plan.

Another law, the Newborn Infant Hearing Screening and Intervention Act of 1990, provided for funding for state grants for newborn hearing screening and intervention programs (Joint Committee on Infant Hearing, 2000). Although there are benefits and harms of universal newborn hearing screening compared to selective screening of high-risk newborns, this federal legislation is expected to provide for earlier detection of hearing loss so that parents can be informed early of choices in educational placement and communication (Thompson, McPhilips, Davis, Lieu, Homer, & Helfand, 2001) (see Chapters 8 and 12 of this book).

Among the consequences of these laws and court decisions, deaf children are to receive earlier and more appropriate services. For example, prior to the enactment of Section 504 and PL 94-142, children who had been excluded from public schools due to IQs below 70, behavior disorders, or multiple physical disabilities now had to be admitted to these schools and educated. Today, in a residential facility such as the Florida School for the Deaf and Blind, 10 percent of the student body is classified as educationally mentally handicapped, physically impaired, or emotionally handicapped based on very strict criteria (Turrentine-Jenkins, personal communication, January 15, 1999). The influx of these multiply disabled children created a demand for school psychologists and mental health professionals able to provide services.

By 1977, 178 people were working as school psychologists with deaf children, based on a survey by Cantor and Spragins (1977). However, only 9 percent of these persons had credentials as school psychologists. Of these, none had any special training in deafness.

In response to this obvious need for qualified professionals, Gallaudet University established programs to prepare both school psychologists and school counselors for work with deaf and hard-of-hearing children. As graduates of these and other programs have gone out into the field, a nucleus of well-qualified educational psychologists and counselors now exists.

These individuals are providing clinical services, some are doing research, and a number have gone on to complete doctoral work and serve on university faculties. One such individual, Dr. Jeffrey Braden, has also done extensive research on deaf people and intelligence, which is reported in his book *Deafness, Deprivation, and IQ* (Braden, 1994). As a treatise on the implications of deafness for IQ differences between groups, it represents a milestone in the literature on deafness.

As the supply of psychologists increased, it reached a level that would have become sufficient to meet the needs of deaf children who were in state and private residential and day schools for the deaf. However, the trend is for deaf children to be placed in local public school settings rather than residential or specialized day schools. Although this trend in actually started after World War II (Moores, 2001a), Public Law 94-142 (which mandates an appropriate education in the least restrictive environment, whatever that may be) and a series of court decisions based on it has favored the placement of deaf children in their home school districts. There may be only one or a few students with profound hearing losses in an entire school system. In these situations, critical decisions are made regarding these deaf children by psychologists, teachers, and administrators who have little or no experience with deafness and who cannot communicate with them. In such situations, the results are likely to be catastrophic for the child, both educationally and psychologically.

The practice of letting professionals with little or no experience or competence in the field of deafness diagnose and determine educational placement has been challenged peripherally in the courts and the literature, but more and stronger test cases need to be brought to court before the practice will be stopped (Raifman & Vernon, 1996a, 1996b).

PSYCHOLOGISTS AND EDUCATIONAL POLICY

From 1880 until around 1967, deaf youth in the United States and most of Europe were educated orally for the most part (Moores, 2001a). Sign language was strictly forbidden in classes and discouraged or taboo in residence halls, dining rooms, and recreational areas. Parents were routinely told that signing was bad for their children and that sign language was actually not even a language, but merely a group of ugly, primitive gestures.

Dr. William Stokoe, a professor of English at Gallaudet University, did a definitive research analysis of sign language that resulted in his classic *Sign Language Structure: An Outline of the Visual Communication Systems of the American Deaf* (1960). This work and his other research and publications (Stokoe, 1975, 1980; Stokoe, Casterline, & Croneberg, 1965) showed conclusively that American Sign Language (ASL) was a language having the syntactic and vocabulary properties of other languages, such as French, German, and English. Stokoe was vilified for his work by oralists who opposed the teaching of signs, as well as by many of his faculty colleagues at Gallaudet (Stokoe, 2001b). However, his work generated intense interest among a group of bright, young scholars who were fascinated with the origins of language—people such as Eric Lenneberg, Robbin Battison, Ursula Bellugi, Noam Chomsky, Charlotte Baker-Shenk, and Bob Johnson. Many of these individuals did research that further verified and amplified Stokoe's findings and generated increased knowledge of and attraction to ASL by both academics and the lay public.

The profound impact this work had on the education of deaf children was followed by a book, *They Grow in Silence,* written by child psychiatrist Eugene Mindel and myself (Mindel & Vernon, 1971). It was published by the National Association of the Deaf, which felt that it articulated the views of many professionals and persons who were deaf on the role of ASL in the education of deaf youth and its role in facilitating communication within families in which there was a deaf member.

Publication of *They Grow in Silence,* along with investigations in the United States and Great Britain by such researchers as Richard Conrad, Kay Meadow, G. Montgomery, Ross Stuckless, McCay Vernon, and S. Koh, further established that using sign language with deaf youth could facilitate educational achievement and psychological adjustment (see reviews in Mindel & Vernon 1971; Vernon & Andrews, 1990; and Moores, 2001a).

Because of the new perspectives coming from education, psychology, psychiatry, and psycholinguistics, a good number of oralists, especially the young professionals, were beginning to reconsider the role of sign language in the education of deaf children. I remember many instances during this period when, after speaking before groups of teachers and administrators on what the data clearly showed to be the advantages of using signs and finger-spelling along with speech and lip-reading, the controversy over the use of sign would be studiously avoided during the discussion that followed. However, after these discussion sessions ended and the meeting was formally closed, there would always be administrators and teachers employed in schools requiring oral-only education who would come to me when no one else was around to say, "Keep up the good work," "I agree with the data you presented," or other comments in this same vein.

Over time, as bright, younger people have come into the profession with new ideas about educating deaf children, the educators in the field have moved toward greater acceptance of ASL. In fact, today there is more interest and importance given to arguments over the relative merits of bilingualism, total communication, and signing systems based on English usage, as well as the role of speech and listening within these approaches than to the controversy between oralism only versus the use of signed communication in combination with speech.

PROFESSIONAL TRAINING

In addition to its programs to prepare psychologists and counselors at the master's level to work in schools with deaf children, Gallaudet University now has an accredited doctoral program in clinical psychology in addition to accredited graduate school psychology, social work, mental health, and counseling programs. The National Technical Institute for the Deaf at Rochester Institute of Technology has added a new graduate certificate program in school psychology. The California School of Professional Psychology at San Diego has a number of faculty experienced in deafness and is preparing a few doctoral students for work in deafness. Increasingly, more of the students completing these programs are deaf.

A large percent of the social workers and some doctoral-level psychologists with experience in deafness are going into mental health clinics and hospitals. This has resulted in much needed improvement in services, particularly for adult deaf patients using these facilities. However, the number of hospital inpatient units serving deaf adults throughout the United States is currently between 12 and 15 (Schonbeck, 2000). This is very low for the number of deaf adults needing specialized services. For teenagers with serious mental illnesses requiring inpatient care, there is an almost total lack of adequate, appropriate inpatient care (Willis, 1999; Willis & Vernon, 2002). One has to search hard and long throughout the country to find inpatient psychiatric wards for deaf children.

PROFESSIONAL ASSOCIATIONS

In the 1970s, psychologists within the American Psychological Association (APA), the premier organization of psychologists in the United States, began advocating for more attention to disabilities issues, including issues pertinent to deafness (Pollard, 1996). This also included improving accessibility for deaf psychologists within the organization. Barbara Brauer, a deaf psychologist, participated in this endeavor as part of the Task Force on Psychology and Handicaps. The Committee on Disability Issues in Psychology was a direct result of the task force, and deaf psychologists have regularly served on this committee, which has been chaired at different times by Tovah Wax, Allen Sussman, and Irene W. Leigh, all deaf psychologists who have worked to influence APA's sensitivity to people with disabilities as part of the diversity spectrum. Interpreter services have regularly been provided. Additionally, Robert Pollard, recipient of the American Psychological Association's prestigious Distinguished Contributions to Psychology in the Public Interest Award in 1994, who is hearing, spearheaded the APA Special Interest Section for psychologists working in deafness. Both he and Barbara Brauer were on the APA Board for Psychology in the Public Interest, which has a direct influence on APA projects. As a consequence, psychologists in deafness are becoming more a part of the mainstream. Increasingly, papers on deafness are appearing in the association's journals and convention programs.

A similar transformation occurred in the American Psychiatric Association. This goes back to the 1970s, when psychiatrists involved in deafness research, such as Kenneth Altshuler, Eugene Mindel, John Rainer, Franz Kallmann, and Roy Grinker, contributed seminal papers on mental health and deaf people, the first of their kind, to major psychiatric journals and books. Today, the American Psychiatric Association also has a special section for psychiatrists working in deafness with a newsletter edited by Barbara Haskins and several recent publications in American Psychiatric Association journals by research clinicians, such as Annie Steinberg.

PSYCHIATRY AND MENTAL HEALTH

Prior to the mid-1950s, a late-deafened Danish psychiatrist, V. C. Hansen (1929), reported the only research study to appear in the psychiatrist literature on deafness up to that date. Although he did not know sign language, Hansen gathered data on 36 deaf patients in psychiatric hospitals in Denmark in the 1920s. He reported that this represented a 10 times greater prevalence of deaf inmates in Danish psychiatric hospitals than would be expected based on the prevalence of deafness in his country. Hansen also found deaf patients to be significantly more chronic than hearing patients. For example, their average hospital stay was 20 years. Almost one-third (31 percent) of the deaf patients were undiagnosed. This is understandable, considering that there was no hospital staff able to communicate with them in sign language.

In the late 1960s and 1970s, there was a sudden increase of psychiatric interest in deafness in this country and Europe. Major studies were conducted in the United States by Rainer, Altshuler, Kallman, and Deming (1963), Rainer and Altshuler (1966), Grinker (1969), and Robinson (1978). In Great Britain, John Denmark (Denmark & Warren, 1972) pursued similar research. In Scandinavia, major researchers were Terje Basilier of Norway (1964) and Jørgen Remvig of Denmark (1969, 1972). These and later studies are reported in some detail in a 1999 paper (Vernon & Daigle-King, 1999). They were landmark studies that have had a profound impact on our knowledge of deafness and mental health and on the care these patients receive.

A major finding was that when mental patients are placed within a general hospital population and provided no staff or therapists who can communicate in sign language, their stays are much longer than those of hearing patients. More recent studies (Daigle, 1994; Trumbetta, Bonvillian, Siedlecki, & Haskins, 2001) indicate that when provided care by psychologists, psychiatrists, social workers, and nursing staff who can sign and/or when provided round-the-clock sign language interpreting services, deaf patients are no more chronic than their hearing counterparts. It is this access to sign language and professional staff knowledgeable about deafness that has been legislated by the Americans with Disabilities Act of 1990 (ADA) and other civil rights laws. Unfortunately, such services have been provided in only a minority of states. Consent decrees have had to be used to force compliance (Katz, Vernon, Penn, & Gillece, 1992).

Another finding from the studies reporting symptoms that mental health patients demonstrated on admission to psychiatric facilities was that these symptoms generally involved impulsive acts of violence or self-destruction, such as fighting, hitting a family member, destroying property, making suicidal gestures, and so on. Most of the studies noted that organic brain damage was more prevalent among deaf patients, which is understandable in view of the consequences of some etiologies of deafness.

With the exception of the New York State work (Rainer & Altshuler, 1966), the earlier studies did not report cases of the dual diagnoses of substance abuse and mental illness. The New York study found alcoholism to be far less common in deaf patients than in their hearing counterparts. More recent work by Guthman, Lybarger, and Sandberg (1993) and Daigle (1994) indicate substance abuse and mental illness in combination is widespread in both the deaf and hearing populations, but no specific comparative data are provided.

Earlier studies reported more mental retardation among deaf psychiatric patients. A lot of this was due to misdiagnoses by psychologists and psychiatrists (Pollard, 1994, 1996; Vernon, 2001) and therefore felt to be an invalid finding. Pollard (1994) has pointed out some of the problems involved in diagnosing deaf patients, especially when the diagnostician cannot sign and the patient depends on sign language to communicate. This makes some of the data on types of mental illness reported to be present in deaf patients based on past research open to question.

Even though deaf people generally have not been well served by the mental health system, deaf members of minority ethnic backgrounds have been even more poorly served (Pollard, 1994). In the psychiatric studies reported in the literature, minimal attention has been paid to the relationship between ethnic background and diagnostic categorization for these individuals (Leigh, 1999c).

In these psychiatric studies, one conclusion was generally agreed upon: The repression of sign language in schools and the limited ability to understand communication were partially responsible for both the type and amount of psychopathology seen in deaf patients and in the educational retardation and lack of general knowledge found in these individuals (Vernon & Daigle-King, 1999). John Denmark, the British psychiatrist who grew up in a school for the deaf where his father was superintendent, felt strongly about the need to use sign language in the educational process. Thus, in addition to his writings in psychiatric journals, he stated his views in an educational publication (Denmark, 1973).

The only psychiatrist to do a significant amount of research with deaf children was Hilde Schlesinger who, with sociologist Kay Meadow, conducted a series of studies of deaf children and their families (Schlesinger & Meadow, 1972). Their clinical research focused on three primary areas: language acquisition using sign language, mother/child interaction comparing deaf and hearing children, and a comparative study of children whose parents were deaf with those deaf children having normally hearing parents. Among their conclusions were that the controversy then raging over methods of communication was detrimental to the mental health of the children involved. They recommended that a combination of manual communication and speech and lip-reading be used. This recommendation is being implemented today in both the bilingual and total communication programs within the educational setting.

Schlesinger and Meadow also found that when families used sign language with their young deaf children, acquisition generally paralleled milestones in spoken language acquisition. Knowledge of sign language did not interfere with speech acquisition. Instead, spoken words and lip-reading facility increased with sign language acquisition. In addition, the level of communication frustration was decreased in the families they observed who used both oral and manual communication in combination (Schlesinger & Meadow, 1972). Among their other findings were distinct advantages deaf children with deaf parents enjoyed versus deaf children with hearing parents. The difference manifested in areas such as educational achievement, family climate, maturity, and a number of other variables.

Finally, it is important to note that even though inpatient and outpatient services have increased in the United States and Europe over the last few years, most of the significant and relevant research was done more than two decades ago (Vernon & Daigle-King, 1999).

DEAF CULTURE

Over the last decade, an interesting psychological dynamic has arisen. Today, there is a strong reaction by some deaf people to the perception of deafness as a pathology. This is the result of a number of influences. One was the repression and exclusion of deaf people by the majority society (Vernon & Makowsky, 1969), as Stewart (1972) so powerfully delineated in his *New York Times* article, "A Truly Silent Minority." This repression manifested in denying deaf youth the right to use sign language (Lane, 1992; Mindel & Vernon, 1971; Vernon, 1969b). Another factor was that deaf people were not permitted to teach in most schools for the deaf (Andrews & Franklin, 1996/1997; Vernon, 1970). There were no deaf educators serving as heads of schools, for the deaf, and only a few managed to attain lower level administrative jobs (Vernon, 1970; Vernon & Makowsky, 1969). Deaf applicants were refused admission into teacher training programs and graduate schools, even at Gallaudet, an institution of higher learning for the deaf. The rationale for this discrimination was that deaf people would not be able to emphasize articulation (speech) training because they could not hear (Winefield, 1987).

Harlan Lane, a specialist in the psychology of language and linguistics, entered the field of deafness primarily as an observer and historian. A brilliant scholar, recipient of a MacArthur Fellowship, and a prolific author, he found himself offended and angered by the treatment of deaf people by society and by professionals in the field. It was he who early on made the argument that deaf people who chose to interact with others who were deaf formed a cultural minority, different in many respects from hearing people's culture, but not in a pathological manner (Lane, 1992). This supported Carol Padden, a deaf linguist who, in 1980, wrote a seminal article arguing for the existence of an American Deaf culture (Padden, 1980), followed by *Deaf in America: Voices from a Culture* coauthored with Tom Humphries (Padden & Humphries, 1988). Lane made this argument persuasively in his writing, using emotionally laden language to express feelings and thoughts that meshed with the perceptions of deaf leaders and the deaf community. Many of them had harbored those same convictions for years, even though they were not openly expressed. Lane was often polemical and made assumptions that were not always factual (Moores, 1993a, 1993b; Lane, 1993), but he spoke and wrote with a deep conviction that, in addition to its profound impact on deaf people, resonated strongly with young professionals entering work with deaf people.

Lane (1992) was sharply critical of the literature under the rubric of "psychology of the deaf." He lambasted studies that encouraged the perception of deaf people as deviant, deficient, and pathological—studies that were all too often based on questionable methodology and that did not sufficiently take into account numerous factors that might have differentially influenced study results. He has denied the existence of a psychology of the deaf, pointing out that there are no books or scientific studies focusing on the psychology of minority groups. However, it is important to understand how deaf people function psychologically. To emphasize this, courses that examine the interaction between psychology and deafness, with titles such as "Psychology and Deafness," are included within training programs for professionals working with deaf people.

Lane was sharply critical of professionals in the field. In essence, he said that professionals demonstrated insufficient concern for the viewpoints and experiences of deaf people themselves (Lane, Hoffmeister, & Bahan, 1996). This criticism had considerable merit and validity, but it implied all such professionals were guilty of his charges, which was not true. However, Lane's overall contribution to the field of deafness has been in the direction of sensitizing professionals to the need to listen to deaf people themselves and to scrutinize the implications of their research work with deaf people more carefully.

The criticisms and challenges to oralism mentioned earlier were instrumental in bringing about two major changes in deafness: One was the increased use of ASL in schools and classes as part of a total communication or bilingual method of teaching deaf students. The other involved increased opportunities for deaf professionals to become teachers and administrators.

The Gallaudet University teacher-training program opened its doors to deaf applicants in the early 1960s out of the desire to provide deaf students with opportunities equal to those of hearing students (Moores, 2001a). In the early 1970s, a time when most colleges were still refusing to admit deaf students into teacher-training programs, McDaniel College (formerly Western Maryland College) opened its doors to deaf applicants and supplied them with interpreters and some deaf instructors. By the late 1970s and early 1980s, the college had graduated and certified far more deaf teachers than any other program in the United States, including Gallaudet. This pioneering effort put large numbers of deaf professionals in schools and classrooms all over the United States and Canada and set an example now followed by most teacher-training programs nationally.

The climactic culmination of all these changes occurred in March 1988, when a deaf psychologist with the regal name of I. King Jordan was named president of Gallaudet University (Christiansen & Barnartt, 1995). A week earlier, in a well-meaning but demeaning decision, the Gallaudet Board of Trustees had selected a normally hearing woman with no experience in deafness or ability to sign as Gallaudet's new president. This 124-year-old college for the deaf had always had hearing presidents, but this time the deaf student body, deaf faculty, and deaf alumni erupted in open rebellion at what they rightly perceived as an outrageous insult to the competency and integrity of deaf people. After a week of strong protests covered in great detail by national television, newspapers, and other media, the trustees backed down and named Dr. Jordan as president.

This victory by deaf people gave tremendous impetus to the Deaf Pride movement and the feeling by many deaf people that they are a cultural minority who choose to use sign language and associate primarily with other deaf people. They want deafness to be seen not merely as a disability, but more as a human difference.

The issue of whether deafness is a disability has collided with the perception of deafness as a cultural difference. It is true that many of the cultural dimensions of deafness—such as the use of sign language and facial expressions to communicate, a sometimes lack of subtlety in interpersonal relationships, overt ways of getting the attention of others, and so on—have often been perceived by society and professionals in the field as pathological instead of as human differences that represent effective communication from the perceptions of deaf people themselves. However, there are some aspects in which deafness is a disability. When it comes down to reality, most deaf people realize this and accept the fact as evidenced by their fight for their rights under the Americans with Disabilities Act of 1990, Social Security Disability and Supplementary Income provisions, and the Vocational Rehabilitation Act of 1978.

The point to be made is that the hearing population, including professionals, need to focus on and recognize the assets and positive aspects of deaf people. Psychologically, the pendulum has swung from a time when deafness was viewed as a pathology so severe that Alexander Graham Bell, in a paper published by the prestigious National Academy of Science, proposed that stringent eugenics should be applied to eradicate deafness through genetic and reproductive restrictions (Bell, 1883). This bears testimony to the conditions and attitudes deaf people have faced in the past. It makes understandable their desire to have their culture respected and the focus placed on their abilities, not limitations.

CONCLUSION

Psychologists, psychiatrists, and psycholinguists have played an important supporting role in changing the ways society perceives deaf people and their culture, and in facilitating the ability of deaf people to realize their potential and demanding more equality. In the final analysis, this may be the greatest contribution of these disciplines to the mental health and well-being of those who are deaf and hard of hearing.

SUGGESTED READINGS

Maher, J. (1996). *Seeing Language in Sign: The Work of William C. Stokoe.* Washington, DC: Gallaudet University Press.
  This biography of William Stokoe traces his work as an English professor at Gallaudet and chronicles his struggles in getting his idea on the linguistic structure of American Sign Language accepted by both hearing and deaf communities.
Morton, E., & J. Christensen (Eds.). (2000). *Mental Health Services for Deaf People: A Resource Directory.* Washington, DC: Department of Counseling, School of Education and Human Services, Gallaudet University.
  This directory provides program descriptions for mental health services in the United States and Canada. Listed by state, it provides names of directors and agencies, addresses, phone numbers, types of services, accreditation, fees, program size, and accessibility. Copies can be ordered from Gallaudet Research Institute, HMB S-444, Gallaudet University, 800 Florida Avenue, NE, Washington, DC 20002 (phone: 202-651-5000).

CHAPTER TWO

THE DEAF COMMUNITY
A Diverse Entity

*The voice of Deaf people of the modern age is one of cultural explicitness and
self-consciousness and a centeredness around a signed language that is not
reflected in previous images of the Deaf self. However, the level of tension
within communities of Deaf people across the country reflect that, as always,
there is no peace or serenity among ourselves about who we are. "What is
American Sign Language (ASL)?" "What is Deaf culture?" "Am I Deaf or
deaf?" Deaf people ask these pointed questions of each other, of scholars, and of
themselves. There are no answers, of course, because the questions themselves
are born of evolving images of self and self-representation.*

—Humphries, 1996, p. 100

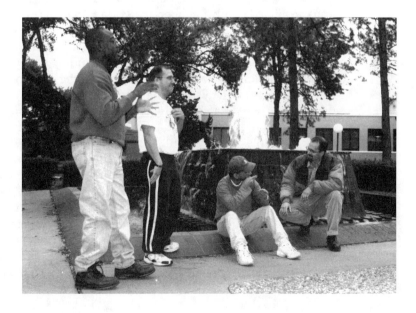

The deaf community has a vibrant history. It provides many deaf people with a place they can call "home." It is a fluid, evolving community. We view the deaf community and Deaf culture as valuable resources for professionals in the fields of medicine, hearing health, psychology and social sciences, and education, as well as for hearing and deaf parents and deaf children.

CHAPTER OBJECTIVES

In this chapter, we provide demographics to help explain what the deaf community is. We show how deaf communities are geographically dispersed, bilingual, and multicultural. We examine the medical and cultural models and challenge negative stereotypes of socially isolated and deprived deaf people. While describing the Deaf culture—its history and heritage, its art and literature, its customs and values—we suggest the advantages this information might hold for understanding and working with deaf and hard-of-hearing people.

DEAF PEOPLE

The *deaf community* is a term that represents a very diverse entity with demographic, audiological, linguistic, political, and social dimensions. There are international, national, regional, and local deaf communities that share and work together to achieve common goals (Van Cleve & Crouch, 1989). The deaf community includes deaf children of hearing parents, deaf children of Deaf parents, hearing members who participate as parents of deaf children, marriage or life partners, siblings, extended family members, coworkers of deaf people, and hard-of-hearing as well as "oral deaf" persons (Singleton & Tittle, 2000). The term *deaf* is used to denote individuals with hearing loss that precludes the understanding of speech through hearing alone, with or without the use of auditory amplification. In contrast, the term *Deaf culture* refers to individuals within the deaf community who use American Sign Language (ASL) and share beliefs, values, customs, and experiences (Padden, 1980). These Deaf individuals are not only deaf offspring of Deaf parents; they are also deaf individuals with hearing family backgrounds who learn about Deaf culture in adolescence or adulthood, if not earlier.

Deaf Americans—children and adults—are as ethnically diverse as the general population (2000 Census). When we say that Deaf Americans are multicultural, we mean that they differ in more ways than just skin color or ethnic heritage. They differ across a variety of dimensions: degree, age, extent of hearing loss, etiology, gender, geographic location, country of birth, communication preference, language use, use of vision, use of technology, educational level, occupation, and socioeconomic background. Most important, many Deaf people have a unique Deaf perspective, commonly referred to as the *Deaf Way*, based on their backgrounds and experiences.

DEMOGRAPHICS

An estimated 28 million Americans in the United States are deaf or hard of hearing (Blanchfield, Feldman, Dunbar, & Gardner, 2001). It is difficult to arrive at accurate estimates. There is a lack of uniformity in defining the term *hearing loss.* There are also multiple data sets, such as self-reports and audiometric results including recent newborn screening statistics. The overall prevalence estimates are roughly 1.1 in 1,000 live births for congenital sensorineural hearing loss. Researchers using current data from universal newborn screening programs have reported data to be 2 to 3 with hearing loss per 1,000 live births. Otitis media (middle-ear infection) accounts for 24.5 million doctor visits and is the most frequently cited reason for taking children to the emergency room. Approximately 10 million Americans have permanent, irreversible hearing loss from noise or trauma. Researchers have reported that people are losing their hearing earlier in life. Men in the 35- to 60-year-old age group are more frequently affected now than in the past (Blanchfield et al., 2001; Fujikawa, 2001).

The numbers of persons over age 65 with hearing loss in the United States is growing and will reach almost 13 million by the year 2015. About 29.1 percent of this population have hearing loss, compared to 3.4 percent of the population ages 18 to 34. The overall prevalence is 10.5 percent for males and 6.8 for females. Males at all ages are more likely than females to be deaf or hard of hearing, with the gap widening after age 18. In the adult population, the prevalence is greater for those who are not high school graduates than for high school graduates. The prevalence of hearing loss for all ages decreases as family income increases. Overall, those with a family income of less than $10,000 are twice as likely as those with a family income of $50,000 and over to have a hearing loss (Blanchfield et al., 2001; Schein, 1996).

An estimated 735,000 persons have vision problems combined with hearing loss that is either congenital or acquired. People with combined vision and hearing loss represent a heterogeneous population of children and adults who may have minimum combined vision and hearing loss or, in the most extreme cases, complete deaf-blindness. The fastest growing segment of the population to be affected by combined vision and hearing loss are the elderly.

Schein (1996) reported the overall prevalence for deafness is 9.4 percent for whites compared to 4.2 percent for African Americans and 4.2 percent for Hispanics. Based on early estimates, there are approximately two million African Americans with hearing loss, of whom 22,000 are profoundly deaf (Hairston & Smith, 1983). However, in a study carried out in Atlanta, Georgia, researchers reported that African American male children had the highest rate of congential deafness, 1.4 per 1,000 (Van Naarden, Decoufle, & Caldwell, 1999).

Approximately 60,000 Asian/Pacific Island (Asian/PI) Deaf persons live in the United States; other estimations are that as many as 600,000 Asian/PI Americans with hearing loss live here (Christensen, 1993). We do not have estimates of Latino adult Deaf Americans. We can infer from national statistics and school-age Hispanic deaf demographics that the Deaf Hispanic American population is increasing.

Large numbers of deaf and hard-of-hearing American Indian populations reside in the states of California, Oklahoma, Arizona, New Mexico, and Alaska. Deaf Native American children pose unique educational, linguistic, and social challenges. For example, more than 200 languages and dialects are spoken within the different tribes, the poverty level is high, and the graduate rate from high school and postsecondary program is low. There is great diversity among American Indian tribes in cultural values, religious and spiritual beliefs, and how tribal identity is developed and maintained (Busby, 2001). There is also great diversity within the Asian American category (e.g., Korean, Japanese, Chinese) and the Hispanic population (e.g., Mexican, Puerto Rican, South American, Spanish). Therefore, simple generalizations regarding the educational, linguistic, and cultural needs of deaf children of color are not possible.

In contrast to the total figures of Americans with hearing loss, it has been estimated that only about 400,000 Deaf Americans and Canadians use ASL and consider themselves part of Deaf culture (Schein, 1996).

Data from Gallaudet Research Institute's Annual Survey of deaf school-age children represent an estimated 60 to 65 percent of all deaf and hard-of-hearing children receiving special education. Due to increases in immigration, the demographic changes among deaf school-age children are dramatic.

Table 2.1 shows three 10-year spans from 1973 to 2001. Deaf children of color increased by almost 10 percent each decade, and in four years (1995 to 1999), we see another 10 percent increase. Deaf children of color already outnumber white children in Texas, California, and New York. Hispanic deaf children, mostly of Mexican heritage, constitute almost 22 percent of the deaf school-age population nationwide. These children of color are assimilated into Deaf culture when they attend a state residential school or, if in the mainstream, later when they join a deaf club or sport organization (Stewart, 1991).

Deaf individuals from multicultural backgrounds often have to live in four worlds: the world of their families, the world of the dominant white culture, the world of the dominant Deaf culture, and the world of Deaf American Latinos, Asians, African Americans, Native Americans, and so on. To meet these challenges, Deaf multicultural Americans have established national organizations to advocate for deaf and hard-of-hearing individuals from culturally diverse communities. These are listed in Chapter 10. Also see the appendix for listing of web addresses.

LABELS OF DIFFERENT PERSPECTIVES

The terminology used by the medical and deaf communities to label deaf Americans reflect different perspectives. Deaf people often differentiate between upper-case *Deaf*, which refers to an affiliation with Deaf culture or the Deaf World, and lowercase *deaf*, which refers to the medical/audiological descriptions of being deaf. Most members of Deaf culture prefer to be referred to as *Deaf* or *hard-of-hearing Americans.* They do not like terms such as *auditory handicap, handicapped* or *disabled, hearing-impaired, hearing-handicapped, hearing-disabled* or *having a hearing loss* because

TABLE 2.1   Race/Ethnic Background of Deaf Children in the United States, 1974 to 2001

RACE/ETHNIC BACKGROUND	1973–74 (n = 43,794)	1983–84 (n = 53,184)	1993–94 (n = 46,099)	1999–2000 (n = 43,861)	2000–2001 (n = 43,416)	PERCENT CHANGE
Total Known Information	41,070	52,330	46,099	42,738	42,603	
White	31,115 76%	35,069 67%	27,779 60%	23,384 55%	22,992 54%	–22
Black/African American	6,407 16%	9,337 18%	7,935 17%	6,945 16%	6757 15.9%	–1
Hispanic	2,987 7%	5,720 11%	7,381 16%	8,903 21%	9,299 21.8%	+14.8
Asian-Pacific Islander	278 .7%	1,130 2%	1,760 4%	1721 4%	1,681 3.9%	+3.2
American-Indian	177 .4%	297 .6%	312 .7%	370 .9%	350 .8%	+.4
Other	106 .3%	479 .9%	638 1%	692 2%	727 1.7%	+1.4
Multiethnic	Not reported	298 .6%	294 .6%	723 2%	797 1.9%	+1.3*

* Percent change from 1983–84.

Source: 1973–74 to 2000–01 Annual Surveys of Deaf and Hard of Hearing Children & Youth. Washington, DC: Gallaudet Research Institute, Gallaudet University. Reprinted with permission.

these terms focus only on the disability and not who they are or how they live (Stewart, 1991). Such medical terms imply a condition in need of "correction" or repair, which many Deaf Americans see as stigmatizing. These individuals do not think of themselves as needing to be auditorily "fixed" or "cured, " because they can rely primarily on vision as an alternative approach to communication. Rather, they prefer to view themselves as a distinct linguistic and cultural group, seeking equal access to communication, education, and employment opportunities, just like other diverse Americans (Lane, Hoffmeister, & Bahan, 1996; Padden & Humphries, 1988).

On the other hand, professionals often use the generic term *hearing-impaired*, utilizing the term *deaf* only for children or adults who have a profound hearing loss of 91 decibels (db) or greater. The terms *deaf and dumb* and *deaf-mute* were used in times past, and deaf children were placed in asylums. But deaf people are not mute—they can speak and communicate, and the term *asylum* connotes a care-taking facility for mentally deficient or mentally ill persons, not a school where children are educated.

Many Deaf Americans prefer to use descriptions based on a communication mode using these designations: *Strong-deaf, deaf, encultured deaf, oral, deaf-deaf, high-sign,* and *strong-oral.* These labels point to the diversity of communication modes Deaf Americans use—ASL, English in a sign, spoken, or written mode, or a combination. These designations provide more information about communication than the term *hearing loss,* but they give an incomplete picture of the person's individuality, feelings, interests, strengths, special talents, and so forth (Corker, 1996).

There are some persons with hearing losses who do not adopt the norms and beliefs of Deaf culture (Stewart, 1991; Van Cleve & Crouch, 1989). They consider themselves *oral deaf.* Although they may not use ASL openly or join Deaf culture organizations, oral deaf persons will utilize the technology that the deaf community can take advantage of—*visual* technologies such as visual alerting devices, vibro-tactile devices, TTYs (text telephones used to facilitate visual communication using telephone lines), closed-captioned TV, real-time captioning, speech recognition software, and so on, as well as *auditory* devices such as hearing aids, and assistive listening devices such as audio loops, and, more recently, cochlear implants. Other communication technologies that provide a bridge between individuals include two-way pagers, telecommunication relay services, video interpreting services, videoconferencing, email, instant messaging (text and sign video), and handheld wireless devices. Gallaudet University's Technology Access Program (TAP) researches accessibility issues using technology (www.tap.gallaudet.edu).

Oral deaf Americans and those who identify with Deaf culture recognize common needs and have worked together, as part of the deaf community, on joint projects such as TTY dissemination ventures and teacher certification standards for CED (Council on Education of the Deaf). But these groups view themselves in different ways (Leigh, 1999b), and we now explore these perspectives.

TWO MODELS

In the popular media, much has been written on how the medical/disability and the cultural/linguistic models of explaining social perspectives of deafness collide and clash. However, little has been written about how each model affects deaf Americans in their everyday lives.

The Medical/Disability Model

The conventional medical view of deafness is important to most deaf Americans. For instance, they may see a physician for medical complications related to their auditory systems (e.g., earwax buildup, infections, earaches, and tumors) or for cochlear implant surgery. Deaf Americans will use audiological diagnostic services at certain junctures of their lives to attain eligibility for educational services, vocational rehabilitation, disability benefits, auditory and visual assistive devices, interpreting services, and otherwise to obtain all the protections and services provided by the American with Disabilities Act and other legislation.

Physicians and audiologists focus on hearing loss as a disability or pathological condition that should be detected, cured, and rehabilitated with remedies such as surgery and amplification (Gonsoulin, 2001). Users of ASL use a sign, made outside the ear, to illustrate what they see as a focus on the ear. This sign, with its English translation of "pathological model," encompasses their feeling that the medical/disability view imposes restrictions on them by overly focusing on their access to communication through sound instead of through vision. Physicians, audiologists, and other professionals, however, do not see the medical/disability view as limiting. They see it more broadly in the context of the health of the entire human body, since many auditory disorders have medical correlates (e.g., vascular, renal, and heart problems; nervous and immune-system disorders; vestibular dysfunction; syphilis; tumors; fungal, bacterial, and viral infections of the cochlea; ototoxity) that require medical treatment and management. Not all auditory disorders, of course, have medical correlates. Many deaf Americans enjoy good health, hearing loss notwithstanding. In fact, the National Association of the Deaf (NAD), the world's largest advocacy organization of and for deaf people, uses the term *wellness model* to emphasize that deaf people can be perceived as "healthy" (National Association of the Deaf, 2001).

Increasingly, adult deaf professionals are being included as part of the team that plans the individualized family service plan (IFSP) for children birth to age 2 or the individualized education plan (IEP) for children between ages 3 and 21. State residential schools, such as those in Texas and Maryland, employ Deaf adults to serve in this capacity to counsel parents, furnish sign language instruction, and provide deaf role modeling.

It is when parents are *not* informed about the benefits of sign language and Deaf culture when told about different approaches that concerns many adult Deaf Americans. They view themselves as the "end product" of auditory rehabilitation plans, which traditionally have not optimally included visual components, such as the use of sign language or other visual enhancements to facilitate language acquisition. Today, this is changing, with more audiologists incorporating signing in therapy plans in view of empirical evidence that shows the use of sign language not to be detrimental to the development of speech skills (see Wilbur, 2000, for reviews).

Some professionals encourage parents to place their deaf children in public schools with hearing children in the interest of "helping" deaf children "overcome their handicap" and fit into mainstream society. Deaf Americans, though, view interpreters, captioned TV, relay centers, hearing aids, and so on simply as tools for accessing auditory and visual information (Stewart, 1991), just as, for example, hearing persons use microphones, amplifiers, and telephones to access auditory information. Additionally, some professionals view deaf persons as not being able to "function independently in the hearing world without significant help from another person as an interpreter" (Blanchfield et al., 2001, p. 184). In contrast, deaf persons view the use of an interpreter as allowing them to function very independently in the hearing world. For example, with an interpreter, a deaf lawyer can fully participate in the trial of his or her client, a deaf Ph.D. researcher can easily participate in a group discussion about theoretical linguistics or any other scholarly discipline, and a deaf person can use an interpreter when getting services from a doctor, lawyer, real estate agent, and others, so that he or she does not have to depend on friends or family members. Such are the different views.

Although the medical/disability model is important for its concern with overall health, it focuses primarily on medical and audiological intervention. In the view of many Deaf Americans, the model does not adequately take into account their early cognitive and linguistic needs and social-identity issues. These individuals would like physicians, audiologists, and speech-language pathologists to learn about their Deaf culture and to share this information with parents and other professionals. Thomas Gonsoulin, M.D. (2001), asks his fellow otolaryngologists to think philosophically about these different perspectives and maintain dialogue with Deaf-World members who would prefer to be viewed from a multifaceted sociolinguistic/cultural perspective.

The Sociolinguistic/Cultural Model

For many deaf persons, etiology, type and degree of hearing loss, and even age of onset make little difference to them in the ways they function as adults in the deaf community. Being a deaf person has more to do with one's identity as a "whole person." It involves their shared experiences, language, culture, attitudes, social obligations to each other, quality-of-life issues, and how they cope in daily life (Padden, 1998; Padden & Humphries, 1988).

Although ASL is of great value for those in the Deaf World, it is more the shared experiences involved with being deaf that encourage diverse deaf persons, including oral-deaf people, to explore the community. Deaf culture is primarily transmitted by ASL users (Stewart, 1991). Many Deaf persons will also not just use ASL exclusively, but also Contact Signing, to communicate with other deaf people or with hearing people (Lucas & Valli, 1992). Contact Signing is described as ASL signs in English word order.

Deaf persons will also use a signing system of English and/or written English and, if possible, spoken English, with hearing friends, family, and coworkers. Consequently, they are more often described as being bilingual, or users of two languages, than monolingual in, for example, spoken English or ASL.*

Within the sociolinguistic/cultural model, sign language is viewed as a natural language equal to spoken languages. Socialization with other Deaf persons is encouraged and supported. Deaf adults are viewed as positive role models, and involvement with Deaf people as a group is seen as "working with Deaf people" to promote access to the same rights, opportunities, and privileges other diverse Americans enjoy (Jankowski, 1997). Later in the chapter, we expand the sociolinguistic/cultural model. Deaf history and heritage, literature, drama, art, and Deaf Studies are discussed.

Bilingual is defined as having the functional use of two languages, but not necessarily having native proficiency in both languages (Grosjean, 1998). We cover the topic of deaf bilinguals in Chapter 7.

BELIEF SYSTEMS

Professionals have historically tended to overlook the importance of visual orientation and its potential for language learning in deaf children. Understandably, these professionals tend to focus on auditory processes and strategies, including amplification, implants, and auditory training. Visual strategies may not be introduced into the deaf child's life until language delay becomes evident. Critical years of early language acquisition through the visual-spatial channel may be lost if delays are not addressed early (Wilbur, 2000).

Psycholinguists today consider language acquisition to be a dual-channel activity involving both auditory and visual processes. Neurocognitive scientists and linguists have reported that age of ASL acquisition is important. The earlier the deaf child is exposed to sign language, the better it is for the child's cognitive and linguistic development (Corina, 1998; Mayberry & Eichen, 1991). The language-learning capacity of the brain includes both auditory and visual capabilities. Focusing only on auditory stimulation will not consistently guarantee language acquisition for deaf children. Yes, unquestionably, there have been deaf adults who have successfully acquired spoken English based on the use of speech-reading with or without auditory amplification (e.g., Lang, 2000). But there also are deaf adults who have written about their difficulties in acquiring language through oral methods alone (Mindel & Vernon, 1971; Nover & Moll, 1997).

Generally, there is limited professional awareness about the daily lives of Deaf people (Gonsoulin, 2001; Lane et al., 1996). Most professionals have rare contact with Deaf adults, including those who are well educated (Andersson, 1994). Thus, they are more susceptible to describing Deaf culture members as lonely and isolated rather than socially fulfilled through interactions with deaf peers (Stewart, 1991). This is understandable, given the low incidence of deafness in the population.

Consequently, the ability to inform parents about the many successful Deaf adults who use alternative visual communication strategies such as signing, with or without ancillary auditory strategies, suffers. Often, parents have to seek out this information about sign language and Deaf culture on their own (Christiansen & Leigh, 2002). By the time parents learn about these facts, their children may be teenagers who are struggling due to inadequate mastery of English. However, recent evidence indicates that more parents are using sign language with their deaf children than previously thought (Christiansen & Leigh, 2002).

Low reading levels have been ascribed to the use of sign language and attendance at state residential schools for deaf students. The fact is that variability in English proficiency among deaf persons is broad, with many graduates from state schools learning to read very well while many deaf children in mainstream public schools do not and vice versa (Marschark, 1993). Although it is true that, on the average, many deaf youth leave school between the ages of 16 and 21 reading at the third- or fourth-grade level (Moores, 2001a), the low reading achievement cannot be solely attributed to the use of sign language or school placement. On the contrary, deaf children of deaf parents typically have continuous exposure to sign language, and tend to read better than deaf youth with less or no exposure to ASL. Admittedly, reading proficiency is dependent on many complex psycholinguistic variables, which we examine in Chapter 5.

Instead of viewing the deaf community as a haven for the unsuccessful or as an isolating, separatist lifestyle, Deaf Americans see their culture as providing positive opportunities to learn, grow, and expand their interests and hobbies; to serve as mentors for younger deaf people, particularly those with hearing parents and those in mainstream education programs; to develop friendships; to develop wider links to deaf communities at the local, national, and international levels through its networks of organizations and institutions; and to manage their own affairs (Stewart, 1991). Deaf people in more than 90 countries have formed national and international organizations that arrange regular events such as congresses, festivals of arts and crafts, theater presentations, and seminars (Andersson, 1994). In 1989, Deaf Way, an international cultural festival for Deaf people, attracted more than 5,000 deaf persons from around the world to Washington, DC, for lectures, theatrical performances, and professional presentations about Deaf culture (Erting, Johnson, Smith, & Snider, 1994). In the summer of 2002, people from all over the world attended Deaf Way II in Washington, DC. At this cultural event, there were presentations of Deaf theater, art, history and heritage, education, linguistics, and other issues relevent to the deaf community. Counteracting the separatist perspective, these organizational activities require working with hearing people in the larger society at varying levels.

But as in mainstream society, not all succeed. There are some Deaf Americans who are uneducated, underemployed, or unemployed who lead, in Deaf culture vernacular, a "no good" life (Buck, 2000). Based on three nationally representative data sets, Blanchfield and colleagues (2001) reported that of the severely and profoundly deaf population over the age of 17, about 44 percent did not graduate from high school, compared to 19 percent of the general population. Further, only 46 percent of those who graduated from high school attended some college, compared to 60 percent of the general population. Only 5 percent of the deaf students graduated from college, compared to 13 percent of the general population. In another survey, researchers reported that vocational degree recipients were more at risk of underemployment than academic degree recipients and that underemployment is no longer a serious problem for college graduates at entry levels (Schroedel & Geyer, 2000). Unquestionably, the problems listed here are in large part related to society's failure to provide deaf people with equitable educational and employment opportunities or to the fact that the individuals concerned, for whatever reasons, fail to achieve their human potential.

Communication-disorder specialists may view Deaf people as uninterested in audiologists and speech pathologists who emphasize the need for spoken language and amplification. It is true that some Deaf people express anger at having been denied sign language when growing up, having had to go through speech therapy and wear hearing aids with little benefit (Jacobs, 1989; Nover & Moll, 1997). But there are also Deaf Americans who benefit from speech and audiology services, including hearing aids and cochlear implants, and are appreciative of the help. There exists a diversity of opinion, depending on individual experiences and the extent to which deaf persons may or may not have had the hearing needed to benefit from some of these services.

Professionals in audiology, rehabilitation, and medicine refer to electronic equipment used to assist deaf people in communication as *adaptive devices* or *auxiliary aids* (visual and auditory) to compensate for a deaf persons' inability to hear. In line with the cultural view, these are enhancement devices rather than compensatory devices. Many people prefer to refer to these devices as *visual alerts* and *electronic devices* for communication and signaling. These include hearing ear dogs, flashing signalers, TV and movie captioning, computer-assisted note taking, sign language interpreters, TTYs, the Internet, electronic mail, hand-held wireless pagers, audio and video relay services, and so on. This view reflects many deaf people's emphasis on the importance of vision for communication.

DEAF CULTURE: THE ANTHROPOLOGY VIEW

As with other cultures, Deaf culture can be viewed anthropologically as an adaptive coping mechanism though which Deaf people have developed a language to accommodate their necessarily visual orientation. Deaf people use their language to pass down social norms, values, language, and technology to younger generations (Van Cleve & Crouch, 1989). Deaf culture, though, is both similar to and different from other cultures. Even though Deaf people are geographically dispersed in cities and rural areas (Schein, 1996), most live near large populations of other Deaf Americans, usually near a residential school or university such as Gallaudet University in Washington, DC, the world's only liberal arts university for deaf people, or the National Technical Institute for the Deaf/Rochester Institute of Technology in Rochester, New York (recently introduced as *Sign City* on a CBS Sunday Morning show (2002, January 13 & 20).

In some communities, hearing persons have learned sign language in order to incorporate deaf citizens into the economic, religious, and social milieu of their communities. There are historical accounts of large numbers of deaf and hearing people in the eighteenth century who all used sign language with each other, living in communities such as Martha's Vineyard, Massachusetts; Heinneker, New Hampshire; and Sandy River Valley, Maine (Lane, Pillard, & French, 2000). Such bilingual societies of hearing and deaf persons have also been reported and documented in the Little Cayman Islands, Ayent, a Swiss commune, Lancaster County in Pennsylvania, a clan of Jicaque Indians in Honduras, Adamarobe in Ghana, the Guntar area of Andhra Pradesh in India, a Scottish clan, Jewish communities in Britain, cultural units in Israel, a Mayan Indian village of Nohya, villages of Providence Island in the Carribbean, and the Yucatec Mayan village in Mexico (cited in Jankowski, 1997).

VALUES AND CUSTOMS

Deaf Americans do not have their own architecture and furniture, as is typical in other cultures, although Deaf houses often have more lighting and use visual alerting devices to signal sounds (e.g., door bell, baby crier, alarm clock). They are more like Native Americans, Asian Americans, or African Americans who live as a minority within a larger culture (Vernon & Makowsky, 1969). The Deaf culture has its own folklore—including ABC story-poems, ASL stories, stories and narratives, literature, puns, riddles, jokes, theater, and visual arts—that provides avenues for the expression of feelings about the Deaf experience (Baldwin, 1993; Erting et al., 1994; Peters, 2000).

Many professionals unfamiliar with Deaf culture are usually puzzled by the split Deaf people make between *Hearing* and *Deaf* culture. In comparing mainstream American culture and Deaf American culture, Stokoe (1989) described the differences when using vision instead of hearing for getting vital and incidental information. For instance, Deaf people use sign language; hearing people use a spoken language. Hearing people use telephones and alarm clocks; members of the deaf community use TTYs (and email) and flashing light or vibrating alarm clocks, and so on. These reflect different approaches to daily life.

More fundamental differences stem from how children acquire their culture. Auditory experiences in general play a huge role in the ways culture is transmitted through conversations, social rules and routines, songs, poems, radio, television, and family stories. Hearing children learn from listening to their parents, teachers, and friends and from incidental conversations around them, and deaf children try to follow as well. Hearing people may wonder why some Deaf people do not maximize the use of auditory technology devices. These individuals, though, perceive what is around them visually, and as they accumulate these visual experiences into a visual memory, they use these visual experiences to think, communicate, problem solve, and generally relate to other people.

Deaf people use their eyes, their expressions, spatial relationships of signs, body movement, and touch far more than hearing persons do in everyday conversations. A high value is placed on American Sign Language and how the hands are used (Padden & Humphries, 1988). Deaf people vary in their use of speech. Some consider it to be a restriction and denial of the need to communicate comfortably in their own language (Padden & Humphries, 1988). Others use speech freely and many will "mouth" some English sounds silently while signing.

One of the strongest features of Deaf culture is an emphasis on social relationships with other deaf persons who share similar experiences. American Sign Language storytelling is an art. Themes often center on success stories of deaf persons (Padden & Humphries, 1988). Other values include the rituals of introduction. When persons are introduced, information such as the place of birth and the name of the school attended are often included (Padden & Humphries, 1988). The assigning of name signs is another custom unique to Deaf culture (Supalla, 1992).

MEMBERSHIP

Deaf of Deaf Parents

Unlike most people who are born into their culture, Deaf children who have Deaf parents represent the minority in this culture. Deaf children of Deaf parents most often grow up learning ASL, attend deaf schools, deaf clubs, and picnics, and, through everyday experiences, learn the values of Deaf culture (Padden & Humphries, 1988). Deaf persons from Deaf families enjoy a special status in Deaf culture and often become leaders in the community. For example, the four student leaders of the 1988 Deaf President Now movement were from Deaf families, as were many of the faculty who supported the movement (Christiansen & Barnartt, 1995).

Deaf of Hearing Parents

In contrast, most deaf persons come from hearing families and learn about Deaf culture later in life when they meet Deaf adults at school, go to a summer camp with other Deaf youth, join a sports team of deaf players, attend a deaf club, church, or Deaf cultural festival, or find work with other Deaf persons, even if they have been completely mainstreamed growing up (Lane et al., 1996; Stewart, 1991). They may enter Gallaudet University or the National Technical Institute for the Deaf, or they may enter a college or university that enrolls deaf students and employs sign language interpreters. In these ways they learn about Deaf culture. Many become comfortable in the culture, whereas others may stay on the fringe, and many will remain comfortably within their hearing communities.

Hearing Members in Deaf Families

There are groups other than deaf people who consider themselves part of the deaf community, such as hearing persons who marry deaf spouses, hearing children of deaf parents, and siblings of deaf people. These hearing individuals with deaf family members often live in hearing-deaf cross-cultural environments, depending on the level of Deaf culture involvement of the deaf family members, similar to those who live in bilingual and bicultural families (Singleton & Tittle, 2000).

Growing up as a hearing child with deaf parents can involve complex communication, socialization, and cultural issues within the home and within the extended family. As children, these hearing individuals might acquire ASL and internalize Deaf culture to varying degrees depending on family interest and background. They also learn English as a second language. For example, there have been studies of hearing toddlers of deaf parents in Puerto Rico who learned Puerto Rican Sign Language as their first language and Spanish as their second language (Rodriguez, 2001). Studies show they acquire both languages on the same time table as other bilingual children do (Pettito, 2000).

Deaf parents, even if they rely primarily on signing, will also use speech in addition to signing with their hearing children (Rodriguez, 2001). This is particularly true if these parents come from hearing families. Deaf parents will also expose their hearing children to hearing neighbors, relatives, TV, teachers, and peers in preschool for speech development. Those who grow up bilingually also internalize two identities and learn to navigate between them. On the other hand, if deaf parents communicate with their hearing children using only speech, these children will more likely develop English as their primary language (Singleton & Tittle, 2000).

Often, the hearing family member becomes the "go-between" between the deaf family and the hearing society. This can be a burden, especially for a young child of deaf parents. In some cases, it is a source of conflict, as parents may depend on the child to be the family interpreter. However, because of recent developments—such as telephone relay services, facsimiles, electronic mail, hand-held wireless communication devices, and TV captioning—these burdens are less common. In adulthood, some will leave their deaf heritage behind as they enter adulthood, never to return; whereas others leave and return.

Hard-of-Hearing Children of Deaf or Hearing Parents

The term *hard of hearing* refers to the individual with a hearing loss who can use audition as the primary channel for receiving speech (Vernon & Andrews, 1990). Hard-of-hearing children with Deaf parents naturally become part of Deaf culture. Hard-of-hearing children with hearing parents may also belong, depending on the extent of exposure to the deaf community. Most of these hard-of-hearing individuals are educated in public schools but experience difficulty with language development, much like children with early onset profound hearing losses. This is especially true if their hearing loss was prelingual (occurring before language was acquired) (Grushkin, 1998). Hard-of-hearing children in hearing families may meet deaf peers in high school or college and get involved in Deaf teams or clubs, particularly if they have the ASL skills to move back and forth between the hearing and Deaf worlds. They will often learn ASL and use it as a second language, although some will reject ASL because they do not wish to mix with signing deaf and hard-of-hearing people (Stewart, 1991).

Deaf Adoptive and Foster Children

Many hearing and deaf individuals are adopting and/or taking in foster deaf children from places such as the United States, Korea, the Philippines, Viet Nam, China, South America, Russia, and Bosnia. For a deaf child, it can be enormously beneficial to be adopted into a hearing or deaf signing family who understand the psychological, social-emotional, communicative, cultural, and educational ramifications connected with being deaf. In a study of 55 deaf parents of adopted children, a major finding was that deaf adoptive parents perceived much stronger social support from natural social networks within the deaf community than from formal service providers, primarily because of inaccessible communication and social workers' lack of awareness of the needs of deaf clients (White, 1999). Deaf parents in the sample demonstrated an unconditional sense of entitlement to their deaf adopted children, including those with language delays who were older at the time of placement. White (1999) explained this by saying that deaf parents and deaf child dyads formed a "goodness of fit" for adoptive placements.

Like other transracial adoptions, deaf adoptees must grapple with physical differences compared to their adoptive families. Deaf adoptees may want to learn more about their biological families and home countries as they get older. Adoptive issues related to bonding and identity compounded with hearing loss can become acute, especially during adolescence and early adulthood. More research is needed into the experiences of deaf adoptees and their families (White, 1999).

Late-Deafened Persons

It is estimated that more than 10 million people in the United States have acquired a hearing loss after age 18, due to disease, noise, trauma, or other causes (Fujikawa, 2001). Many will benefit from amplification or cochlear implants because of their memory for spoken language. Some retain speech skills, although distortions and tone variation can occur due to difficulty in monitoring vocal production and volume (Vernon & Andrews, 1990). Late-deafened adults may rely on speech-reading. However, many find speech-reading fatiguing and inadequate. Disruptions in career and family life are typical if communication adjustments are not made. Many late-deafened adults will also learn ASL as a second language or use simultaneous communication (signs and speech). There is a lot of variation in how much speech and how many signs late-deafened people use. It is often dependent on their social networks and jobs. Some late-deafened persons will associate with deaf people to a greater extent because of the difficulty of lip-reading and the ease of signing. Some will enter the deaf community and enjoy its networks of clubs and sports teams (Stewart, 1991). Some choose not to, but prefer to communicate with hearing persons. Many will join a support group called ALDA (Association of Late-Deafened Adults). See the appendix for web addresses.

Deaf-Blind Persons

Persons who are deaf-blind have their own communication preferences. Depending on the etiology and age of onset of hearing and vision loss, those individuals may use amplification, cochlear implants, magnifying devices, and braille, while others may use sign language. For instance, those with Usher syndrome, a genetic condition that leads to blindness (see Chapter 3), may have been born deaf and brought up using sign language. On the other hand, an elderly person who gradually loses hearing and vision may use hearing aids and magnifying devices. The deaf community may shun deaf-blind persons due to fears and prejudices. This is understandable, given the deaf people's dependence on vision for communication and fears of losing that vision. Deaf-blind Americans have their own societies, organizations, and periodicals (Duncan, Prickett, Finkelstein, Vernon, & Hollingsworth, 1988). They have their own adaptive technologies, too. Special equipment includes desktop and laptop computers with glare-reduced computer screens, braille output devices, voice output devices, text enlargement programs, closed circuit televisions (CCTV), large print or braille watches, vibrating or flashing alerting systems, large print TTYs, amplified or large-button telephones, braille telephones, computerized braille note-taking devices, and magnifying devices, to name some. *Orchid of the Bayou* is a moving memoir of a deaf-blind woman who grew up in Louisiana and lost her vision due to Usher syndrome in young adulthood. This story is also informative about the high incidence of Usher syndrome in people of Cajun descent (Carroll & Fischer, 2001).

Ethnic Differences

Deaf Americans, like hearing Americans, have differences based on ethnic background, gender, alternative lifestyles (gays and lesbians), and disabilities, among others (Christensen, 2000; Erting et al., 1994; Lane et al., 1996; Leigh, 1999c). Recent autobiographies and biographies of Deaf Americans of color have provided insight into what it means to grow up with a double or a triple minority status. For example, Mary Herring Wright, an African American woman deafened by age 10, tells her story of going to the North Carolina School for the Deaf and Blind during the racial segregation in the 1920s. Wright points out the painful injustices she felt when observing how well the schools for white students were equipped and furnished , compared to her African American school (Wright, 1999).

The cultural forces that draw deaf people together have also created institutional racism in the Deaf World. Deaf people, like their hearing counterparts, often discriminate against other deaf people who differ across dimensions of skin color, sexual orientation, gender, disability, or age (Gutman, 1999; Lane et al., 1996; Stewart, 1991). Because of inadequate education and limited access to information and having been socialized toward "being normal," some Deaf people are intolerant of group differences and thus discriminate against "multiple minorities" just as does the hearing majority (Erting et al., 1994).

TRANSMISSION OF DEAF CULTURE

Unless the family is Deaf, Deaf culture is transmitted mostly through peer socialization (Meadow-Orlans, 1996; Padden & Humphries, 1988). This can start as early as elementary school or as late as middle age. It often occurs in residential schools where Deaf culture is introduced informally through Deaf peer and adult interaction and/or formally through the direct teaching of Deaf culture as a subject in the curriculum. Transmission can also occur through Deaf journalism and periodicals, in Deaf clubs, athletic groups, churches, political organizations, and at Deaf festivals and other events (Jankowski, 1997).

Deaf culture can also be transmitted through organizations such as the American Sign Language Teachers Association (ASLTA); the National Fraternal Society of the Deaf (FRAT); the Captioned Media Program (CMP); American Society for Deaf Children (ASDC); Convention of American Instructors of the Deaf (CAID); Conference of Educational Administrators of Schools and Programs for the Deaf (CEASD); the National Association of the Deaf (NAD); state deaf associations across the 50 states; Deaf art, theater, sport groups, and organizations (Stewart, 1991), Deaf religious groups, and Deaf hobby groups.

Accounts of the transmission of Deaf culture can be found in written histories of deaf people forming their own communities to minimize isolation, to establish a system embodying their own values and beliefs, to preserve sign language, to chronicle their achievements, and to transmit Deaf culture. Such accounts are often available in historical descriptions of the founding of schools for the deaf as well as in the controversies surrounding the question of oral versus manual communication (Gannon, 1981; Van Cleve, 1993). Some writers have attempted to chronicle the history of the deaf experience over a period of time, and to place events and controversies in a wider historical context (Van Cleve, 1993). For example, the repression of sign language during the early 1900s can be understood within the context of Darwinism and evolutionary theories, which fostered the perception that sign languages were "primitive" and inferior to spoken languages (Baynton, 1993). In 1991, the first International Conference on Deaf History took place at Gallaudet University, and subsequent conferences continued to bring together scholars who enlighten us about deaf history.

Culture can also be transmitted through literature. The literature of Deaf Americans incorporates poetry, stories, plays, oral storytelling, and stories in films and on videotapes, CD-ROMs, and DVDs that reflect the biculturalism of being deaf (Cohn, 1999; Peters, 2000). Deaf literature is ASL stories passed down through the years as folklore, or "Deaf lore." Deaf literature can also be stories and poems written in English, such as the works of Robert Panara and others (Peters, 2000), or through adaptations of literature into sign language, such as a play or poem by Shakespeare. There are also new, complex poetic forms using the linguistic parameters of ASL in playful and meaningful ways, as illustrated by the ASL poetry of Dorothy Miles, Ella Mae Lentz, Clayton Valli, Patrick Graybill, Debbie Rennie, Peter Cook, and Jim Cohn. The ASL stories of Ben Bahan (e.g., "Birds of a Feather"), Sam Supalla ("For a Decent Living"), and the VisMa mythology, a folkloric story of the history of deaf education written in English by Charles Katz (1994), are other examples.

Deaf literature also includes the performing arts, such as drama and mime for theater and television (Baldwin, 1993). In the book, *Pictures in the Air: The Story of the National Theater of the Deaf*, Steve Baldwin (1993) tells the history of the National Theater of the Deaf (NTD) from 1959 to 1993. Early deaf drama groups in America consisted of weekend skits, mime shows, and signed songs and poems at local deaf clubs. The NTD was started at the O'Neill Theater in Waterford, Connecticut, in 1965, having evolved from the collaboration of hearing and deaf people in writing grants for funding. It has become a versatile touring company that travels all over the world. *My Third Eye,* an original drama (1971–72), exemplifies the life as seen from the perspective of deaf persons. There are many role reversals between hearing and deaf characters. Deaf company members wrote, directed, and designed the sets and costumes for *My Third Eye.*

Deaf actors have also performed in plays, on TV, and in soap operas, movies, and commercials. In 1975, Brian Kilpatrick a deaf actor, and Charles St. Clair, a hearing actor, founded the Fairmont Theater of the Deaf in Cleveland, Ohio. This theater produced many innovations in bilingual and bicultural entertainment, theater scripts for other audiences, the use of professional translators who prepared scripts in both American Sign Language and English prior to the rehearsals, combining a deaf-signing actor and hearing-voicing actor into one character, and collaborations with a Cleveland television station to disseminate several of its productions. Original works dealt with deaf-hearing intercultural conflicts, the oppression of deaf people in medieval times, innovative concepts of sign language and voice theater, and the creative use of ASL in a circus format (Bangs, 1987). In the 1990s, the Fairmont Theater changed its name to SignStage Theater. More recently, Deaf West Theater of Los Angeles, founded by Ed Waterstreet, a Deaf actor and director, received a large federal grant to enhance its artistic programs and to train deaf and hard-of-hearing performers.

During the 1950s and 1960s in television, hearing actors were used to portray deaf people. Deaf characters were portrayed as "mute dummies" or "mute imposters" or perfect "lip-readers." Only recently have deaf actors been given the opportunity to play deaf roles. They have distinguished themselves in television production, ranging from soap operas to TV serials and to children's shows such as *Sesame Street.* After deaf actors protested of discrimination in using hearing performers in deaf roles, casting and script writing changed. By the 1980s, television programs began to explore the complexity of deaf persons (Schuchman, 1988) and teach more about Deaf culture, through programs such as the Hallmark movie for television, *Love Is Never Silent.* The television series *Deaf Mosiac,* produced by Gil Eastman and Jane Wilk at Gallaudet University, provided the public with valuable information about Deaf culture and deaf people. Topics handled on this show included deaf adoptions; Deaf organizations; clips from television shows such as *Cagney and Lacey, Sesame Street, and Love Is Never Silent;* the role of deaf people in film, theater, television, and dance programs; and interviews with well-known deaf persons, among other topics. Television and radio celebrities such as Nanette Fabray and Rush Limbaugh have used the television medium to openly discuss their deafness, all of which has contributed to the public's sensitivity and understanding of hearing loss.

Art enlightens deaf and hearing audiences by presenting visually rendered experiences seen through deaf eyes. A specific genre called Deaf View/Image Art has been developed by deaf painters who use their art to express cultural aspects of the deaf experience, including sign language and difficulties with hearing aids or speech training. Deaf artists who support the Deaf View/Image Art make use of formal elements such contrasting colors, intense colors, and textures. This artform may focus on facial features such as the eyes, mouths, and ears (Erting et al., 1994).

There have been traveling art shows from Northeastern University and the National Technical Institute for the Deaf that show deaf artists' work. Many residential schools also showcase the sculpture, paintings, woodcuts, and drawings of deaf artists.

Deaf artists have created many visual works, such as sculpture, woodcut printing, portraiture, painting, woodcarving, photography, wildlife art, scientific illustrating, commercial art, landscape painting, dry point etching, silhouettistry, folk art, and architecture. Jack Gannon provides a comprehensive listing of some of these deaf artists, and the origins and the highlights of their major works in *Deaf Heritage* (1981). Deaf scholars also have written biographies of accomplished artists (Lang & Meath-Lang, 1995) and a comprehensive history of deaf artists and their work from colonial to contemporary times (Sonnenstrahl, 2002).

Deaf Studies Programs

The scholarly field of Deaf Studies pulls together Deaf history and heritage, politics, ASL literature, art, and theater into one discipline. The field of Deaf Studies is concerned with the study of the preservation of Deaf history and heritage. The late Fred Schreiber, Executive Director of the NAD, made this statement:

> If deaf people are to get ahead in our time, they must have a better image of themselves and their capabilities. They need concrete examples of what deaf people have already done so they can project for themselves a brighter future. If we can have African-American Studies, Jewish Studies, why not Deaf Studies? (Schreiber, 1981)

Bachelor's degree programs in Deaf Studies have been established at Boston University, at California State University at Northridge (CSUN), Gallaudet University, and McDaniel College (formerly Western Maryland College). Deaf Studies encourages students to look at the *whole person* rather than focus on the hearing loss. Within this study, students can develop new theories and views to explain the rich diversity of the characteristics of the deaf community (Katz, 1999). Deaf Studies courses can be found in other curricula and disciplines, such as education, interpreter training, vocational rehabilitation, social work, psychology, nursing, special education, and the like. Most sign language classes will also incorporate Deaf Studies components (Katz, 1999).

DEAF COMMUNITIES

Historical research published on local deaf communities is virtually nonexistent. Deaf people have been marginalized in many historical writings about culture. The tendency is to focus on a few highly literate and successful late-deafened deaf people rather than everyday members of the deaf community. Thus, one rarely gets a broad view of what it means to be part of an average deaf community (Katz, 1996).

History shows that deaf communities in America typically emerge where there are deaf schools and deaf churches. For example, the New England Gallaudet Association was formed in 1853 during a reunion at the American School for the Deaf. Many organizations of the deaf were established during various functions at residential schools for the deaf as well as in deaf religious organizations. Deaf ministers, such as Reverend James Fair in Beaumont, Texas, other itinerant deaf ministers, and Father Tom Coughlin, a Roman Catholic priest, have also played an important role in providing religious services that bring deaf people together in their communities for religious education and fellowship.

One historical study provides a microscopic picture of how a small deaf community was formed in Beaumont, Texas. This study may be representative of how other small deaf communities have been found all over the United States. In Beaumont, the local deaf club, a school, and a church organization held deaf people together in this small community and also provided networks for deaf community members through state organizations, national organizations, the National Association of the Deaf, and the American Athletic Association of the Deaf (AAAD) (Katz, 1996). Katz found that as the active club members got older and as younger members left Beaumont to attend Gallaudet University never to return, the membership dwindled, mirroring trends across the nation. Unlike the earlier deaf generations, the new generation gets together less often in person at clubs to exchange news, ideas, signs, and stories. With the proliferation of captioned television, captioned movies, TTYs, VCRs, electronic mail, hand-held wireless telecommunication devices, relay services and mainstreaming, small regional and local Deaf clubs have diminished in numbers across the country. Yet the preservation and promotion of the psychosocial aspects of the deaf and hard-of-hearing community still exists but through alternative means: home entertainment, conferences sponsored by organizations such as Deaf Senior Citizens, sports competitions, Deaf festivals, alumni meetings, and electronic communication (Erting, Johnson, Smith, & Snider, 1994).

CONCLUSION

Whatever their race, color, ethnicity, religion, gender, socioeconomic background, lifestyle, cultural orientation, mode of communication and language use, hearing status, education background, and use of communication technologies, deaf Americans function in two worlds—the Deaf and the hearing worlds. Many deaf Americans utilize a diversity of communication and languages depending on their family background, education experiences, and with whom they are communicating.

Members of the deaf community gravitate between being "included" and being "excluded" in the hearing world. When deaf people are with hearing people and have no interpreter or captioning, or cannot understand what is being said, they are "excluded." On the other hand, they can be "included" in the hearing world when they do have appropriate auditory and visual access to communication through technology and sign language interpreting with colleagues in the workplace or with their hearing families at home. By the same token, if they understand their deaf peers, whether oral or signing, they are included instead of excluded. Every day of their lives, deaf people negotiate these differences and tensions by using different communication modes—whether it is sign language, spoken language, written language, technology aids, or a combination—similar to the hearing bilingual/multilingual and multicultural person who code-switches between two or more languages and cultures (Grosjean, 1998).

SUGGESTED READINGS

Bahan, B., & S. Supalla. *ASL Literature Series.* (One 60-minute videotape of two classic stories based on the Deaf experience.)
Ben Bahan's fable, *Bird of a Different Feather,* explores the differences of a bird within a family of eagles. Rather than accepting the bird's differences, the eagle family tries to apply a pathological approach to raising the unusual bird, an odyssey familiar to many deaf people. Sam Supalla's *For a Decent Living,* a boy is searching for his deaf identity. He escapes from his hearing family and goes on a journey to prove himself to his family, the Deaf community, and the world. (www.dawnsign.com)

Buck, D. (2000). *Deaf Peddler: Confessions of an Inside Man.* Washington, DC: Gallaudet University Press.
Peddling is deplored by the National Association of the Deaf because it reinforces negative stereotypes of deaf people who are not capable of finding employment. Dennis Buck reveals the inside story of how he exploited his deafness to earn easy money. He provides a chronicle of his life as a deaf peddler. He also provides a history of deaf peddling, as a way for uneducated people to make money. Buck reveals how vulnerable rings of deaf workers are to deaf and hearing peddler overseers and provides a fascinating study of the cultural phenomenon of panhandling in U.S. society.

Chuck Baird 35 Plates. (1993). San Diego, CA: Dawn Sign Press. (www.dawnsign.com)
Deaf artist Chuck Baird has been commissioned by schools and universities to do murals, paintings, and three-dimensional wood sculptures. His themes range from political art with Deaf themes to whimsical paintings of animals and objects that incorporate sign language. This book contains 35 of his paintings in color. A short biography of the artist is also included.

Lang, H., & B. Meath-Lang. (1995). *Deaf Persons in the Arts and Sciences.* Westport, CT: Greenwood Press.
The authors provide biographies of the accomplishments in the arts and the sciences of hundreds of deaf Americans.

Ogden, P. (1992). *Chelsea: The Story of a Signal Dog.* Boston: Little, Brown.
Paul Ogden has written a love story about his best friend—his dog, Chelsea. Chelsea is a dog who has been trained to respond to signs and to alert his master to sounds in the environment. Throughout the book, Ogden writes about the barriers deaf people encounter in their daily lives.

CHAPTER THREE

WHERE DOES IT ALL BEGIN?

Deafness is not silent; it isn't anything describable in a single word or phrase. Rather, it's a range, a spectrum of conditions.
—Ogden, 1996, p. xi

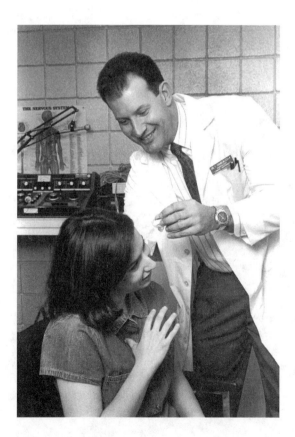

For most people, "deaf" begins at the moment of diagnosis, when hearing loss is identified. The reactions to this process carry the baggage of typical cultural perceptions of deafness. Essentially, these perceptions involve the concept that "beyond sound are no human relationships, no government, no equality of existence, no inkling of knowledge" (Brueggemann, 1999, p. 106). In the eyes of those who rarely encounter deaf people, sound is life and the lack of sound is the death of human connection. For this reason, many parents grieve when they realize their child is diagnosed as deaf, and adults who could hear grieve as they see their ability to hear others diminishing. There is a full life after diagnosis, but it takes time for parents and others to realize this.

CHAPTER OBJECTIVES

This chapter explains why etiology is important, and outlines the major causes of deafness. We discuss the explosion of genetic information and the implications of genetic counseling for deaf and hearing people. Readers will become aware of the psychodynamics surrounding the diagnostic process with particular focus on the reactions of both hearing and deaf parents. Having sensitive professionals who can appropriately provide service to parents during the period after diagnosis—a difficult phase during which these parents are confronting the critical decisions they will need to make about audiological, communication, and educational interventions—is emphasized as important.

ETIOLOGY: THE CAUSES OF HEARING LOSS

The Significance of Etiology

If a person cannot hear, it means that the ear, auditory nerve, or brain is not doing the job it was designed to do. Multiple causes affect hearing abilities, and the patterns of onset have implications for the psychological development and functioning of deaf children and adults. For example, if a child was born hearing and two years later contracted spinal meningitis that resulted in hearing, vision, and balance losses, that child's psychological experiences will differ from those of a child who is born deaf to deaf parents. Many deaf people are, to some extent, molded psychologically not only by the functional effects of their hearing but also by physiological or neurological involvement depending on their specific etiology.

Recognizing the various ways in which each etiology and its potential consequences may interact with the environment and affect child development will therefore contribute to constructive audiological, linguistic, and educational approaches that can enhance psychological adjustment and educational progress. For this reason, differential diagnosis is of critical importance. It is facilitated by a good medical history that includes information about the hearing loss as well as the age of onset and other related factors. In the end, whatever the etiology, habilitative and educational needs for the deaf child often are complex, extensive, and require long-term commitment (Diefendorf, 1996).

In our discussion of deaf people, we are basically looking at individuals with *sensorineural hearing loss,* defined as a hearing loss most commonly situated in the inner ear or, less frequently, in the auditory nerve, or both (Martin & Clark, 2000). Sensorineural deafness can be congenital (dating from birth) or can occur at any time after birth. Often there are delays in identifying deaf children, particularly when etiology is unclear (Pal Kapur, 1996), the child is under age 2, and there is a time lag between the hearing loss and the time of diagnosis. The physician must then retrospectively consider factors such as family history, medical history, and the site of the auditory dysfunction in determining cause. Sometimes there are several possible causal conditions, such as deafness in the family and maternal exposure to diseases causing hearing loss. Often the cause is unknown, but recent evidence indicates the importance of genetic factors, with at least 50 percent of cases attributable to genetic causes (Marazita et al., 1993; Willems, 2000).

Medical factors influence prevalence figures. For example, the rubella epidemic in the mid-1960s resulted in a temporary dramatic increase in the deaf population. Vaccines and medical advances not only have reduced incidences of hearing loss due to certain conditions, such as complications of Rh factor and rubella (Pal Kapur, 1996), but they have also increased incidences of hearing loss due to improved survival rates for infants, especially those born prematurely. For example, antibiotics help people survive meningitis, but the individuals often end up with hearing loss (Chase, Hall, & Werkhaven, 1996).

Here, we briefly present various leading causes of deafness to illustrate the complexity of etiological factors and the potential psychological and educational consequences for the developing child.

Major Nongenetic Causes of Deafness

Infections.   *Rubella,* or in popular terminology, *German measles,* is usually harmless except when the rubella virus infects a pregnant woman. Usually, the expectant mother is unaware that she has been affected, since there may be few overt symptoms of infection (rash, fever, etc.). Although rubella can affect the fetus any time during pregnancy, more damage to the fetus is possible when infection occurs during the first trimester. The invading virus attacks fetal tissues and reduces cell division. Damage can occur in the developing ear, eye, brain, and heart. Hearing loss occurs in 60 to 80 percent of these infants (Meyerhof, Cass, Schwaber, Sculerati, & Slattery, 1994) and there has been a high incidence of deaf-blind children as well (Moores, 2001a). Learning disabilities and other neurological difficulties may also be present. Since the last major rubella epidemic of 1964–1965, during which over 12,000 infants were born with hearing loss (Trybus, Karchmer, & Kerstetter, 1980), an effective immunization program has drastically reduced the incidence of maternal rubella in the Western world (Pal Kapur, 1996). In the United States, this etiology is more prevalent in deaf adults born during the 1960s and earlier; few children are currently affected.

Generally, post-rubella deaf children and youth do not do as well educationally as their deaf peers. The mean IQ (95.3) of the rubella group is significantly below the average IQ of 100 in the general population (Vernon, 1969a). Specifically, there is a higher chance of lower intellectual functioning in this group, although many do score above average or higher in intellectual functioning. Compared to other deaf and hard-of-hearing children, post-rubella youth have relatively large amounts of residual hearing (Hardy, Haskins, Hardy, & Shimizi, 1973). However, some of them cannot benefit from auditory amplification, whereas others with more profound losses are able to understand speech remarkably well. Although auditory training and the age at which it began may have some bearing on results, the varied, almost idiosyncratic way in which the rubella virus affects the auditory mechanism makes it difficult to predict potential benefit from residual hearing (Vernon & Andrews, 1990).

In terms of language and communication, there is a greater chance that individuals in the rubella group may have more difficulty with language processing in comparison to children with similar congenital hearing losses and IQs (Vernon & Andrews, 1990). The incidence of autism is greater than might generally be expected. Nonetheless, there are cases of post-rubella individuals who have exceptionally good language skills. Relative to psychological functioning, it is important to note that the majority of prenatal rubella deaf persons are within the normal range and have gone through life with no special difficulty. Research does indicate that behavior problems such as impulsivity, distractibility, and rigidity occur disproportionately within this group (Vernon, 1969a).

Cytomegalovirus (CMV), a member of the herpes group of viruses, has recently been identified as the most common cause of congenital viral-induced hearing loss (Schildroth, 1994; Strauss, 1999). This virus is so pervasive that 44 to 100 percent of adult sample populations have had previous exposure to CMV. Infections tend to result in mild symptoms except during pregnancy, when the virus is passed across the placenta to the fetus, or when the fetus is passing through the birth canal where the virus is being shed, or through infected breast milk or saliva. The extent of the problem in developing countries is likely much higher (Pal Kapur, 1996).

Symptoms of CMV in children depend on the timing of the infection during pregnancy and may include low birth weight, prematurity, small head size, increased intracranial pressure, spasticity, mental retardation, jaundice, hemorrhagic areas on the skin, and visceral abnormalities (Strauss, 1999). Out of approximately 40,000 infected infants, 30 to 60 percent of those born with symptoms can have hearing loss, and 6 to 24 percent of those without symptoms may exhibit hearing losses that progress throughout childhood (Meyerhof et al., 1994). Up to 10 percent of newborns born with CMV may develop varying degrees of perceptual, behavioral, psychomotor, or other neurological problems such as hyperactivity, ataxia, or hypotonia with clumsiness (Strauss, 1999). Schildroth (1994) reports that in a sample of deaf children with an etiology of CMV, there were significant percentages of mental retardation, cerebral palsy, orthopedic needs, learning disabilities, behavioral problems, and visual impairment, including blindness. Emotional problems may be progressive or appear later. Since late-onset hearing loss is possible, universal screening of hearing in newborns born with CMV infection will detect less than half of all cases that result in hearing loss (Fowler, Dahle, Boppana, & Pass, 1999). Ongoing hearing evaluations are critical for this group of infants.

Other viral causes include the herpes simplex virus and the human immunodeficiency virus (HIV). Based on a survey to identify the etiology of hearing impairment among Saudi children, a high prevalence of hearing impairment was found for those children with herpes simplex virus infection (Al Muhaimeed & Zakzouk, 1997). According to Dahle and McCollister (1988), as cited in Chase and colleagues (1996), the herpes simplex virus may have nearly the same effects as CMV for infants born to infected mothers. Although children born with HIV appear to have a greater incidence of middle-ear diseases compared to noninfected children, the possibility of sensorineural hearing loss exists (Chase et al., 1996). Pediatric HIV cases are also at risk for developmental language and perceptual delays, as well as motor and cognitive deficits (Madriz & Herrera, 1995).

Meningitis is an infection of the membranes surrounding the brain. *Viral meningitis* may occasionally result in deafness, but *bacterial* meningitis is a leading cause of deafness (Chase et al., 1996; Pal Kapur, 1996; Stein & Boyer, 1994). Interestingly, susceptibility to hearing loss as a result of meningitis may have a genetic component (Collins, 2001).

The meningitic syndrome often will result in intracranial pressure from accumulation of exudates, clotting, or rupturing of blood vessels, and generalized hemorrhaging. These conditions can result in severe neuropsychological sequelae in addition to abnormalities in body physiology and biochemistry (Vernon, 1969a). Since older children can verbalize the symptoms of the disease, such as headache or stiff neck, this facilitates earlier diagnosis and treatment with vaccines before significant damage occurs (Epstein, 1999; Stein & Boyer, 1994). Consequently, the incidence of deafness in older children has decreased where vaccines are available.

The diagnosis of meningitis in infants and young children may be delayed until the child becomes phlegmatic, convulses, or develops a very high fever (Vernon & Andrews, 1990). At this advanced stage, if the child survives, there is a significant chance that hearing loss and damage in brain functioning will occur, with hearing loss a likely consequence for up to 40 percent of this group (Stein & Boyer, 1994). Severe to profound sensorineural hearing loss occurs in 5 to 10 percent of children with bacterial meningitis (J. Niparko, personal communication, September 6, 2001). Post-meningitic children have the most severe hearing losses among the major etiologies for deafness (Vernon, 1967). If maximum amplification is of minimal help, cochlear implants may be of benefit if inserted before extensive cochlear ossification (new bone) sets in (Ng, Niparko, & Nager, 1999). Language development may be additionally affected by aphasia due to cerebral damage, although there is much individual variation. Behavioral problems such as hyperactivity, poor impulse control, and distractibility are possible consequences of meningitis. If there is damage in the vestibular system, which affects one's sense of balance, young post-meningitic children will be delayed in their ability to walk.

Congenital Toxoplasmosis.   Congenital toxoplasmosis is a parasitical infection caused in large part by improper handling of cat litter pans or contact with soil or sand (in playgrounds, for example) that may be frequented by cats. Congenital toxoplasmosis occurs only when pregnant women are infected during gestation or when they have a compromised immune system (Chase et al., 1996). About 30 percent of infants with congenital toxoplasmosis may have symptoms ranging from jaundice to hydrocephalus and cerebral calcifications, microcephaly, motor and intellectual retardation, eye scarring, and seizures. Prevalence studies indicate that roughly 15 to 26 percent of infected children could have some degree of hearing loss, either stable or progressive (Pal Kapur, 1996; Stein & Boyer, 1994). Differential diagnosis can be difficult because many manifestations of this disorder occur in other perinatal diseases, especially those caused by CMV. Audiological follow-up is recommended due to the possibility of progressive hearing loss. With early diagnosis, medical treatment can alleviate some of the symptoms (Stein & Boyer, 1994).

Erythroblastosis Fetalis.   Commonly known as the *Rh factor,* erythroblastosis fetalis is caused by blood incompatibility between mother and fetus, which can result in hearing loss after birth. It used to be a leading cause of deafness, but currently is controllable with Rh factor immunizations for the Rh– mother and blood transfusions for the Rh+ infant after birth. More than 70 percent of Rh factor children may present with additional disabilities such as cerebral palsy, difficulties in coordination, seizures, and language problems (Vernon & Andrews, 1990).

Ototoxic Drugs.   Drugs in the ototoxic category potentially may cause symptoms of hearing loss, tinnitus, imbalance, or vertigo (Pappas & Pappas, 1999). Whereas particular care must be taken with aminoglycosides (a specific group of antibiotics including streptomycin, gentamycin, and neomycin among others) (Chase et al., 1996; Martin & Clark, 2000; Pappas & Pappas, 1999), a study done by McCracken (1986) indicates that out of 1,300 infants receiving aminoglycosides, findings of hearing loss were infrequent. However, Pappas and Pappas (1999) comment that detecting hearing loss in young children based on audiometric data is difficult. Also, it is not always clear whether it is the disease or the drug used to treat the disease that causes hearing loss. Frequently, a medicine known to be ototoxic must be used in order to save a patient's life. Interestingly, it has recently been noted that some of those who lose their hearing subsequent to administration of aminoglycosides may have a genetic vulnerability for hearing loss (e.g., Fischel-Ghodsian et al., 1997).

In recent years, new possible causes of congenital or early-onset hearing loss have been identified, including drugs such as alcohol and cocaine ingested by the mother during pregnancy (Gerber, Epstein, & Mencher, 1995). These drugs have the potential to put infants at risk for developmental delays. Fetal alcohol syndrome (FAS) occurs in roughly 2 out of every 1,000 births. Preliminary findings on 22 FAS patients studied by Church, Eldis, Blakley, and Bawle (1997) indicate that 77 percent had intermittent conductive deafness due to recurrent ear infections, 27 percent had sensorineural hearing loss in addition to conductive hearing loss, and 55 percent presented with central hearing deficits. Additional complications include mental retardation, language deficits, and facial anomalies. Learning, behavioral, and emotional difficulties are often seen in this group of children.

When a mother has a history of ingesting cocaine, this may result in several factors that can cause birth asphyxia, hearing impairment, and behavioral differences such as hypersensitivity, high-pitched crying, and difficulty in orienting to visual or auditory stimuli (Gerber, Epstein, & Mencher, 1995). Further study is warranted to determine the actual impact of FAS and cocaine on hearing levels.

Prematurity.   To consider prematurity as a causative factor for deafness is debatable (Moores, 2001a). This is because, in part, prematurity can accompany other conditions causing deafness, such as ototoxic medication, meningitis, or other congenital causes of deafness (Vernon & Andrews, 1990). However, it has been found that 10 percent of premature infants (defined as having a birth weight of less than roughly 3.3 pounds) will have sensorineural hearing loss (Chase et al., 1996; Pal Kapur, 1996). For premature as well as full-term babies, anoxia and trauma during delivery can affect not only hearing but also vision as well as cognitive and neuromotor development. Although medical advances have raised the survival rate for prematurely born infants, the risk of multiple disabilities is present.

Noise-Induced Hearing Loss.   The etiology for approximately 36 percent of the total population with hearing loss can be attributed to damage from exposure to loud sounds (Einhorn, 1999). Hearing loss resulting from such exposure tends to take place over time and it is not often that one finds children with noise-induced hearing loss.

Genetic Causes of Deafness

It is highly likely that many individuals who attribute their deafness to unknown causes may have a genetic etiology. At present, it is known that genetic factors are responsible for approximately 50 to 60 percent or more of children diagnosed with hearing loss (Marazita et al., 1993; Willems, 2000). Considering that approximately 400 types of genetic deafness have been identified (Gorlin, Toriello, & Cohen, 1995), deciphering the specific type of genetic deafness is a complex endeavor, to say the least. Also, a complicating factor is that very often the child with an inherited hearing loss is the only such person in the family, therefore making it difficult to identify the cause of hearing loss. However, newly developed genetic testing procedures have improved this situation (Willems, 2000). Considerable progress has been made in understanding the biochemical and molecular characteristics of the genes involved in the composition of the hearing mechanism and the clinical effects of many types of hereditary deafness. This has resulted in practical applications of this new knowledge, improved genetic testing, and better access to genetic counseling for deaf individuals and their families (Arnos, 1999).

One-third of all genetic deafness is syndromic (characterized by hearing loss in combination with other medical or physical characteristics) (Willems, 2000). The rest is nonsyndromic (with only hearing loss). In other words, most individuals with genetic deafness inherit only the trait of hearing loss.

Genetic Transmission of Deafness

Each nucleated cell in the human body contains a copy of DNA (deoxyribonucleic acid), which is inherited (Arnos, Israel, Devlin, & Wilson, 1996). This biochemical material is organized within the nucleus of the dividing cell into structures called *chromosomes*. There are 46 chromosomes organized into 23 pairs in the nucleus of each cell. One pair of chromosomes is called the *sex chromosomes;* females have two X chromosomes and males have an X and a Y chromosome. One of each pair of chromosomes is inherited from the father, the other from the mother.

Each chromosome is composed of thousands of genes, which provide the biochemical instructions that "program" body development. The hundreds of genes that determine the structure and function of the ear are not isolated to a single chromosome but are spread across all the chromosomes. One change in a single gene in the pathway controlling the development of the hearing organ, or other parts of the body, can result in a variety of physical manifestations, including hearing loss in isolation or with other characteristics.

Genetic deafness is inherited in specific patterns that vary such that the deafness may be congenital (at birth) or occur any time after birth, even in the third or fourth decade of life or later (Gorlin, Toriello, & Cohen, 1995). Recently, it has been shown that some types of deafness may possibly be caused by the interaction of specific genetic and environmental factors (Usami, Abe, & Shinkawa, 1998).

Since chromosomes come in pairs, the genes that control particular traits or functions also come in pairs, one from each parent (Arnos et al., 1996). One of each pair of chromosomes is contributed to the child through the mother's egg cell and the father's sperm cell. Since each parent contributes one of each of their pairs of chromosomes, they also give one of each pair of genes on those chromosomes. There are four inheritance patterns: autosomal dominant inheritance, autosomal recessive inheritance, x-linked recessive inheritance, and mitrochondial inheritance.

Autosomal Dominant Inheritance.   When only a single copy of the gene is required for the trait to express itself, the mode of inheritance is dominant. Dominantly inherited traits are usually, but not always, inherited from one of the parents, and account for approximately 20 percent of hereditary types of deafness (Marazita et al., 1993). If neither of the parents has the trait, this can cause a new mutation (gene change) that can occur during any of the cell divisions that happen when egg and sperm cells are formed. *Autosomal* means that the gene is located on one of the 22 autosomes, or nonsex chromosomes. As shown in Figure 3.1, the per-

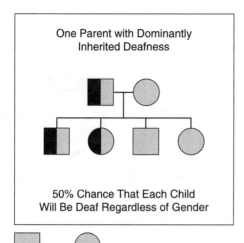

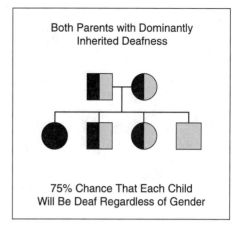

■ Male   ⬤ Female

FIGURE 3.1   Autosomal Dominant Conditions of Deafness

Source: Adapted from M. Vernon and J. Andrews, *The Psychology of Deafness* (New York: Longman), p. 23.

son with dominantly inherited deafness usually has only one copy of the deaf gene and one copy of the hearing gene. Consequently, there is a 50 percent chance of passing the deaf gene to each child. The hearing status of each child does not affect the hearing status of the next child; the chance is still 50 percent for each pregnancy. If both parents have a dominant gene for deafness, there is a 75 percent chance that each offspring will be deaf. In some families, even if all family members have the same gene for deafness, the hearing loss itself can range from mild to profound and can vary in age of onset. This is called *variable expression.* Some family members can even have the gene and still not have a hearing loss (*reduced penetrance*). Variable expression and reduced penetrance can appear in both syndromic and nonsyndromic types of deafness that are dominantly inherited (Arnos et al., 1996). In syndromic types, the associated physical and medical characteristics can even vary from one family member to another.

Autosomal Recessive Inheritance.   The inheritance pattern for genetic deafness is autosomal recessive in approximately 80 percent of identified cases of hereditary deafness (Marazita et al., 1993). In order for the trait to be manifested, a person must receive two copies of the gene, one from each parent. As shown in Figure 3.2, in a situation where the parents are hearing, both are carriers of one gene for deafness. With each pregnancy, there is a one in four possibility, or 25 percent, that the child will be deaf. Since most types of recessive hearing loss are nonsyndromic, it is often difficult to diagnose recessively inherited hearing loss when there is only one deaf child in the family. However, this situation is changing with the recent discovery of a common recessive nonsyndromic gene for deafness for which testing is now available (Willems, 2000). If one parent is deaf from recessive genes and the other

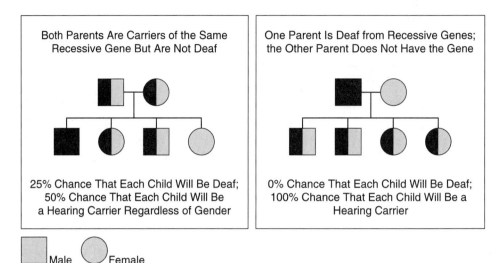

Both Parents Are Carriers of the Same Recessive Gene But Are Not Deaf	One Parent Is Deaf from Recessive Genes; the Other Parent Does Not Have the Gene
25% Chance That Each Child Will Be Deaf; 50% Chance That Each Child Will Be a Hearing Carrier Regardless of Gender	0% Chance That Each Child Will Be Deaf; 100% Chance That Each Child Will Be a Hearing Carrier

☐ Male   ○ Female

FIGURE 3.2   Autosomal Recessive Conditions of Deafness

Source: Adapted from M. Vernon and J. Andrews, *The Psychology of Deafness* (New York: Longman), p. 23.

parent is a carrier of that same gene, they have a 50 percent chance to have deaf children. Although many hearing people are carriers for recessive types of deafness, the parents must carry the exact same gene for the 25 percent chance of having a deaf child to apply.

The recent identification of *connexin 26* represents a significant development in the investigation of genes for nonsyndromic deafness (Arnos, 2002; Denoyelle et al., 1997). This gene codes for a protein that helps form tiny pores between support cells of the inner ear through which small molecules and chemicals critical for cell functioning are exchanged. To date, researchers have identified over 50 mutations in the connexin 26 gene that can alter the protein (Van Camp & Smith, 2001). Depending on the form of the connexin 26 anomaly, the onset and progression of the hearing loss varies. One mutation, which is very common, accounts for about 70 percent of deafness related to this gene (Arnos, 2002; Green et al., 1999). Most deafness caused by changes in the connexin 26 gene is inherited as a recessive trait. Following the recessive gene pattern for inheritance, when an offspring inherits a specific mutation in the connexin 26 gene from each parent, that person will be deaf. Current estimations are that mutations in the connexin 26 gene are the cause of deafness in at least one-third or more of individuals who have congenital, moderate to profound hearing loss (Arnos, 2002; Green et al., 1999). Mutations in connexin 26 are also estimated to be the cause of deafness in 50 to 80 percent of individuals with deaf siblings and hearing parents (Denoyelle et al., 1997). Rarely, a single mutation of the connexin 26 gene that is associated with deafness will be passed through families in a dominant pattern (Van Camp & Smith, 2001). Interestingly, in families with deaf parents and all deaf children, it is very likely that the etiology can be attributed to connexin 26 deafness, with the parents both having two copies of a recessive connexin 26 gene mutation, not necessarily the same mutation. Due to the molecular characteristics of connexin 26 mutations, testing for connexin 26 is relatively easy in comparison to other more complex genes for deafness (Arnos, 2002). Many genetic laboratories now offer connexin 26 testing on a research or clinical basis.

X-linked Recessive Inheritance. In approximately 2 to 3 percent of cases of hereditary deafness, the hearing loss is due to genes that are located on the X chromosome (Marazita et al., 1993). A female with a recessive gene for deafness on one of her X chromosomes (Xx) most often is hearing, and each of her sons has a 50 percent chance to inherit this X chromosome and be deaf (xY) (Arnos et al., 1996), as indicated in Figure 3.3. Each of her daughters has a 50 percent chance to be a carrier (Xx). If the father is deaf from an X-linked recessive gene, his daughters will be hearing carriers. All the sons will be hearing noncarriers of this gene, since they inherit the Y chromosome from their father.

Mitrochondial Inheritance. Mitochondrial transmission involves *mitochondria,* which are tiny cellular structures containing one circular DNA piece in the cytoplasm that produces energy for cellular activities. Mitochondria are transmitted from mother to child through the egg cell; there is no transmission from the father. Several rare types of deafness caused by mutations in mitochondrial genes have been identified (Van Camp & Smith, 2001). In addition, recent research indicates that the combined interaction of a mitochondrial gene mutation with an environmental variable can cause hearing loss. A mutation of a mitochondrial DNA gene has been implicated in some individuals who lose their hearing subsequent to low

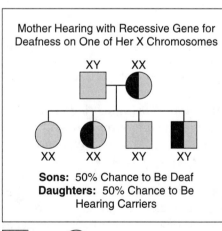 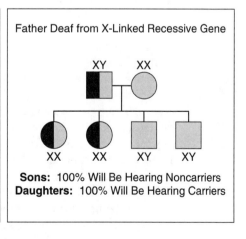

FIGURE 3.3   Sex-Linked Recessive Conditions of Deafness

Source: Adapted from M. Vernon and J. Andrews, *The Psychology of Deafness* (New York: Longman), p. 23.

dosages of aminoglycosides antibiotics (mentioned earlier in the Ototoxic Drugs section) (Fischel-Ghodsian et al., 1997).

Major Genetic Syndromes Involving Deafness

Several common types of syndromes will be discussed here. These syndromes were selected because of their relative frequency, because they represent conditions having psychological correlates, or because there are serious consequences. If identified and understood, appropriate treatment sometimes becomes possible.

Branchial-Oto-Renal Syndrome (BOR). The branchial-oto-renal syndrome is now recognized as one of the more common forms of autosomal dominant syndromic hearing impairment, with a prevalence of 2 percent or fewer of profoundly deaf children (Smith & Schwartz, 1998). Common features include malformed external ears, skin tags on the ear, ear pits (tiny holes) usually in front of the ear, tiny holes of the neck, kidney anomalies, and conductive, sensorineural, or mixed hearing impairment (Gorlin, Toriello, & Cohen, 1995; Smith & Schwartz, 1998). Individuals with BOR may have one or more of these features. This is an example of variable expression of a dominant gene, as discussed earlier. Identifying these individuals is important because of the need for screening family members and identifying potential kidney problems.

Jervell and Lange-Nielsen Syndrome. In the Jervell and Lange-Nielsen syndrome, which is inherited as an autosomal recessive trait, profound congenital hearing loss is associated with a heart condition (involving the electrical activity of the heart), which leads to fainting episodes that can range from several per year to several per day (Gorlin, Toriello, & Cohen, 1995). Sudden death is possible, and for this reason, early identification is critical to treat the heart abnormality. Carrier parents are also at risk for cardiac arrythmia (Smith, Green, & Van Camp, 1999). Any deaf child with a history of fainting spells should be referred for a genetic and/or cardiac evaluation (Smith, Schafer, Horton, & Tinley, 1998).

Neurofibromatosis Type 2 (NF-2). *Neurofibromatosis Type 2* is an inherited type of bilateral acoustic neuroma or nonmalignant tumors of the eighth cranial nerve and other brain sites that arise from the covering cells (Schwann cells) (MacCollin, 1998). It is inherited as an autosomal dominant trait, and the gene has been identified on chromosome 22. Associated symptoms—which can include progressive hearing loss, disturbances in balance and walking, dizziness, and tinnitus—may emerge during childhood, adolescence, or early adulthood. Surgery is resorted to if tumors reach large enough sizes or become malignant. After surgery for an NF-2 acoustic tumor, the eighth cranial nerve is divided and not amenable to cochlear implantation. Auditory brain stem implants have been placed in approximately 200 patients to date, with varying levels of success (J. Niparko, personal communication, September 6, 2001).

Pendred Syndrome. Pendred syndrome is an autosomal recessive condition that includes a combination of sensorineural hearing loss, usually congenital, and problems with iodine metabolism that leads to thyroid enlargement and goiter (Smith & Harker, 1998). Even though the gene for Pendred syndrome has been identified, genetic testing is made more difficult by the fact that this gene has many possible mutations and that clinical testing for Pendred syndrome is not widely available. Many individuals with Pendred syndrome will display cochlear malformations, usually characterized as Mondini aplasia or enlarged vestibular aqueduct. According to Ng, Niparko, and Nager (1999), Mondini aplasia may also be found in other syndromes, such as Waardenburg and Treacher Collins, and in some environmental forms of deafness. These authors cite studies that indicate the possibility of cochlear implantation in cases involving Mondini aplasia. Treatment is available for individuals who have secondary thyroid hormone imbalance.

Stickler Syndrome (SS). The Stickler Syndrome, or hereditary progressive arthro-opthalmopathy, is an autosomal dominant syndrome that results in variable symptoms that can include flattening of the facial profile, cleft palate, vision problems such as myopia or retinal detachment, musculoskeletal and joint problems occurring over time, and hearing loss (Nowak, 1998). The hearing loss can be attributed to Eustachian tube dysfunction secondary to cleft palate, or less often to high-frequency sensorineural hearing loss, which may be progressive. Mitral valve prolapse is possible; therefore, cardiology consultations are recommended for this syndrome. However, due to symptom variability SS is often underdiagnosed. Because of the multisystem impact, a multidisciplinary approach is critical to minimize the risk for associated problems.

Treacher-Collins Syndrome. The Treacher-Collins syndrome, also called *mandibulofacial dysostosis* and *Frenceschetti-Klein syndrome,* is a dominantly inherited condition that is associated with conductive (bone) hearing loss and malformations of the external ears, downward sloping eyes, flat cheekbones, and other facial features (Gorlin, Toriello, & Cohen, 1995; Reich, 1996a). It occurs in at least one of every 10,000 live births (Reich, 1996b). This is another example of a syndrome with variable expression of symptoms; the symptoms can also vary in severity. The conductive hearing loss can be treated with surgery or hearing aids. Because of the physical appearance, severely affected individuals often require psychological support for the psychosocial problems that can result from their physical appearance (K. Arnos, personal communication, January 22, 2002). Although facial surgical corrections are possible, these are complex and need to be tailored to the individual (Reich, 1996a).

Usher Syndrome. Usher syndrome is the cause of deaf-blindness in more than half of all deaf-blind adults, and its psychological and social effects can be devastating (Keats & Corey, 1999; Miner, 1999). There are three different forms, all of which can result in blindness by adolescence or early to late adulthood. Individuals with Type I have severe to profound congenital deafness, balance difficulties, and retinal degeneration due to retinitis pigmentosa beginning in childhood. *Retinitis pigmentosa* is an eye disease that proceeds from night blindness to retina pigment changes, loss of peripheral vision, and eventually to blindness in many individuals. About 3 to 6 percent of children born deaf will have Type I. Cochlear implants may be helpful for this group of individuals, in order to provide additional sensory input to compensate for vision loss. People with Type II, which may be relatively more common, have moderate to severe hearing loss, normal balance function, and later onset of retinitis pigmentosa in comparison to Type I. Type III, which is not as widely recognized clinically, involves progressive hearing loss and retinitis pigmentosa.

The progressive loss of vision necessitates ongoing readjustment in communication for those who have relied on vision (Miner, 1999). Activities of daily living become more difficult. Navigating the world becomes very stressful and new techniques have to be learned to maintain as much independence as possible. Since there is no medical treatment, schools for the deaf have developed screening programs to facilitate early identification and modifications in the environment to lessen the impact of vision loss on educational and psychosocial development (K. Arnos, personal communication, January 22, 2002). The recent identification of the myosin VIIA gene in one type of Usher syndrome (Keats & Corey, 1999) offers hope for future medical management in preventing vision loss.

Waardenburg Syndrome.   The Waardenburg syndrome is a common dominantly inherited condition that consists of several features, including sensorineural hearing loss, vestibular dysfunction, wide-set eyes (which can be of different colors or bright blue), white forelock of hair, a broad nose, and skin depigmentation (Gorlin, Toriello, & Cohen, 1995; Smith & Harker, 1998). Not all are necessarily present in any one case. Intelligence tends to be in the normal range. Hearing loss may be present in only 20 to 50 percent of all cases. Because of the dominant genetic transmission, it is typical to see Waardenburg syndrome in several generations within families, with many not knowing they have the gene because the features are so variable (Smith, Kolodziej, & Olney, undated).

Genetic Counseling

It is increasingly important for professionals who work with deaf persons and their families to have some understanding of genetic conditions and traits, and their social, psychological, educational, and medical impact, and to know when to make referrals to genetic counselors (Arnos, 1999). Genetic counseling can assist families in getting accurate information about the causes of deafness, related medical or psychological complications, the chance for future children to have syndromic or nonsyndromic deafness, and reproductive options (Arnos, 1999). Even though an exact etiology cannot always be determined through genetic counseling or testing, parents can feel reassured if they are informed that the possibility of additional medical complications is low or nonexistent. This information can be very helpful for families as they try to plan their future. Additionally, families can be informed about new technologies in genetic testing and programs that offer testing for specific genes for deafness. Effective genetic counselors will assess the emotional state of the people seeking genetic counseling and help them with issues that emerge in dealing with the results of genetic testing and making decisions that will impact the family (Arnos, 1999; Vernon & Andrews, 1990). This is particularly important for individuals who are overwhelmed by information that their child may have symptoms related to their genetic make-up that require specialized medical or educational attention.

Genetic counseling is often useful not only for hearing couples with deaf children but also for deaf adults. The etiology of deafness generally is not of major concern to people who have grown up deaf, since basically they adjust to life as deaf persons and do not dwell on why they are deaf. Also, they often do not have other physical or medical conditions that warrant special attention. However, it is natural for deaf persons to wonder about the cause of their deafness and about the possibility of having deaf or hearing children as they approach reproductive age (Arnos, 1999, 2002). Culturally deaf adults may prefer to have deaf children (Middleton, Hewison, & Mueller, 2001) and therefore seek genetic counseling. This is understandable, considering the fact that deaf persons, particularly culturally Deaf individuals who are very comfortable with their Deaf way of life, may be more comfortable having deaf children, just as hearing persons will be more comfortable having hearing children. Other deaf adults have health problems and want to know about the possibility of syndromes associated with deafness that may be impacting the ease of their lives (Arnos, Israel, Devlin, & Wilson, 1996).

The genetic counseling process generally involves an evaluation by a team of professionals, including a medical doctor specializing in clinical genetics, a Ph.D. medical geneticist, genetic counselors with master's degrees, social workers, and nurses (Arnos, 1999). For the evaluation, information is obtained about family history, medical history, physical examination results, and medical testing as needed.

Family history is very important, as it provides details about family patterns of hearing loss or medical features of family members. Information about the health and hearing status of close and distant relatives is collected, as well as information about the blood relationship among relatives and the ethnic background of the family. However, if there is nothing in the family history, this does not necessarily mean the etiology is not genetic (Keats, 2001). Some genes can be passed on with no one being affected for generations. The medical history covers birth history, serious illnesses, or chronic health problems, and also includes audiograms for the deaf person and other family members. This information can provide clues indicating the presence of a genetic syndrome or environmental cause. The physical examination—done by a board-certified M.D. clinical geneticist trained to recognize specific traits and features, as well as additional medical testing such as chromosome or metabolic testing—will contribute to a genetic diagnosis when combined with the family and medical history.

The final part of the genetic evaluation involves discussion of diagnosis, inheritance pattern, prognosis, and treatment options. This information must be provided to clients in a way that is sensitive to their emotional and family needs, since there may be profound consequences for individual lives depending on the type of genetic conditions identified during the evaluation. The team can also make appropriate referrals to educational programs, medical facilities, or organizations specializing in specific genetic conditions as needed, particularly in cases where families need follow-up help.

In this era of expanding genetic technology, particularly as a consequence of the well-known Human Genome Project, which is in the process of mapping the thousands of genes that exist, genetic testing and genetic counseling will likely become more widely available. There are moral and ethical considerations that have to be taken into account, since the possibility for genetic manipulation is increasing. The implications of this process for altering human life are profound.

In the case of genetic deafness, the values attributed to a hearing child in comparison to a deaf child (depending on parent reactions) may differ and eventually affect reproductive decisions that can have repercussions for the future of Deaf culture and the deaf community (Arnos, 2002). This is an area where medical perspectives of what it means to be deaf may collide with Deaf cultural perceptions (see Chapter 2). Lane and Bahan (1998) state that the healthy diversity of people relies on the preservation of minority cultures, of which Deaf culture is one. The possible eradication of genetic deafness can be viewed as an ethical move to alleviate the difficulties of being deaf in a hearing society, or alternatively perceived as denigrating the value of the lives of Deaf people and as leading to cultural genocide. Lane and Bahan (1998) define this latter aspect as unethical.

During the late 1880s, a eugenics movement supported selective breeding and/or the elimination of undesirable genes (Friedlander, 1999). This eventually culminated in the Nazi Germany doctrine of racial purity that condoned the sterilization and killing of victims who carried hereditary diseases, including deaf people (Biesold, 1999). Arnos (2002) recommends that in order to counteract the mistakes of the past—when the misuse of genetic information caused people to lose their humanity—more members of the deaf community should empower themselves through being educated about the genetics of deafness and form their own judgments about emerging genetic technology and its potential impact on the lives of deaf people.

THE DIAGNOSIS OF DEAFNESS

Hearing Screening

Screening for hearing loss has emerged as an important aspect of neonatal care. Early diagnosis of deafness will enhance the child's opportunities to develop environmental awareness, communication, and academic and social skills (Diefendorf, 1999). In the United States, universal newborn hearing screening is now mandated in an increasing number of states, and there are ongoing efforts to implement such screening in more hospitals (ASHA, 1999). However, one must not forget that this screening may miss children with, for example, progressive or central hearing loss (involving the central nervous system) (Tucker & Bhattacharya, 1992).

In studies soliciting opinions about neonatal hearing screening, the overwhelming majority of parents of children with varying degrees of hearing loss who responded would have welcomed this screening had it been available (Luterman & Kurtzer-White, 1999; Watkin, Beckman, & Baldwin, 1995). In a 1991–93 prevalence study of children with serious hearing impairment in metropolitan Atlanta, the mean age for diagnosis was 2.9 years old (Van Naarden, Decoufle, & Caldwell, 1999). Christiansen and Leigh (2002) report that in their parent sample, age of diagnosis was more common between ages 12 and 24 months. Universal newborn hearing screening should lower this mean age considerably.

The Diagnostic Phase

For most parents,* the diagnostic process tends to be a complicated one, unless there is a major illness causing the deafness or an infant screening picks up on the deafness. When new parents do not recognize poor responses to sound, deny suspicions about hearing loss, have pediatricians who minimize parent concerns about their child's inability to hear, and get inaccurate information from audiologists after testing, it takes that much longer to diagnose the deafness and deal with its implications (Christiansen & Leigh, 2002; Mertens, Sass-Lehrer, & Scott-Olson, 2000; Vernon & Andrews, 1990).

Pediatricians are usually the first resource that parents use when there is suspicion about hearing loss. Parents are then referred to otologists and audiologists for hearing evaluations. The time lag from suspicion to final diagnosis is often six months or more (Mertens, Sass-Lehrer, & Scott-Olson, 2000).

Some parents may experience relief that there is not a worse diagnosis, but for most, this information comes as an emotional shock or as an intense disappointment, the full depth of which is rarely sensed by the professional making the diagnosis (Christiansen & Leigh, 2002). Parents new to deafness often cannot immediately assimilate the irreversibility of deafness and the implications of having a deaf child. They are dealing with the loss of the "normally hearing child" dream and substituting the vision of a child who cannot hear the parents' words of comfort, their singing, or their spoken language.

Luterman (1999) writes that it is a mistake for professionals to give extensive information to parents at the time of diagnosis, for parents need time to process what often is devastating news. The emotional pain can be intense before subsiding into a dull ache, as parents acknowledge that their lives as parents will not be what they had expected. More information can be absorbed during follow-up visits, though parents will experience grief reactions of varying intensity and varying duration (generally 6 to 12 months) (Kricos, 1993; Luterman, 1999). These grief reactions are not pathological; rather, this is a normal process that allows the entire fam-

---

* In referring to parents, we recognize that they are part of many different family constellations, including single parent families and families with nontraditional structures.

ily to come to terms with the deafness and move ahead in exploring ways to cope with a deaf child in the family. Parents feel supported and less alone when they meet with other parents who have been in similar situations (Hintermair, 2000; Kampfe, 1989; Luterman & Kurtzer-White, 1999).

During the grieving process, many feelings—most often guilt, anger, and/or depression, either separately or simultaneously—are expressed (Kampfe, 1989; Luterman, 1999). Parents may feel guilty that they did not protect their child and wonder what they did to contribute to the child's deafness, particularly when there is no clear cause. For example, the mother may reenact each step of her pregnancy to ascertain what might have happened. For this mother, genetic counseling may help to deal with the guilt.

Depending on the family's background, cultural explanations may predominate over Western medical interpretations. Eldredge (1999) presents several such examples for Native Americans, including one in which the mother, having seen an owl (an evil omen) during her pregnancy, was believed to have caused the baby's deafness. The deafness may be seen as punishment for previous transgressions or as an act of God, both fatalistic attitudes that prevail in many Latino cultures (Hernandez, 1999; Steinberg, Davila, Collazo, Loew, & Fischgrund, 1997). The punishment perspective may hold in some Asian/Pacific cultures, based on a variety of beliefs about the cause of disabilities, such as parents' wrongdoing or pregnant women looking at scissors or rabbits (Cheng, 2000). Therefore, deafness is seen as a curse, though that is slowly changing.

If parents feel cheated by not having a normally hearing child, this can lead to anger, because of the burdens they may feel that a deaf child brings. They do not realize the joys they may experience as they watch their child learn and grow. Parents' anger reflects a loss of control; it also acts to mask fear about the loss of a supposedly secure future with their child (Luterman, 1999). Some parents may run from doctor to doctor, searching in vain for a different diagnosis or cure. It takes energy to be angry—energy that can be channeled into constructive action when parents are able to acknowledge their fears and frustrations. Anger can also turn into depression if the parents feel that everything they do is futile. As a normal part of the grief reaction, bouts of depression may emerge. Depression is pathological if it becomes chronic and the parent cannot act in the interest of the child.

Grandparents, siblings, and other family members are also emotionally affected by the diagnosis (Luterman, 1999; Morton, 2000). Some grandparents are able to provide warm support even when they are sad; others may be stuck in denial, offer well-meaning advice, or try to make the parents feel better by putting a positive spin on the diagnosis. This only encourages the parents' denial of their emotional pain.

Siblings have to adjust to a new set of family circumstances that may include changes in priorities as more attention is paid to the deaf child. For example, all of a sudden, the sibling has to go with mom and new baby to parent intervention programs instead of staying home and playing with neighborhood friends. Changes in how family members communicate may be perceived as another added burden.

Parents may experience feelings of inadequacy when faced with the task of learning how to raise a deaf child. In this situation, they may be overly willing to entrust hearing specialists, educators, or other helping professionals, and allow them to make critical decisions about how to direct their child's life. Some of these professionals may make the mistake of accepting this responsibility, which Luterman (1999) calls the *Annie Sullivan Effect*.* To counteract this, professionals should take utmost care to help the parents increase their own feelings of confidence about their capacity to parent. When that happens, the end result more likely will be a well-adjusted child.

When the emotional feelings surrounding the diagnostic phase are cathartically expressed in a safe environment over time, parents can begin to psychologically let go of the "normal" child they had expected and internalize the fact that they have a deaf child—a child who is not hearing but who can still enrich their lives in different and equally satisfying ways (Leigh, 1987). They then are more able to accept and enact the necessary changes in the life situation of their family. A positive attitude facilitates the family's ability to grow together in this new situation (Luterman, 1999; Vernon & Andrews, 1990).

Parents from relatively affluent, middle-class backgrounds tend to use services more effectively (Moores, Jatho, & Dunn, 2001). There is a critical need for comprehensive services that meet the needs of less educated and less affluent families. Whatever the family situation, all professionals must be sensitive to family dynamics in order to facilitate adaptations that will facilitate both the acceptance of the diagnosis and the healthy development of the deaf child. Professionals need to recognize the resiliency of many families who can "rise to the occasion" in the process of surmounting crises (Leigh, 1987; Moeller & Condon, 1998; Moores, Jatho, & Dunn, 2001). Corollary to this, Pipp-Siegel, Sedey, and Yoshinaga-Itano (2002) conclude from an ongoing longitudinal study that the stress levels of mothers of children with hearing loss enrolled in early intervention programs do not differ from the typical stress levels of mothers with hearing children, further affirming the resiliency factor when support is available. The researchers found that for those mothers exhibiting stress, risk factors include lower income, lower perceived support from others, negative perceptions of daily hassles, presence of additional disabilities, language delays, and less severe hearing loss (possibly due to the underestimation of communication difficulties).

One of the best enabling types of interventions is to ask the parents or family members about what interventions would work for them, keeping in mind that these families are heterogeneous with respect to culture, language, economic resources, genetic make-up, and family structure, and no two children are alike (Mertens, Sass-Lehrer, & Scott-Olson, 2000). Moeller and Condon (1998) recommend setting up a collaborative parent-professional partnership that incorporates talking together, clarifying parent needs and concerns, identifying questions and

*As the teacher of deaf-blind Helen Keller, Annie Sullivan took over all responsibilities for Keller, thereby minimizing the role of Helen's parents.

supports, designing a plan of action, deciding who does what so that parents as well as professional partners share responsibilities, and evaluating the process.

Deaf Parents

For deaf parents, the diagnostic phase takes on different overtones (Lane, Hoffmeister, & Bahan, 1996; Leigh, 1987). Many deaf parents will say that the most important thing is to have a healthy child, with hearing ability being secondary (Leigh, 1987). For this reason, they are not as focused on the diagnosis of deafness per se, preferring to ascertain their child's hearing status through careful observation. However, with universal newborn hearing screening, it is more likely that clarification of hearing status will happen shortly after birth.

Deaf parents are more open to the possibility of having a deaf child, primarily because of their experience and comfort with being deaf. They also see the deaf child as a reflection of themselves, just as a hearing child is a reflection of hearing parents. Some culturally Deaf parents may experience temporary disappointment if their child is deaf, considering that the child may face many extra challenges in life, but this reaction usually does not last (Lane, Hoffmeister, & Bahan, 1996). Studies have reported positive results for interactions between deaf children and their deaf parents (Meadow-Orlans, 1997).

However, the reality is that approximately 80 to 90 percent of deaf parents have hearing children (Schein & Delk, 1974). They have to cope with a different set of realities relative to socialization, communication, and education needs. Other things such as socioeconomic and educational levels being equal, deaf parents are as capable of parenting children, deaf or hearing, as their hearing peers, and this is increasingly recognized in today's society (Lane, Hoffmeister, & Bahan, 1996). Preston's (1994) comprehensive study of hearing adult children with deaf parents indicates that their views about their childhood experiences are as diverse as those of other groups. Hearing children of deaf parents are generally not considered to be at risk for developmental problems. However, some deaf parents can benefit from support services to increase their level of comfort and efficacy in parenting hearing children. This is especially true if they have had limited communicative experiences with hearing family members while growing up (Meadow-Orlans, 1997). This is analogous to the problem hearing parents new to deafness face in raising deaf children.

The Aftermath of Diagnosis and Psychological Considerations

This period involves the recognition that there is a bewildering array of complex decisions that parents have to make about communication approaches, language choices, amplification (including hearing aids and cochlear implants), and type of education (Christiansen & Leigh, 2002; Leigh, 1987; Stewart & Kluwin, 2001). Early intervention is critical in helping parents develop effective approaches, particularly in communicating with their newly diagnosed child. Parents may feel overwhelmed and confused, considering the plethora of communication, language, and educational approaches to choose from, as well as various amplification options. We discuss these issues throughout the book. Research indicates that parents want unbiased information from professionals (Christiansen & Leigh, 2002; Mertens, Sass-Lehrer, & Scott-Olson, 2000). This will empower parents in gauging what may work best for their family situation.

Whether hearing aids or cochlear implants are selected as the primary amplification tool should depend on the level of hearing loss, age of onset, and other related factors. Audiologists evaluate whether the loss is mild, moderate, severe, or profound, and recommend specific types of amplification depending on medical and audiometric results. It is not possible to predict speech or spoken language reception based on degree of hearing loss alone, since there are other factors such as age of diagnosis, environmental noise, how much hearing there is for the different frequencies that are part of the speech range, and the ability to use auditory aids. See the appendix at the end of this chapter for additional information on audiological aspects.

Children with mild hearing losses are currently identified as a group requiring services such as assistive listening devices, since they may demonstrate inconsistent responses to sound and do miss softly spoken speech (Maxon & Brackett, 1992). Hard-of-hearing children fall into the category of those with moderate to moderately severe hearing loss. They generally have the capacity to use hearing as the primary mode for understanding speech and acquiring language when appropriately fitted with hearing aids (Maxon & Brackett, 1992), and can supplement their listening with information perceived through vision, such as speech-reading or signs (Diefendorf, 1996).

For deaf children with severe and profound hearing losses, sound is a secondary and supplemental channel to vision, or to touch if there is a vision problem (Diefendorf, 1996). Most often, vision is the primary channel for environmental awareness, communication, and language learning. Amplification by itself is rarely sufficient for understanding spoken communication, but it is of value in supplementing vision. Although hearing aids are often of considerable help, cochlear implants (see Chapter 7) are increasingly being recommended for those children whose hearing losses preclude benefit from hearing aids (Christiansen & Leigh, 2002). Parents presented with this option have to decide whether to have their young child undergo the surgical procedure for a cochlear implant. For many of them, this can be an agonizing process, and they do not make this decision lightly. In retrospect, most see the implant as beneficial because of increased environmental awareness or communicative competence.

Other decisions involve language and communication choices (spoken English or spoken language in the home if not English, ASL, signed English, cued speech, etc.). Parents face the pressure of deciding how to communicate with their child, and then need to learn how to maximize their child's ability to understand them. This means learning specific techniques or learning signs or cued speech, all of which take time for parents to master. If parents work, they may have to be resourceful in juggling time to cope with an avalanche of new requirements for helping their child. Educational programs have different communication and language approaches, and parents must select which program best meets their child's needs, depending on what is available in their area. As time goes on, parents face the need to consider whether to place their deaf child in a specialized school for deaf children or in a mainstream/inclusion setting (see Chapter 6). It helps parents if they are aware that children can change programs, since their communication and educational needs will change as they develop. Parents are understandably fearful of making mistakes when facing this myriad of necessary decisions. They need reassurance that they are doing the best they can for their child and that any decision they make is not necessarily irrevocable.

By selecting specific educational placements, parents are making choices about whether their child will interact with hearing or deaf peers, or both. This represents an additional factor that parents must face. Bat-Chava and Deignan's (2001) review of the literature indicates that deaf children can be lonely or isolated if there are problems socializing with hearing peers. Parents who are relatively comfortable with having a deaf child will be more comfortable with their child having deaf friends. Exposure to the gamut of deaf adult role models, ranging from oral deaf adults to members of Deaf culture, will help increase the comfort level of parents (Hintermair, 2000). Parents do not often meet signing deaf adults, and when they do, they usually feel intimidated initially because of their limited signing skills (Christiansen & Leigh, 2002). Professionals can help facilitate this process of interaction when parents are ready and willing.

In the case of deaf parents with deaf children, the aftermath of diagnosis is less intense. Deaf parents are aware of language and communication options, educational options, and amplification choices. They make decisions depending in large part on their own experiences growing up, what is available in their area, and what they perceive their children's needs to be. Many will opt for specialized schools for deaf children, which they see as providing full communicative accessibility and optimal socialization opportunities with deaf peers. Others are comfortable with mainstream settings. The literature provides ample evidence of the fact that deaf children of deaf parents tend to fare better overall than deaf children of hearing parents in language development and educational achievement (Marschark, 2001), although many deaf children of hearing parents also achieve success.

CONCLUSION

If the "beginning" is handled in ways that facilitate parental adjustment to the presence of a deaf child in the family, the end result can be a deaf adult who functions effectively in society. When professionals help parents understand etiology and all the complex factors, including communication, that need to be considered in making child-rearing decisions, parents are better enabled to do the best they can for their deaf child.

SUGGESTED READINGS

Gerber, S. (Ed.). (2001). *The Handbook of Genetic Communicative Disorders*. San Diego, CA: Academic Press.

    This book contains two excellent chapters related to genetics and deafness. Chapter 5, titled Genetic Deafness, is authored by Robert J. Ruben. Dr. Ruben provides a succinct history of the genetics of hearing impairment. He provides a classification of genetically based hearing disorders. He also gives a description of 10 genetic syndromes associated with deafness with clinical applications and recommendations for management. The last chapter, Treatment and Prevention, written by Sanford Gerber, provides an excellent discussion on gene therapy. He raises provocative questions on the ethics of gene therapy and its implications for professionals working with the deaf community.

Waltzman, S., & Cohen, N. (2000). *Cochlear Implants:* New York: Thieme.

    This book contains chapters on a wide variety of topics associated with implants: engineering of the implant, medical and surgical aspects, device programming, variables affect speech and language, educational implications, and future trends.

Schwartz, S. (Ed.). (1996). *Choices in Deafness*. Bethesda, MD: Woodbine House.

    This book provides information about medical evaluation of hearing loss, audiological testing, and amplification options, including hearing aids and cochlear implants. Additionally, it includes chapters about the various communication options that parents will be considering. The information is presented in a nonjudgmental way. There is a comprehensive list of national organizations serving individuals who are deaf and hard of hearing.

■ ■ ■ ■ ■

THE BASICS OF AUDIOLOGY

Audiology covers the science of hearing (Martin & Clark, 2000). So exactly what does an audiologist do? With appropriate professional qualifications, an audiologist provides services related to the assessment and habilitation or rehabilitation of persons with auditory and vestibular impairments, as well as services directed at preventing these impairments (American Academy of Audiology, 1997). Audiologists work in a variety of settings, including private practice, schools, ENT offices, government agencies, university training programs, and hospitals. The American Speech-Language and Hearing Association, the national organization for professional audiologists, maintains updated lists of certified individuals and sites where audiologists can be found (www.professional.asha.org).

THE HEARING MECHANISM

Let's begin with the ear itself. How do people hear?* What is described here is a very simplified explanation of the process, which starts at the outer ear (pinna or auricle) when the sound is channeled down the ear canal (external auditory meatus) to the first part of the middle ear—specifically, the eardrum (tympanic membrane). Sound causes the eardrum to vibrate. This sets in motion a chain of vibrations transmitted sequentially by three tiny bones (ossicles) called the *hammer* (malleus), *anvil* (incus), and *stirrup* (stapes).

   The movement of the stapes into the oval window, which separates the middle ear from the inner ear, sets the stage for the next part of this sound transmission system. The inner ear holds the vestibular system (involved in balance) and the cochlea. The cochlea contains auditory receptor cells with hair-like structures (cilia), often called *hair cells*. These hair cells convert the mechanical energy set up by the middle-ear system to electrical energy. This energy then travels via the auditory nerve (the eighth cranial nerve) on to the auditory centers of the brain, thus resulting in the perception of sound.

*Note: The condensed information in this appendix is based on the section "How We Hear and Hearing Loss," published in J. Lucker, "Cochlear Implants: A Technological Overview," in *Cochlear Implants in Children: Ethics and Choices*, by J. Christiansen & I. W. Leigh (Washington, DC: Gallaudet University Press, 2002), pp. 45–64. Used with permission.

TYPES OF HEARING LOSS

If the components of the outer and middle ear are operating inefficiently, the related hearing loss is said to be *conductive*. Interference with sound transmission going through these two parts of the ear can come from many sources, including wax buildup in the ear, ear infection, or anatomical malformations. Conductive hearing loss is often temporary and generally can be corrected by medical treatment, including surgery, such as, for example, the draining of middle-ear fluid or reconstructing the middle-ear bones. When the hearing loss is caused by problems within the inner ear, it is called *sensorineural hearing loss*, which tends to be permanent. Sensorineural hearing loss can be caused by environmental factors, such as noise, toxic medications, or head injury, and can also be genetic and progressive in nature. With sensorineural hearing loss, hair cells do not perform their role in the transmission of sound stimuli to the brain. This happens when hair cells do not develop normally, are damaged, or have deteriorated secondary to aging or disease. Last, mixed hearing loss reflects problems that occur simultaneously in both the conductive and sensorineural mechanisms (Martin & Clark, 2000).

THE MEASUREMENT OF HEARING

Traditional hearing tests use calibrated equipment to determine the type and degree of hearing loss and to assess communication potentials. During one portion of the hearing test, the equipment generates pure tones within a restricted range of frequencies, usually in discrete intervals from 125 to 8,000 Hz, with Hz (hertz) representing cycles per second. The equipment can also vary the loudness level of each frequency. Pitch, a subjective term reflecting how high or low sounds are, is related to frequency. Specifically, pitch rises as frequency increases. Examples of low pitch would be men's voices, drums beating, doors closing, and vowels in words. High pitch examples include women's voices, bird sounds, telephones ringing, and consonants in words.

   The technical term for loudness is expressed in dB (decibel), which represents the unit of measurement of sound intensity. The audiologist charts the loudness level (dB) where individuals just barely detect each pitch or frequency (Hz) presented. This represents the threshold level and is plotted on an audiogram (see Figure 1).

   During the pure tone evaluation procedure, sound is directed to the ears via earphones (air conduction) and via a vibrator held at either the forehead or mastoid part of the skull (bone conduction). An individual's air and bone conduction threshold responses are compared. This provides information about the type(s) and degree of hearing loss that may be present.

   Figure 1 shows a sample form that audiologists fill out when conducting hearing evaluations. The audiogram on the form is designed to show both frequency and decibel information. The broken line at the 15 dB hearing level (HL) reflects the

Name:_____ Date:_____ Age:_____ Sex:_____ **Audiologist:** _____

DOB: _____ Referred by:_____ **Transducer: headphones insert**

AUDIOMETER:_____**IMMITTANCE METER:**_____ **Response Reliability:** good   moderate   poor

AUDIOGRAM
FREQUENCY (PITCH) IN HERTZ (Hz)

LEGEND

		Right	Left
Air:	Unmasked	◯	✗
	Masked	△	▢
Bone:	Unmasked	◁	▷
	Masked	▢	▢

No Response ↓ _____
Best Bone ▢ _____
Vibrotactile Response ★ _____
Unaided Sound Field **S** _____

Narrow Band Noise
Warble Tone

PURE TONE AVERAGE (R: / L:)

	Right	Left
AIR	dBHL	dBHL

TYMPANOMETRY (daPa)

ABBREVIATIONS

C1 Canal Volume
CNA Could Not Average
CNE Could Not Establish
CNT Could Not Test
DNT Did Not Test
HL Hearing Level
MLV Monitored Live Voice
MTS Monosyllable, Troches, Spondees Test
MCL Most Comfortable Listening Level
NR No Response
PB% Word Recognition
SC Static Compliance
SDT Speech Detection Threshold
SRT Speech Recognition Threshold
S/N Signal To Noise Ratio
UCL Uncomfortable Listening Level

	daPa	
	Right	Left
C₁ =		
SC=		

ACOUSTIC REFLEX MEASUREMENTS

Ear	Right				Left			
Stimulus	.5K	1K	2K	4K	.5K	1K	2K	4K
Contra (HL)								
Decay								
Ipsi (HL) (SPL)								

SPEECH AUDIOMETRY (dBHL) MLV ▢ RECORDED ▢ LIST:_____

	SDT	SRT	MCL	UCL	PB% / HL	PB% / HL	PB% / HL	SIGNAL____ NOISE____ HL	MTS Categ% / Recog%
R								%	
L								%	
SF UNAIDED								%	
AIDED								%	

TEST INTERPRETATION:

TYPE:	R	L
▢ No Hearing Loss	_____	_____
▢ Conductive	_____	_____
▢ Mixed	_____	_____
▢ Sensorineural	_____	_____

DEGREE

R:_____

L:_____

RECOMMENDATION(S)

▢ Medical Referral
▢ Recheck Following Consultation
▢ Special Tests_____
▢ Hearing Aid Evaluation

▢ New Earmold(s)
▢ Hearing Aid Check
▢ See Hearing Aid Worksheet
▢ Annual Reevaluation
▢ Other (Specify):_____

COMMENTS: _____
_____
_____
_____

_____   _____
Supervising Audiologist, CCC-A   Graduate Clinician

FIGURE 1   Sample Audiogram Form
Source: Reprinted with permission of the Gallaudet University Hearing and Speech Center.

upper limit of normal hearing sensitivity. The degree of hearing loss is often indicated by the average of the responses obtained at three different frequencies (500, 1,000, and 2,000 Hz). Hearing loss levels are classified into the following categories (Clark, 1981, as cited in Diefendorf, 1996, p. 9):

0–15dB	Normal
16–25dB	Slight or minimal hearing loss
26–40dB	Mild hearing loss
41–55dB	Moderate hearing loss
56–70dB	Moderately severe hearing loss
71–90dB	Severe hearing loss
>90dB	Profound hearing loss

Readers must be aware that even if two people both have a 90 dB hearing loss, it cannot be anticipated that the audiogram will look the same, because the three pure tone hearing threshold levels for each person may be at varying points, even if the end result is an average of 90 dB. People with a 90 dB hearing loss do not necessarily hear things in the same way, which is why they may prefer different types of hearing aids that are better suited to their individual audiometric configuration.

Figure 2 provides some examples of where ordinary environmental sounds may fall on the audiogram when considering their decibel level and frequency range. Someone with a hearing loss of 85 dB HL at 500 Hz will be unable to hear a dog barking, as indicated in Figure 2.

Returning to Figure 1, note a section on Speech Audiometry. This involves assessing the individual's ability to identify, recognize, and discriminate speech. Standardized tests are administered using the same calibrated equipment used for pure tone testing. There are many different tests that an audiologist can use to assess communication potentials. Results can often be very consistent with the type and degree of hearing loss. Measurements are obtained in both unaided (no amplification) and aided listening conditions.

In the Figure 1 audiogram, there is a chart labeled Tympanometry. *Tympanometry* is an objective test that evaluates middle-ear status—more specifically, how well the eardrum moves. This is determined by using specialized equipment that measures eardrum movement with the introduction of a tone and various amounts of positive and negative pressure in the external ear canal. The individual just has to remain quiet during the procedure—no volitional response is required. Abnormal readings can suggest conditions such as fluid in the middle-ear space, Eustachian tube dysfunction, perforation of the eardrum, or disarticulation of the ossicles.

Other procedures have also been developed to predict the presence or absence of hearing sensitivity. These include Auditory Brainstem Response (ABR) testing (like an EEG) and measurement of Otoacoustic Emissions (OAE), both of which are useful for children and difficult to test populations. Both procedures are noninvasive, although administering ABR sometimes requires sedation.

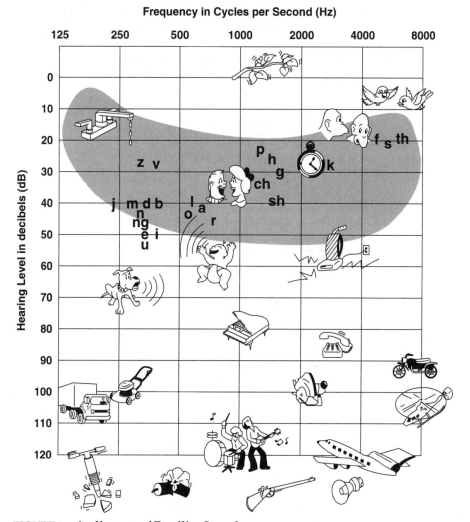

FIGURE 2   Audiogram of Familiar Sounds
Source: Reprinted with permission of the American Academy of Audiology.

AMPLIFICATION SYSTEMS

Once it has been determined that hearing loss is present and medical consultation has ruled out any medical or surgical intervention, there are various amplification options to consider. The final decision depends on what may be the best match between individual needs and the options being considered. Since there is a wide range of amplification choices, the audiologist will facilitate the process of selecting the type of amplification that best fits the person.

The most basic option is the hearing aid worn behind the ear or in the ear canal. This device amplifies sounds at various frequencies. Analog and digital hearing aids offer several different circuit options, which provide the listener with different sound processing strategies that can be adjusted by the audiologist to suit the person's needs. Digital hearing aids can be programmed to adjust gain, frequency response, and output to the individual person's needs, as opposed to analog hearing aids, which have less flexibility. The frequency transpositional hearing aid is a body worn type of instrument that offers some individuals more access to higher frequency sounds. There are also bone-conduction hearing aids that stimulate hearing by vibrating the skull behind the ear instead of sending amplified sound down the ear canal.

There are also different types of surgically implanted devices. Middle-ear implantable hearing devices have been developed in an attempt to maximize sound transmission and enhance sound quality when behind-the-ear and in-the-ear devices are less than satisfactory. The purpose of cochlear implants is to electronically stimulate the eighth nerve, and is suitable for those sensorineural hearing losses with extensive hair cell damage in the cochlea so severe as to preclude benefit from traditional hearing aids. Some individuals have damage beyond the cochlea at the site of the auditory nerve, such as in the case of people with neurofibromatosis Type 2 (NF-2) who have acoustic neuromas. Surgical auditory brainstem implants have sometimes been recommended since these implants bypass the damaged auditory nerve.

Vibrotactile aids convert everyday sounds into vibratory patterns that end up as tactile stimulation on the surface of the skin. Microcomputers in these aids facilitate the production of vibratory patterns that are related to specific sounds. Unfortunately, these signals alone cannot be interpreted as speech. Usually, the listener must combine this information with other modalites for effective communication.

The usefulness of amplification systems varies. Both objective measures and subjective perceptions are required. It is necessary to evaluate gain at each frequency covered by the device as well as the extent to which environmental and speech stimuli are recognized. Audiologists have developed procedures to evaluate the types of benefit individuals can obtain from their devices. The final determination rests on subjective perceptions of how the device is performing, and whether it meets the needs and expectations of the individual.

Assistive listening devices (ALDs) were developed to overcome three major room acoustic deterrents to listening to speech: (1) noise, (2) distance, and (3) reverberation (echo). Some technologies are used in conjunction with hearing aids. These are not a replacement for hearing aids. There are many personal systems on the market that are hard-wired or wireless and can be used in small- to large-group listening situations. Some operate on specially designated radio frequencies, whereas others use infrared light systems or induction loops. These devices transmit acoustic signals directly to the listener's hearing aid(s) or earphones.

Alerting devices use flashing lights or vibrators to indicate the presence of sound. Examples include baby crier signals, alarm clocks, doorbells, smoke alarms, and telephone-ringing signals. The audiologist can assist individuals in selecting the most appropriate technology to meet their everyday listening needs.

CHAPTER FOUR

LANGUAGE, COGNITION, AND THE MIND

*Hands are real—not abstractions—and they are so thoroughly connected
to brains that their use literally makes impact after impact on cognition.*
—Stokoe, 2001a, p. 13

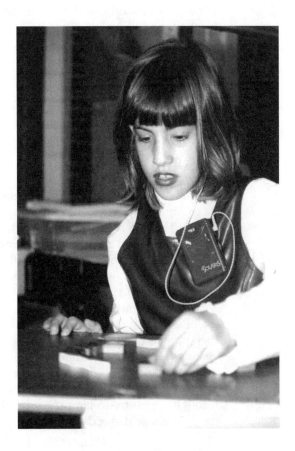

How do deaf students think, learn, and use logical reasoning? Researchers and educators have asked this question for centuries. Deaf people have demonstrated thinking abilities on nonverbal intelligence performance tasks (Chapter 1). But even though deaf students use their cognitive skills for easy and rapid acquisition of sign language, applying them to the mastery of English is another matter (Vernon & Andrews, 1990). Can English, a sequential, phonetic language, be mapped on ASL, a spatial language? Is timing a factor? In other words, because deaf persons may learn ASL and English on different timetables, does this affect their ASL and English language learning? Or is it their lack of auditory experiences that alters how the brain processes language? Do deaf children have the same cognitive capacities for memory, creativity, and attending to stimuli that hearing children do? Can they benefit from instruction in cognitive skills? If so, how can they transfer these skills to improve the learning of language and academic content? Overall, what is the psychological impact of learning primarily through vision rather than audition? We explore these issues in this chapter.

CHAPTER OBJECTIVES

We begin by examining the way infants use gestures to develop cognition, communication, and language. The chapter then shows how hearing and deaf children develop different language pathways depending on their family, sensory strengths, and modality preference. Next is a discussion on the structures of English and ASL and how both languages are processed in the brain. The effects of environment and cognition on language learning in atypical populations is also discussed. Finally, the chapter explores how educational researchers have created methods to help teach deaf students cognitive strategies for improving their academic achievement.

EARLY GESTURAL ROOTS

The hands and the eyes are at the heart of early cognition, the mind, and language. Reaching, grasping, waving, holding, pointing, and gesturing—the hands have many uses. The baby's hands clench and open, reach and grasp for objects, bang spoons, wave and gesture. The eyes gaze ahead, look intently, recognize faces, pay attention, and inspect the surroundings. Hearing and deaf children alike explore their environment with their hands and eyes and develop gestural communication (Volterra & Erting, 1994).

For hearing children, gestural behaviors such as pointing, giving, and showing emerge before speech. These early gestures are often interpreted as words by their parents (Acredolo & Goodwyn, 1994). Researchers disagree on whether these gestures with hearing infants constitute a language or are simply functional communication. In their edited book, *From Gesture to Language in Hearing and Deaf Children,* Volterra and Erting (1994) extrapolate from available research that infants go through a gesture-to-language transition. Babies' gestures become increasingly more symbolic depending on the type of language input. From birth to 7 months, babies exhibit gestures primarily as part of their movement or motor development. From 7 months to 12 months, they use gestures to show what they want. As they use these communication gestures in different situations, the gestures take on symbolic meaning. In hearing infants, gestures will emerge, be used in combination with speech, and then are dropped when speech becomes an easier means of communication (Volterra & Erting, 1994).

Programs have been developed to teach hearing infants as young as 9 months to communicate using ASL. These programs have led to increased communication among mothers, caregivers, and their babies. Interestingly, as these children begin to use spoken words, their use of signs usually diminishes by age 2 (Acredolo & Goodwyn, 1994).

Researchers have also found that sign language builds visual-motor skills in hearing children. In an Italian elementary school, 28 children in a sign language treatment group had significantly higher scores in attention abilities, visual discrimination and visual cognition, and spatial memory than children without the sign treatment (Capirci, Cattani, Rossini, & Volterra, 1998).

In most societies of hearing people, speech is the major form of language, and language origins are believed to evolve from the development of the vocal tract, the eating and breathing organs, and the brain (Poizner, Klima, & Bellugi, 1987; Stokoe, 2001b). The use of sign language by the Deaf community, however, has motivated language theorists to speculate that pointing and gestures were humans' earliest form of language. Speech development came afterward. Grammar is believed to have evolved through the use of gestures (Stokoe, 2001b).

Other language theorists, such as Noam Chomsky and Steven Pinker, take a different position. They argue that language is biologically innate, that it is an instinct. Language is a complete set of abstract rules that are genetically hard-wired into the human brain at birth (Pinker, 1994). Chomsky's linguistic theory proposes an innate language component called the *language acquisition device (LAD)*. Chomsky's framework was used to examine how children created their own child language, which has different rules from adult languages (e.g., *she goed*). In this process, children overgeneralize the grammar of their adult caregivers, but with more exposure and experience children's language becomes more adult-like. Chomsky dismissed the behaviorist view of B. F. Skinner, which held that children learn acquired language through imitating adult speech. Skinner believed that children form associations through classical and operant conditioning (Pinker, 1994).

Related to deaf children's language development, in a fascinating look at how language in Nicaraguan deaf children evolves, even without adult language models, linguists have traced the progression from home signs to a somewhat structured pidgin sign language, and then to a well-structured grammar. In other words, when the deaf children were isolated with their hearing families, they developed a home sign or an idiosyncratic gesture system. But when they began to interact with each other at school, they developed a pidgin which is considered to be an intermediate stage between home signs and a full-fledged sign language. Young children who were exposed to the pidgin took this sign input and restructured it into a more complex grammatical sign language. This fascinating development is linguistically described and chronicled in Emmorey (2002). Such evidence is interpreted as indicative of children's biological capacity to learn the grammar of a language without native adult input.

Today, it is commonly believed that language learning also includes parents' structured input (e.g., child-directed talk) as well as cognitive and social factors (Vygotsky, 1978). Additionally, it includes information processing, linguistic elements, and biological components (Pinker, 1994). Some researchers add that with deaf children, there is an additional language factor—that of modality difference (Newport & Meier, 1985; Poizner, Klima, & Bellugi, 1987). Children's cognitive and social skills affect their language acquisition. In turn, as children develop more language, their cognitive and social skills are changed or modified (Vygotsky, 1978) (see Chapter 5).

Hearing is not always necessary for language acquisition, as shown by deaf children of deaf parents. They follow the same developmental milestones for language that hearing children do, but they acquire language using the visual-gestural modality in signing rather than the auditory/oral modality in speaking (Emmorey & Lane, 2000; Newport & Meier, 1985). The psychological impact of processing language in a visual modality has profound implications for how deaf children learn concepts, language, and social skills. This difference in processing has implications for how to set up early language programs as well as how to structure learning in schools.

Many deaf children of hearing parents will develop a spoken language using amplification devices. But since these devices do not replicate normal hearing, their spoken language development tends to be delayed. This is not to say that deaf students cannot develop oral language. Many do. They develop "inner speech" or an inner phonological awareness that can be useful for analyzing the structures of English words and sentences to aid in reading (Lichtenstein, 1998) (Chapter 5). But learning to speak can be a difficult path to take and requires effort and training (Chapter 7). Sign language, on the other hand, is relatively easy for deaf children to acquire.

Deaf children who use both ASL and English will often mix the two languages. This language mixing is a natural process that second language learners almost always go through (Baker, 2001). With time and repeated exposure, they learn how to separate the languages. Bridging from ASL to English is a common strategy that teachers of deaf children use to teach reading and writing (Grushkin, 1998; Wilbur, 2000). However, the languages are structured so differently that it is hard to map a temporally sequenced phonetic language such as English onto a visually spatial language like ASL. After analyzing some of the structures, one can readily see why.

ASL AND ENGLISH STRUCTURE: A COMPARISON

American Sign Language is a fully developed language with a complex grammar. It has formal structures at the same level as spoken language. Both languages have similar organizational principles and a constrained set of features. In other words, just as a person cannot make up a word with a set of random letters, likewise, a person cannot make up a sign with random handshapes, location, and position. There are linguistic rules governing the way letters are put together in the case of English and the way parameters are assembled in ASL. Both languages have rules at the word level and at the grammar level. Both have what is called recursive grammatical processes. This means that in both languages, one can combine words to create an infinite number of different sentences (Emmorey, 2002; Valli & Lucas, 2000).

English, a sequential, phonetic language, differs from ASL in that the latter organizes its elements in space. Sign language is not done with the hands alone but also with the arms, body, lips, eyebrows, face, head, and eyes. Likewise, spoken languages are rarely localized only in the mouth. Noises are made in the throat and the nose. Gestures, hand and body movements, and facial expressions more often than not accompany and provide meaning to vocal sound patterns (Stokoe, 2001b). There is so much structure happening in speech, writing, or signing that deaf children can get lost if there are no bridging strategies that help them move from one language to the other.

Reading the gestures and signs of a child is often difficult for hearing parents and teachers. The complex use of space by deaf students is often lost on hearing people, because they do not understand the complex nature of ASL. Even those deaf children who are exposed to spoken language or a signed system of English will use gestures and space in ways similar to those that native users of ASL employ (Supalla, 1991).

Understanding how each symbol system works is an important consideration in the teaching of English to deaf students. This understanding allows teachers to recognize the way deaf students code meanings in one language. Teachers can use this information to develop bridging strategies to go from one language to the other. Here, we present some generalities for purposes of our discussion of the difficulties deaf children have in learning the two grammars.

American Sign Language, like English, can be analyzed at the word level and at the sentence or grammar level. Words and signs have a phonology. Words can be analyzed into vowels and consonants, written words into graphemes, and ASL signs into the components of handshape, palm orientation, location, movement, and nonmanual signals (Emmorey, 2002). Looking at the phonology of the word *cat*, we see that it can be broken down into these sounds: /kaet/. It can be written in English as cat or Cat or even CAT. In ASL, CAT can be broken down into hand-shape (F), orientation (palm left), location (cheek) and movement (brush index finger and thumb back toward ear twice). It can also be finger-spelled C-A-T and written in cursive as *cat* or *Cat*.*

Thus, deaf students learn these representational systems: the sign, the finger-spelling, the printed word, and the cursive word. At the word level, these systems

---

*We use the following conventions in this book: (1) capitalized words designate signs and (2) capitalized words with hyphens designate finger-spelled words.

may be easier. But at the sentence level, when words occur in context with other words, meanings shift. Deaf students then often have difficulties in learning how the arrangement of words changes meanings (grammar). On the other hand, hearing children acquire the grammar of their language effortlessly (Chapter 5).

The fact that some signs are iconic has been used to explain why deaf students learn sign language easily. *Iconicity* is a quality that is present at all levels of ASL, at the word, sentence, and discourse or conversational levels. That a sign is iconic means that it resembles the object it represents—for example, the sign BALL. The iconicity of some signs is a feature that makes signs easy for babies to learn. Interestingly enough, iconicity does not play a role in deaf children's acquisition of the rules of their language. Studies of the historical change in sign language over the years show that signs are more symbolic and represent a more symbolic and arbitrary linguistic system (Poizner, Klima, & Bellugi, 1987). Spoken words have an equivalent to iconicity. It is called *onomatopoeia*. This is when words sound like their referent, such *cock-a-doodle doo,* the sound that a rooster makes (Valli & Lucas, 2000).

The phonology structure of English is so different from that of ASL that it can pose challenges for deaf children in learning to speak and read. In learning to speak, deaf children must learn to pronounce all the sounds of English and learn how the sounds change when combined with other sounds. It is a difficult process to learn to speak using your vision to speech read. The ambiguities and fatigue factors make speech reading difficult in itself as well, especially for children who have never heard speech (Chapter 7). In learning to read, the hearing child has the advantage of mapping speech (a phonetic language) onto written language. Even with all the phonetic inconsistencies in English, hearing is a powerful tool that helps the child decode words. For deaf children, vision is not enough to deal with these inconsistencies, and amplification may or may not help sufficiently.

Educators and researchers have looked for creative ways to assist deaf children with this speech-to-print mapping, such as cued speech (LaSasso & Metzger, 1998). *Cued speech* is a system that helps deaf children map speech onto another visual system at the phonetic level to make all its elements visible. There are also signed systems of English, which operate by mapping signs onto morphemes of English (Chapter 5). The downside of these systems are that they are not fully accepted by Deaf people for use in everyday communication (Vernon & Andrews, 1990).

English morphology is another area of difficulty for deaf students (Mogford, 1994). *Morphology* is the study of the way a language builds new words or signs (Valli & Lucas, 2000). Morphemes add grammatical information to a word or a sign. English adds word endings or morphemes in linear order, whereas ASL adds movement and facial expressions. For example, English adds suffixes to show person (e.g., teach + er) and number (cat + s). English verbs have suffixes to show time (walk + ed) or duration (walk + ing) and are sequenced. Sign morphology can be sequenced as well—for instance, making the sign TEACH and the person-agent-maker PERSON. But signs can also be layered to add movement and facial expressions (Valli & Lucas, 2000).

Here is an example of ASL morphemes using movement and facial expression. To the basic sign stem (STUDY), the signer can add movement and facial expression to mean the person is studying continuously, studies regularly, studies for a prolonged period of time, studies over and over again, or studies in a hurry (Valli & Lucas, 2000).*

American Sign Language uses movement and facial expressions (its morphological processes) in numerous ways to form new words. The verb (FLY), for example, can be changed to the noun (AIRPLANE) through the use of movement. In ASL, there are also rules for forming compound words (GIRL SAME means *sister*). In addition, ASL can incorporate number and time into a sign, as THREE-WEEKS-AGO. This illustrates how ASL uses space and movement to show meaning (Valli & Lucas, 2000).

English uses word order to show its relationships or grammar; ASL uses space and movement. For example, using the same words or signs, a person can compose two sentences with different meanings. But when the movement in the sentence is changed, the meaning is also changed:

1. *The dog bit the cat.*
2. *The cat bit the dog.*

In ASL, the signer sets up where the dog is situated and where the cat is situated. The signer then makes the movement from one to the other: DOG CAT BITE or CAT DOG BITE. American Sign Language has many grammatical processes like this that use space and movement to show meaningful relationships among the signs, whereas English uses sequential word order.

Some languages, like ASL, do not use the verb *to be* but instead uses a different predicate system. In ASL, for instance, the sentence CAT SICK consists of a noun and a predicate that is an adjective, SICK. This ASL sentence does not include the verb *is*, but the adjective SICK functions as a predicate; it describes the cat. Verbs, nouns, and adjectives can be predicates in ASL. Many deaf children will often omit the *to be* verbs in their writing because they don't use it in their signing. American Sign Language has a complex verb system made up of classifier predicates, classifier handshapes, and locative verbs. It has a pronoun (*he, she, it*) and a determiner (*the, a, an*) system that are made up of similar pointing signs. The article system is another English structure that deaf children have difficulty with in their writing. The auxiliary verbs in ASL (WILL, CAN, FINISH, MUST, SHOULD) are used at the beginning and end of the sentence instead of internally as in English. Also, ASL does not use prepositions the way English does.

English uses morphemes to express time; ASL uses signs to mark time (NOW, FUTURE, LONG-TIME-AGO, PAST, FINISH) and movement. For example, these sentences have a different time frame:

*See our textbook webpage and companion DVD for examples: http://hal.lamar.edu/~andrewsjf/bookindex.htm.

ENGLISH	ASL
1. The cat walks.	CAT WALK.
2. The cat is walking,	CAT WALK-continuous-movement.
3. The cat walked,	CAT FINISH WALK.
4. The cat *will* walk.	CAT WALK WILL.

In sentence 1, the *s* morpheme means present tense. Sentence 2 expresses the present progressive tense of the duration of the walk. The *ed* in the sentence 3 denotes the past tense. The word *will* expresses the future. The letters *ed* in sentence 3 is pronounced *t*. Spoken words are made up of consonant and vowel segments, and these sounds can change depending on the letters that come before them. English has many words like this that change their sounds, which may be difficult for deaf children. Learning regular tenses (e.g., the rule to add *–ed* to mean past tense) and irregular forms where the whole spelling changes (e.g., *sit/sat; eat/ate, see/saw*) are areas that are problematic for deaf readers and writers. Verbs such as *walk* are regular in their spelling, but English has many verbs that have irregular spellings, all of which have to be memorized by the deaf speller and deaf writer (e.g., *see/saw; eat/ate, hide/hid*). Hearing children may have difficulty reading and writing these forms, but they acquire these forms relatively easily from listening to conversations around them. Deaf children have less exposure to acquire these forms.

The basic order for a sentence found in English, subject-verb-object, is not always found in ASL. American Sign Language allows the signer to place the object in front of the sentence. This is called *topicalization*. Thus, the sentence *The boy loves his cat* can be changed to CAT BOY LOVE. Of course, English arranges its sentences like this sometimes too in complex sentences (e.g., *The coat that belongs to me is in the closet*).

American Sign Language also uses space in role shifting, as in telling a story or signing a narrative involving different characters. A signer may take on the role of a different character. The signer may use body shifts, eye gazes, and head shifts to tell a story. The equivalent of this in English writing is the punctuation of quotations.

English syntax remains a major challenge in deaf students' acquisition of English. In reading, deaf students can often circumvent the grammar of English by concentrating on the semantic meaning of the text by using their background knowledge and experiences. But it is in their written language that understanding the syntax of English becomes very important. Many deaf students master writing to varying degrees, whereas others struggle with writing throughout their lives.

Quigley and associates carried out an extensive study of written English grammar with deaf students (Quigley, Power, & Steinkemp, 1977). They developed the Test of Syntactic Abilities (TSA), a test that can be used to assess the comprehension level of nine syntactic structures that posed difficulties for deaf students ages 10 to 18. On the TSA, even when deaf students understood the concepts in the sentences, they had difficulty with the word order in the sentences. Deaf students showed a delay and a difference in processing sentences. For instance, some of them treated all sentences as having a subject-verb-object word order. They were unable to deal with complex sentences with embedded phrasal structures (e.g., *The girl who kissed the boy ran away*).

We have only scratched the surface of the myriad of differences between English and ASL. The language transfer from the symbol system ASL (or its hybrid forms, including contact signing) to English is not always straightforward in speech, reading, or writing instruction, and this poses difficulties for deaf children (Chapter 5). The fact that many deaf persons can easily acquire the grammar of a visual language but struggle with learning an auditory language leads to the question of how to structure language learning environments in schools (Chapter 7). No doubt, part of the ease of acquisition of sign can be accounted for by the amount of exposure to ASL at home or in school. But as discussed later in this chapter, the ease and rapidity of sign language acquisition may be more related to a number of factors, including timing of exposure, how language is processed in the brain, and the visual learning modality. This is not to say auditory pathways are not useful. They are. But the point is on *emphasis*. Which pathway should teachers emphasize in the classroom? Which pathway should parents emphasize at home? The acquisition literature can provide some guidance.

LANGUAGE PATHS

Deaf and hearing children, depending on their parents' home language and educational experiences, often take different language paths. The visual-gestural and auditory/vocal paths are not mutually exclusive. Deaf children can use either or both. Some deaf parents raise their children using speech; others use ASL or even both. Deaf children with hearing parents may develop competencies in spoken language and/or ASL, depending on skills in picking up either language and on exposure at home and at school.

Deaf mothers, like hearing mothers, use a form of child-directed speech when signing to their deaf infants. Mothers repeat signs, exaggerate them, and present the signs at a slower rate. They make extensive use of touch and vision, mold the babies' hands to make the signs, sign on the child's body, and use exaggerated facial expressions. Deaf mothers have been noted to use positive affect, signing directly in the child's line of vision, and to sign slower to make sure their signs are seen. Mothers also use physical strategies, such as tapping the children's bodies or waving hands to get their attention. Mothers also often use a toy or object that is right in front of the infant as they sign the name of the object (see reviews in Holzrichter & Meier, 2000). Rodriguez (2001) explains that deaf parents of hearing children form a *conversational triangle* or a space for conversation. Thus, at the discourse level, they use space in which to sign to the child, pointing to a book, toy, or food item, all the while maintaining eye contact.

From birth to 9 months, hearing babies babble, whereas deaf babies manually babble or finger babble before they produce their first signs (Petitto, 2000). Hearing babies produce sounds in predictable patterns; deaf babies likewise produce handshapes in predictable patterns and progress to syllable babbling following distinct developmental handshapes. Deaf infants produce sequences of gestures that pho-nologically resemble signing but that are not recognizable as signs. From 9 to 12 months, deaf babies progress to the one-word stage. Their first recognizable signs are produced one at a time in isolation, and this production of one sign at a time continues for several months. Some researchers report that the first ASL signs emerge significantly earlier than the first words in English. But this contention is controversial and not accepted by all researchers (Volterra & Erting, 1994).

From about 9 to 12 months, deaf babies make the signs for pronominal refer-ences (pointing) besides using nonlinguistic points to self and to objects. The first signs are similar to words such as *milk*, *mommy*, and *daddy*—words used by hearing babies in other languages. Deaf babies continue to learn one sign at a time, and by the end of the first year, they have generally acquired 10 or more signs.

Deaf babies then begin to combine their signs into two-word utterances. Dur-ing the second year, the child increases his or her use of pronominal references and begins to use pronouns correctly with first, second, and third persons. From 2 to 3 years of age, deaf toddlers will use classifiers and verbs of motion and location. The first productive use of verb agreement occurs at about age 2½. Classifiers increase in number. Noun and verb pairs are used along with facial expressions, body pos-ture, and movement speed. From age 3 or 3½, classifiers and verbs of motion increase. The children continue their development of complex morphology. At age 4, they use *wh-questions*. At ages 4 and 5, they use more complex sentences and a variety of word order and classifiers (Emmorey, 2002; Newport & Meier, 1985; Pet-tito, 2000). See Table 4.1 for a chart of ASL and spoken language acquisition.

Very early, deaf children of deaf parents learn their pronouns, verb agree-ment, and the use of space to set up sentences. The use of pronouns by deaf children of deaf parents has been used as evidence that pointing progresses from gesture to symbol. Deaf infants at 9 months use their pointing gesture, as hearing children do. But at age 2, when they begin to incorporate many signs into their vocabulary, they stop pointing. At the end of age 2, they use pointing again but as a linguistic symbol. At this stage, linguists have noted some surprising errors of reversal (e.g., the tod-dler signs YOU for ME). Hearing children using spoken language also confuse their pronouns—such as *me* for *you* and vice versa (Pettito, 2000; Poinzer, Klima, & Bel-lugi, 1987).

Linguists have interpreted the acquisition data as demonstrating that the bio-logical structures in the brain show a general human capacity to create a linguistic system even if the child does not hear (Emmorey, 2002; Poinzer, Klima, & Bellugi, 1987). If deaf children can acquire language similarly to hearing children, do their difficulties with spoken language have to do with the timing of exposure to the lan-guage? Or is it how language is processed in the brain? Linguists and neuroscien-tists have come up with some interesting findings.

TABLE 4.1   ASL and Spoken Language Acquisition

AGE	DEAF CHILDREN OF DEAF PARENTS	HEARING CHILDREN OF HEARING PARENTS
Birth to 1 year	Manual babbling	Vocal babbling
1 year to 2 years	Prelinguistic communication gestures Facial expressions Sign phonological errors Baby signs First signs	Prelinguistic communication gestures Facial expressions Word phonological errors Baby words First words
1 year to 2 years	Pass 50 sign milestones Signs for negation Facial adverbs Pronouns	First 50 words milestones Words for negation
2 years to 3 years	Two-sign utterances Correct pronouns Wh-questions with facial expression Verb agreement Some classifier handshapes Fingerspelling	Two-word utterances Beginning of morphemes (articles, pronouns, present progressive, plurals, past tense, contractions, is, auxiliaries, adverbs) Engages in dialogues Wh-questions Overregularization or verb rules
3 years to 4 years	Topicalization and conditions Directional verbs Use of space for location Begin classifier predicates Begin discourse skills Seeks eye contact before initiating conversation	Morphemes become consistent Irregular form of verbs used (*see/saw; eat/ate*) Simple sentences, negatives, imperatives, questions, relative pronouns
4 years and older	Full morphological distinction between nouns and verbs Complex sentences as nominal references, classifier and morphology, aspects of discourse structure, complex verbs of motion, continued refinement of grammar	Relative clauses, passives, and other complex sentences, reflexive pronouns, comparatives and superlatives, adverbial word endings, irregular comparisons, continued refinement of grammar

Source: Adapted from Emmorey (2002) and Newport and Meier (1985).

THE CRITICAL PERIOD

Lenneberg's (1967) *critical period hypothesis* is made up of two related ideas. The first idea is that hemispheric lateralization takes place in an early critical period when the brain is flexible in regard to language development. The second idea is that certain language events must happen to the child during this period if language is to develop. It is commonly theorized that optimal development of the first language, either signed or spoken, depends on this critical period. Research has shown that if language is introduced after this period, learning the language becomes a more arduous process.

Deaf children of hearing parents typically are delayed in their exposure to language, and so they represent a good "test" case for the critical period hypothesis. Deaf children who are not consistently exposed to a spoken or sign language will develop home gesture systems (Emmorey, 2002). These children do not have a language model but instead mold their home gestures in a structured system (Goldin-Meadow & Mylander, 1990). Their language development, however, will not necessarily develop to the extent that it might have otherwise. An extreme example is the case of "Genie" (Curtiss, 1977).

Genie was a hearing child who was kept in a room, physically restrained, punished for making sounds, and neglected for 13 years, starting at 20 months of age. After finally being removed to a more stimulating environment, Genie failed to develop any speech for conversation, but was able to comprehend basic language after five years of work. Her case has been used as evidence for the critical period hypothesis, but it can also be used to argue against the critical period hypothesis given the fact that Genie was able to acquire receptive language even after the age of 13, even though she did not acquire expressive skills.

Studies of deaf adults who learn first and second languages at different periods in their lives have allowed scientists to further investigate the nature of the critical period hypothesis. Emmorey (2002) summarizes the linguistic research on deaf adults who were exposed to ASL at different times in adulthood. She points out that late acquisition of ASL does not appear to affect some aspects of language processing, such as word order and referential processing, but it does affect learning some of the more complex grammatical structures of ASL. This is corroborated by observations of deaf and hard-of-hearing students who transfer from public schools to residential schools (Chapter 6), typically in the late elementary, junior high, or high school years. Although these children tend to have low reading and academic achievement levels, many of them are easily able to acquire ASL rapidly, especially if they live in a dormitory setting and associate with deaf peers. Their fluency is not equivalent to that of native ASL users, but they are able to comfortably communicate and learn using ASL.

The critical period hypothesis is traditionally used to explain why second language acquisition is so difficult for older children and adults. But some researchers have noted that older learners have an initial advantage over younger learners in learning a second language because of their cognitive abilities and motivation (see review by Krashen, Long, & Scarcella, 1982). Younger children, however, have the advantage in learning the phonology or how to speak with a correct accent. The second language learner, whether child or adult, can use the first language to learn the second language. The more traditional pattern is for deaf children to learn English first, and ASL later. But there is an emerging database that shows that those children who learned ASL as a first language can build English literacy skills as a second language (Butler & Prinz, 1998; Chamberlain, Morford, & Mayberry, 2000) (see Chapters 5 and 7).

THE BRAIN AND THE ENVIRONMENT

It is now known that deaf children and adult signers both process language in the left hemisphere of the brain. It was previously believed that, given the spatial nature of ASL signs and grammar, the processing of ASL would occur in the right hemisphere. This is not the case, as shown by deaf signers with brain dysfunction. Neuroscientists have studied these individuals in order to understand how the brain is organized for language and spatial cognition.

In a series of experiments, deaf adult signers were found to process sign-language grammar in the left hemisphere. These experiments used nonlanguage and language tests with deaf aphasic patients, some with damage to the right hemisphere and others with damage to the left hemisphere due to strokes. Results indicated that the left hemisphere was dominant for sign language even though ASL is a language that relies on spatial relations (Hickok, Bellugi, & Klima, 2001; Poizner, Klima, & Bellugi, 1987).

Today, neuroscientists are not limited to studying deaf people with brain dysfunction in order to study the brain. They can use noninvasive scanning technologies, including MRI (magnetic resonance imaging) and PET (positron emitting tomography) to chart brain territories and examine where sign language is processed. Studies of deaf adults given signing tasks have replicated the studies of deaf stroke victims and have added accumulating evidence that sign language is processed in the left hemisphere, as is spoken language, albeit with some differences due to the visual versus auditory processing (Hickok, Bellugi, & Klima, 2001).

The relationships between the environment, various etiologies for deafness, and language learning has been studied with exceptional language learners. These cases provide "natural experiments" to examine the ways cognition and language develop even under unusual circumstances such as in deprived and abusive environments, in families where the parents are deaf and the children are hearing, and in the cases of children who are mentally retarded or have Williams syndrome.

The case of Genie, mentioned earlier, is an example of severe environmental deprivation. Another form of environmental deprivation occurs when preschool children arrive at school with limited or nonexistent language exposure (Vernon & Andrews, 1990). These children often invent their own language and use a spatial syntax. The fact that many of these deaf children will learn sign language, though not as fluently as native signers, in late childhood or even early adulthood challenges the critical period hypothesis, discussed earlier.

The language development of deaf children of hearing parents is highly variable and depends on a host of factors such as age of onset and etiology. Some etiologies, such as cytomegalovirus (CMV), may have neurological correlates that can result in language learning disabilities among other things (Chapter 3). Other factors—such as home language, type of education program, adequacy of auditory amplification, and child motivation—affect language learning. Studies of deaf children have shown English deficits in phonology, semantics, syntax, and pragmatics (Vernon & Andrews, 1990). Nonetheless, many deaf persons do learn English (spoken and written) with varying levels of competence and use it daily.

Many hearing children of deaf parents grow up to be bilingual. They may start with ASL and learn spoken English later. Mogford (1994) has reviewed studies of these children and reports that research findings are not consistent. Some studies show that hearing children of deaf parents develop normal speech, yet other studies show evidence of speech delays. She notes that hearing children do not imitate the speech errors of their deaf parents (e.g., nasal speech) but go through the regular stages of speech acquisition observed in children with hearing parents (Mogford, 1994).

Young speaking-signing bilinguals raise intriguing questions about childhood bilingualism. There are opposing viewpoints about children being exposed to and learning two languages early in life. Proponents of "one language first" believe that if parents expose children to two languages early in life, language confusion and language delays occur. There is also the fear that children will never develop competence in either language (Petitto & Holowka, 2002). But studies of simultaneous childhood bilingualism have shown otherwise. The timing milestones (e.g., first word, first 50 words, first 2-word combinations, and so on) of young signing-speaking bilinguals are similar to hearing monolinguals and bilinguals. Further, the research studies of Petitto and colleagues show that very early simultaneous bilingual language exposure with speaking-signing bilinguals and dual-spoken language bilinguals do not cause young children to be delayed in achievement of the classic milestones nor does it cause children to be confused with their semantic and conceptual learning of language. In other words, hearing children can easily learn both languages early, whether it be two spoken languages or a signed and a spoken language. Pettito concludes from her childhood bilingual research and other studies that it is advantageous for the developing child to learn two languages because there are cognitive, social, and developmental benefits of bilingualism (Pettito & Holowka, 2002).

Language acquisition is generally discussed in relation to cognitive prerequisites. For instance, Piaget's framework for development clearly links language to other aspects of cognition. The child progresses through stages, each building on the last, with language developing at the end of the sensorimotor period, when the child internalizes and uses symbols. One group of children with Williams syndrome, a rare metabolic disorder, challenges this idea. It is a form of mental retardation where linguistic abilities are preserved but there are severe cognitive deficits. When these children speak, they show sophisticated use of language with complex syntax and adult-like vocabulary. However, their cognitive development is below that of a 2-year-old (Bellugi, Marks, Bihrle, & Sabo, 1994). Deaf children, in contrast, have normal cognitive abilities but are severely delayed in their language abilities. Children with Williams syndrome raise fascinating questions about the role of cognition in language learning. Based on Piaget and others, scientists have previously believed that cognitive abilities are necessary. But children with Williams syndrome demonstrate that there are some parts of the brain that can acquire and process language in the absence of higher cognitive abilities previously thought necessary for language acquisition. Bellugi and colleagues are studying these issues at the Salk Institute in San Diego, California.

All of these cases shed light on understanding deaf children's language acquisition. First of all, deaf children do not need speech to learn language. Second, sign language does not necessarily impede the development of speech. From a brain processing perspective, both spoken and signed languages are processed in the left hemisphere, though not in the exact same way. Studies of environmentally deprived children point to the importance of a nurturing environment but show the brain's capacity for acquiring a basic language after the critical period. Studies of adolescents with Williams syndrome show that experts do not fully understand the cognitive mechanism that underlie language acquisition. The highly developed semantic and syntactic skills of these children are present even in the face of serve cognitive deprivation.

BILINGUALISM, INTELLIGENCE, AND THINKING

The study of deaf children and adults has provided scientists with the opportunity to study the effects of deafness on bilingualism, intelligence, and thinking. Related to hearing bilinguals, it was erroneously believed that for many years, bilinguals had inferior intelligence and cognitive abilities. Similar to the historical perspectives that postulated the detrimental effect of sign language on the thinking capabilities of deaf persons, the dominant belief from the early nineteenth century to the 1960s was that bilingualism was generally detrimental to young children's thinking. Like the early research in deafness and cognition, the early research in bilingualism pointed to the negative viewpoint that bilinguals were intellectually inferior (Baker, 2001). But in fact, there is no modern empirical research that states that bilingualism has a detrimental effect on cognition (Baker, 2001). Today, it is generally accepted that there are cognitive benefits to bilingualism, including enhanced creative thinking, cognitive flexibility, and metalinguistic awareness (Baker, 2001).

Metalinguistic awareness refers to one's ability to think about and reflect on the nature and functions of language. The bilingual can reflect on and manipulate spoken (or sign) and written language (Baker, 2001). One can see how deaf people use their metalinguistic awareness of ASL and English in joke telling. For example, see the following translation of the popular deaf joke, "Please But."

One time a Deaf person was driving along and stopped at some train tracks because the crossing signal gates were down but there was no train going by. So he waited for a long time for a train to go by, but nothing. The person decided then to get out of the car and troll the railroad gates. [The controller was sitting there talking on the phone. The Deaf man wrote in his best way (elegantly), "Please b-u-t," and handed the paper to the controller. The controller looked back at the Deaf person quizzically, "Please but? Huh?" He didn't understand that. (Rutherford, 1989)

Rutherford provides a fascinating description on how this joke would not be funny to a nonsigner because the punch line is a play on the sign BUT and the English word *but*. There is a slight change in meaning from "open the railroad gates," and the sign, BUT. Both signs look similar to the viewer. Deaf people can use their knowledge of ASL (the sign for BUT) and their knowledge of English (the word *but*) to make the joke. Rutherford explains that when the joke is signed, the English word *but* is signed as BUT. It has the same parameters for the classifier for railroad crossing gate, with the exception of palm orientation.

Researchers in bilingualism do not agree on which comes first—bilingualism or enhanced cognition. It may be that language learning and cognition work together and one stimulates the other. Most research on bilingualism uses young school children. There is almost no research on the cognitive functioning of hearing bilinguals and monolinguals after the age of 17 (Baker, 2001). Age and experience may give bilinguals and monolinguals similar cognitive skills. Studies of older deaf bilinguals may shed light on this issue and help bilingual theorists refine their theories on the cognitive benefits of learning two languages.

LEARNING HOW TO THINK, REMEMBER, AND LEARN

There is extensive literature on the intellectual abilities of deaf persons (Braden, 1994; Marschark, 1993; Vernon, 1968) (see Chapter 1). Much also has been written on the subjects of learning, memory, and creativity in deaf persons. Deaf people have been found to have both strengths and limitations on memory and creativity tasks, depending on the presence or absence of tasks with verbal language components (Clark, Marschark, & Karchmer, 2001; Marschark, 1993). Deaf individuals are at least equal to hearing persons when the memory tasks are spatial and informational (Parasnis, Samar, Bettger, & Sathe, 1996). People who are deaf use a spatial syntax (Bellugi, O'Grady, Lillo-Martin, O'Grady, van Hoek, & Corina, 1990). But when the tasks require that deaf individuals use verbal encoding of sequential information, their performance is not as good (Bebko, 1998). Parasnis and colleagues (1996) review studies that show deaf signers to demonstrate advantages over hearing signers in a variety of visual spatial tasks, imagery tasks, memory for simultaneously presented shapes, face recognition, and motion detection in the peripheral vision. There have also been numerous studies that show the positive effects of signing on deaf persons' cognitive functioning (see review by Courtin,

2000). Marschark (1993) reviews studies showing that deaf persons were reported to show creativity, spatial cognition, flexibility, and enhancement of episodic memory on tasks where they were allowed to use sign language.

This is all well and good. But the critical issue is how deaf students can transfer these cognitive abilities of thinking, reasoning, and problem solving to the learning of academic subjects, including reading and writing. Several studies with deaf students show that training facilitates the transfer of cognitive abilities to the academic domain (K. Keane, personal communication, February 20, 2002; Martin, Craft, & Zhang, 2001).

TRANSFER OF COGNITIVE ABILITIES TO ACADEMIC LEARNING

Many deaf students enter school without having the ability to "learn how to learn." Regulating one's learning, or knowing when you don't know something and developing a plan to learn what you don't know, is part of what educational psychologists label as *metacognitive abilities.* Metacognitive processes have been explained using a computer menu analogy. The student decides what procedure is next, chooses the procedure from several choices, monitors the effect of the choice made, and then returns to the menu if the results are not satisfactory. Metacognition, or "thinking about thinking," is what students use to control their cognitive processes such as reasoning, comprehension, problem solving, and learning (Baker, 2001).

Metacognition requires the learner to use three skills: planning, monitoring, and evaluation. *Planning* requires that the student ask how much time must be given to the task, when it should be started, what order the tasks should be done, and so on. In the *monitoring* phase, the student asks these questions: "How am I doing?" "Is this making sense?" "Should I change strategies?" *Evaluation* involves making judgments about the outcomes: "Should I change strategies?" For experts, these strategies are automatic. But for some students, the strategies must be taught (Baker, 2001).

Metacognition skills do not depend on hearing per se, but they do depend on students having many experiences and opportunities for incidental learning so they can formulate metacognitive strategies. Many deaf students who come from hearing families with limited communication skills in the home have not had these incidental and formal opportunities to develop metacognitive skills (K. Keane, personal communication, February 20, 2002).

The *Cognitive Modifiability* model has been used with deaf students to teach these metacognitive processes. This model originated with the Israeli scholar and educator Reuven Feuerstein (1980), who worked with low-functioning, culturally disadvantaged adolescents in Europe and Israel. Dissatisfied with traditional IQ tests because he believed the tests did not provide any information on the learning potential of students, Feuerstein developed an assessment tool called the Learning Potential Assessment Device (LPAD). This is a battery of 15 assessments covering a variety of verbal and nonverbal tasks. The LPAD was later developed into a curriculum called the *Instrumental Enrichment (IE)* intervention program and adopted by schools in the United States and Israel. This curriculum provides learning opportunities whereby the teachers can correct the students' deficient cognitive functions and enhance their learning capacity.

The Cognitive Modifiability model is also related to Vygotsky's (1978) socio-cultural learning theory. Feuerstein worked with culturally deprived children who did not have many adults in their environment who could help them learn, problem solve, or interpret their experiences. Vygotsky suggested that cognitive development depended on interactions between children and expert adults or parents who mediate the children's learning experiences by helping them understand their world using the tools of their culture. An important tool, in this case, is language (Vygotsky, 1978).

The essential feature in Feuerstein's approach is not just remediating the skills the students need, such as reading or math, but actually changing the students' underlying cognitive processes in learning the skills. According to Feuerstein, there are two types of learning that affect the students' cognitive abilities: direct learning experiences (DLE) and mediated learning experiences (MLE). *Mediated learning experiences* refers to a student using a "mediating agent"—such as a parent, teacher, or caregiver—who helps him or her with a skill or process and provides meaning to the experience. For example, the mediator sets up the learning experience, draws attention to certain aspects of it by comparing objects or events, focuses the student's attention on important aspects, helps the student label and categorize the lesson, and so on. It is through these so-called mediating learning experiences with a teacher that a student's thinking processes are changed. The learner can go on to monitor or self-regulate his or her own learning in new tasks (K. Keane, personal communication, February 20, 2002).

In a study with 45 severely to profoundly prelingually deaf 9- to 13-year-old students at the Lexington School for the Deaf, a day-school in Jackson Heights, New York, five instruments from the LPAD were used to assess the effects of mediated intervention on the performance of cognitive tasks (Keane, Tannenbaum, & Krapf, 1992). All had hearing parents. Students were randomly assigned to three groups. Group one (*n* = 15, the treatment group) received the maximum support and mediated instruction. For example, after observing a student's performance on one task (e.g., organizing dots into geometric shapes), the examiner modeled the proper way to do the task. Then the student applied what he or she had learned in doing the task again. A test-teach-test approach was used. In the "standard condition," 15 students did not receive any modeling but were simply given directions for doing the task. In the "elaborated condition" situation, 15 students were given the task and received feedback during their performance telling them whether they were right or wrong in their approach. However, they were not given a model of the way to do the task. The students who received the modeling and mediated learning experience outperformed the standard and elaborated condition groups in five of the six LAPD cognitive tasks. The deaf students performed better in the elaborated situation, where they received feedback, than in the standard situation with no feedback, but the performance of the mediated learning group was higher still. The authors reported that students in the mediated learning group were able to transfer their learning, as was indicated on their performance on another cognitive test administered after the experiment. The mediated learning experiences provided to the treatment group contributed to their increase in cognitive abilities compared with the other two groups.

The mediated learning experience model has been integrated into the curriculum in the parent-infant program, elementary school program, and high school program at the Lexington School for the Deaf. Keane (personal communication, February 20, 2002) points out that the diagnosis of deafness was delayed in many of the pupils who often do not have an effective communication system at home. Consequently, they may miss out on many opportunities to have reciprocal communication experiences with their parents. Parents cannot, then, provide mediated learning experiences. Not having enough information in their environment, children may impulsively respond to pieces of information because they have a fragmented view of what information to focus on.

The backgrounds of the students at the Lexington School for the Deaf reflect the changing demographics for deaf children of color nationwide (Chapter 2). The Lexington School enrolls about 380 students. Most of the high school students have transferred from elementary deaf-education programs in the surrounding area. About 80 percent of the students are on the federal lunch program. There are 24 different home languages used by the students' families.

The Lexington School staff has received extensive staff development training in critical thinking, creative problem solving, and mediated language experiences. Through this curriculum, Keane has noted an increase in positive behaviors, in the motivation to learn, and in academic performance on the part of students. After three years of having provided deaf students with mediated learning experiences, 28 percent of the students increased one full grade year level in reading, about 28 percent gained two years, and 16 percent of the students progressed three or more years in reading comprehension level. Math achievement also increased: 16 percent increased one grade level, 20 percent two grade levels, and 32 percent three grade levels on a mathematics achievement test.

Keane points out that the mediated learning experience changes the teachers, too. During staff development, novices learn from experts on how to use this model in the classroom. Teachers must not only know the theory but must also put it into practice. Teachers then become "learners," according to this model. Staff development is very important to this process.

The mediated learning experience approach has also been used at other schools for the deaf and in China and England. In a two-year longitudinal study with deaf high school students at the Model Secondary School (MSSD) at Gallaudet University in Washington, DC, researchers designed an intervention program that adapted materials from Instrumental Enrichment (IE). Six IE instruments (parts-whole, comparison and classification, symmetry, projection of visual relationships, spatial relations, and following directions) were used by teachers who had training in how to use them. Twice a week, teachers added a series of visual, verbal, and geometric activities to the regular subject matter as they helped the students with the activities and engaged them in metacognitive discussions (thinking about thinking). Teachers then discussed with the students how to use these strategies to help them with their other subjects. Deaf students in the experimental group ($n =$ 41) were compared with 41 students in a control group matched by age, hearing loss, sex, degree of hearing loss, and reading ability. Students were tested using four measures: Raven's Standard Progressive Matrices, an observation checklist of cognitive behaviors developed by the authors, a problem-solving situation requiring a narrative solution, and the Stanford Achievement Test (SAT-HI) of reading comprehension, math computation, and math concepts. The researchers reported that the experimental IE group outperformed the control group on the Raven's Standard Progressive Matrices, reading comprehension, math concepts, and problem solving in written situations. These differences reached statistical significance (Martin, Craft, & Zhang, 2001).

This study was adapted and expanded in England and in China. Teachers were provided with training in critical and creative thinking skills based on theories of multiple intelligence, divergent thinking, and Feuerstein's work (1980) on cognitive modifiability. Activities were designed that emphasized the creative problem-solving process. Teachers began a six-month period of using the cognitive strategies in the classrooms. The critical and creative activities occurred three times weekly for 30 minutes each. During each instructional session, the teacher taught the processes on how to solve a problem. Then the teacher discussed with the students what mental processes they might use to solve the problem. Finally, the teacher discussed with the students how they might apply the particular cognitive skill they learned in the session to their content area subjects. For example, a student might learn about categorizing items with similar features in a cognitive strategy session. Then later, the teacher would demonstrate how the student might use those categorization strategies to learn systems of the body in a science class.

Researchers tested groups of deaf students in the 9- to 13-year age range over a six-month time frame. They reported that the IE intervention had a positive effect on students' reasoning abilities as reflected on post-test scores on the Raven's Progressive Matrices. Students also increased their use of cognitive vocabulary to discuss their thinking and problem-solving skills, and increased their ability to consider the viewpoints of others during class discussions. The researchers also noted that the overall attentiveness and classroom motivation to learn improved. Teachers from both countries increased their use of higher-order thinking questions during class. The Martin studies, like Keane's work, illustrate the importance of teacher and staff development training in the use of cognitive strategy instruction techniques.

Another theory, called the *theory of mind*, has been used to understand deaf students' cognitive and language behaviors. This theory is characterized by the ability to break away from "egocentric thought" and to think about and interpret another person's thoughts. It refers to the ability to attribute beliefs, intentions, and emotions to people. The theory is grounded in Piaget's developmental theory of young children who begin to analyze their thoughts. Theory of mind develops in hearing children at about the age of 4 when they can recognize and start to think about the thoughts of others.

Some researchers think children are born with a theory of mind. Others argue that children must build a theory of mind based on their experiences and mediating adults who explain their world to them. The social world plays a part, starting with the family and then with friends. Social cognition develops as children interact with peers and adults, learn how to have conversations, and build up the capacity to communicate. Social behavior and social maturity are important aspects of theory of mind. The theory has also been linked with the ability to benefit from instruction, understanding of stories (Gray & Hosie, 1996), and understanding of scientific reasoning and critical thinking. Teachers can help children make their thinking explicit by talking about it, as in the Lexington School program explained earlier. Children are given opportunities to reflect on their thinking using language. The theory of mind that children can acquire in preschool can give them the conceptual foundation for building metacognitive skills through mediated learning experiences, as demonstrated by the teachers in the schools for the deaf mentioned earlier.

There is some evidence that deaf children do not develop their theories of mind on the same timetable as hearing children do (Peterson & Siegel, 1995, 1998). Such delayed understanding of the task was related to hearing families of deaf children who did not provide conversational support in the home about such topics as mental concepts and beliefs. But this delay is believed to be resolved by adulthood (Clark, Schwanenflugel, Everhart, & Bartini, 1996). Interestingly, Courtin (2000) reports that deaf children's experiences with sign language and perspective taking lead to a change at the representational level that allows signing deaf children to form representations earlier than hearing children. Clearly, this is an area ripe for further exploration.

CONCLUSION

To understand the psychological impact of deafness on cognition, the mind and language, it is necessary to understand the visual ways in which deaf individuals' mental capabilities unfold, develop and are organized. Visual paradigms of learning have been added to auditory paradigms in order to increase our understanding of the ways deaf persons use their cognition, minds and language to learn, think and problem solve.

SUGGESTED READINGS

Deacon, T. (1997). *The Symbolic Species: The Co-Evolution of Language and the Brain.* New York: W. W. Norton.
   The author provides his insights into the significance of symbolic thought by tracing the co-evolutionary exchange between language and the brain.

Emmorey, K. (2002). *Language, Cognition, and the Brain: Insights from Sign Language Research.* Mahwah, NJ: Lawrence Erlbaum.

This book contains a wealth of information of old and new research on the contributions sign language has made to the understanding of cognition, the mind, and language. Thumbnail digital snapshots of signers help the reader understand many of the linguistic descriptions that might pose difficulty for readers who are not linguists.

Stokoe, W. (2001). *Language in Hand: Why Sign Came Before Speech.* Washington, DC: Gallaudet Press.

Published after his death, this book describes Stokoe's views on an evolutionary theory of the origins of language. Stokoe provides an engaging argument with his personal experiences and published research that refutes the commonly held beliefs that humans have a special, innate, learning facility for language.

CHAPTER FIVE

FROM COMMUNICATION TO LANGUAGE TO LITERACY

There are no gimmicks in fostering this development. To become a successful reader, one must enjoy reading and spend time practicing reading. To become a successful writer, one must enjoy writing and spend time practicing writing.
—Tucker, p. viii, cited in Livington, 1997

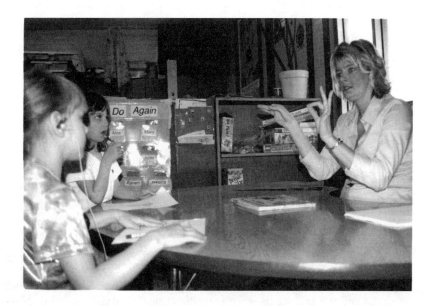

What is the psychological impact of learning to read? What is the psychological impact of *not* learning to read? Both questions are equally profound. No doubt, literacy enhances one's psychological well-being, providing hours of learning, inspiration, vicarious experiences, and armchair travel. It opens doors to higher education and more fulfilling jobs. Not learning how to read severely restricts opportunities for personal growth. Although there are examples of successful people without literacy skills, for most, illiteracy is a handicap and burden.

To understand the impact of deafness on literacy, it is important to understand that many deaf students are learning a language at the same time that they are learning to read. This is no easy task, because reading skills are based on English language skills. For deaf children, sign is acquired easily, but speaking, reading, and writing are generally taught through formal instruction. Despite these difficulties, most deaf persons use English everyday. They make high use of TV captioning, text telephones (TTYs), email, notewriting, faxes—all of which are reading and writing activities.

CHAPTER OBJECTIVES

This chapter examines the perceptual, cognitive, psycholinguistic, and sociocultural processes in learning to read. It explains how deaf students can be viewed as readers who are second language users. The chapter also examines how teachers can set up literacy lessons in the classroom by bridging English to signs, speech, and fingerspelling, and how technology can be used in the reading classroom. Finally, the chapter shows how learning to read by using sign language can explain the reading process not only for deaf children but also for hearing children with cognitive, language, and learning disabilities, as well as those persons who have combined hearing and vision losses.

FIRST CONVERSATIONS

It all begins in the arms of mothers. Early research films show that when infants are actively sucking for milk, gazing, burping, smiling, or vocalizing, mothers are in a rested state. But when mothers actively stroke or talk, their infants are in a rested state. These turn-taking routines of activity and rest during feeding are an infant's earliest conversations. With these routines, prelinguistic infants also use pointing, eye gazing, smiles, vocalizations, and engagement in games with their parents (e.g., patty-cake and peek-a-boo)—all of which build early conversation skills. Whether it be with spoken or sign language, mothers introduce their babies to nursery rhymes and songs, relate family stories, read picture books, give explanations about family events, and so on. It is through these early conversations—in other words, early perceptual-cognitive experiences—within an affectionate and caring family that language learning emerges and flourishes. Such is the foundation of literacy.

Literacy is often thought of as being only a decoding and graphic, perceptual-motor activity. But it is more than that. Reading enables even very young children to think, develop ideas, communicate, and reflect about written language. All of this happens slowly, predictably, and naturally if the right conditions are set up and if adults are able to explain to children what print means, in either sign or spoken language. From perception and cognition to communication and on to language and literacy, such is the path. This path is bidirectional. In turn, literacy learning enhances a person's language, communication, perception, and cognition (Andrews, 1986) (see Figure 5.1).

Early conversations with babies revolve around some shared activity such as eating, reading, playing, or book reading. During these routines, children learn vocabulary and syntax, and the social rules of language. Many parents will talk with their infants, toddlers, and preschoolers about the print they see around them (e.g., Trix cereal boxes, McDonald's, stop signs, M & M candy wrappers, etc.). Children learn that the function of print is to label or name something. They learn that letters have names and can be combined to form words. When children have a book read to them or when they read on their own, they learn how to follow a topic. They learn that stories have a beginning, middle, and end, and contain characters, plots, suspense, and settings. These are reading readiness, or prereading, skills (Andrews, 1986).

Such early parent/child conversations are social and reciprocal. The parent or caregiver forms a scaffold or support. According to Vygotsky (1978), this process creates a *zone of proximal development* in which children depend on parent support to carry out an activity and learn from the process. As the child's language skills emerge, the parent "lets go" of the support. The child is then ready to initiate, maintain, change, and end conversations independently.

A reading lesson is also a conversation or dialogue. Teachers or parents as expert readers provide scaffolding or modeling for the child in how to figure out the meaning of text. The child then tries to read, at first with the expert reader's support. But then slowly the child takes over the reading task and reads independently.

Yet another conversation occurs when one is reading. This conversation is private. Even though written language happens on paper, is permanent, and is constrained by the rules of grammar, punctuation, and so forth, reading is essentially a silent conversation between the reader and the author. Readers bring their background knowledge and expectations to a text. They interact with the author by using what they know to make sense of all the new meanings that the author presents. For instance, in the Harry Potter stories, author J. K. Rawlings talks to her readers through her characters, Harry Potter and company.

As the adult labels objects, food, and persons in the home, the child makes a connection between the object and the name, either spoken or signed. Children

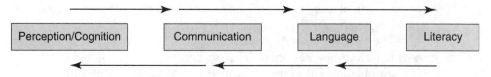

FIGURE 5.1   From Communication to Language to Literacy

quickly acquire vocabulary in this way. As was mentioned in Chapter 4, deaf babies use finger-babbling and go through stages similar to those that hearing babies exhibit with vocal babbling (Petitto, 2000). Many deaf children who acquire sign language in early or late childhood will use finger-babbling in elementary or even junior high school. Finger-babbling skills develop into signs and the finger-spelling of words. In many cases, the first word a deaf child learns to speak or finger-spell, to recognize in print, and to write on paper is his or her name (Andrews & Zmijewski, 1996). The first words children produce in speech or signs are also typically the first words children read and write. In fact, beginning reading should parallel children's speech or signing abilities.

Children's first words are usually names of animals, foods, toys, actions, as well as adjectives and social words such as *thank you, please, no, yes,* and so on (Howell, 1985). When children see the words on paper, they associate the graphemes with a mental representation, such as a picture, an experience, a sign, or a spoken word. Now a sight-word vocabulary begins to develop. The first words a child learns to read are probably learned wholes, as in a first name. Their first finger-spelled words are learned as gestalts or wholes. Soon, though, children learn to match finger-spelling with printed letters. They realize that words are made up of combinations of letters that can be spelled out on their fingers and seen in print (Andrews, 1986).

THE READING PROCESS

Since reading and writing processing involves representations that cannot be observed and measured directly, psycholinguists have used different techniques to infer how readers mentally process print. One tool is to examine models of the ways the brain processes words through the eye and through the ear. Deaf students' reading and writing errors provide further insights into deaf readers' mental processing of print (Ewoldt, 1981; DeVilliers, 1991; Quigley, Power, & Steinkemp, 1977). Studies of eye movements that occur in the watching of captioned programs have also shed light on the deaf reader (Jensema, Sharkawy, Danturthi, Burch, & Hsu, 2000).

A model of "reading by eye" begins when the reader identifies letters by visual analysis and assigns the letters to a graphic code. The resulting graphemes or visual patterns are recognized as whole words and given semantic or meaningful interpretations. The semantic code is then stored in the brain. Some deaf readers also store words in their brains as a sequence of finger-spelled letters. Depending on the tasks, deaf readers will use a combination of signing, finger-spelling, lip-reading, articulation, and the orthographic structure of words to understand, code, and remember English print (see reviews by Marschark, 2000a).

The "reading by ear" model also begins visually with a visual analysis process in which letters are identified (letter recognition) and assigned to a graphic code or set of graphemes. The graphemes are then translated into an acoustic code whereby letters are linked to sounds (grapheme-phoneme correspondence). The reading process is thus linked up with the speech process and the auditory patterns are then recognized as words and semantically interpreted (word recognition) (Crystal, 1997). Of course, this is not true for everyone.

To achieve fluency in reading English, hearing children must master skills such as grapheme-phoneme correspondence rules as well as English orthography or the rules or conventions for using letters to spell words, and all of the exceptions to the rules. The "reading by ear" approach is supported by the fact that beginning readers can easily and naturally associate graphemes with phonemes. Letter name and letter sound recognition occurs rapidly with young children. Children who can phonologically decode words (sound them out) are at an advantage when they come across unfamiliar words.

Both approaches may explain how deaf persons read, although it is likely that *reading by eye* plays a major role in learning to read and managing texts because the phonological code is not fully accessible to prelingually deaf persons. This in not to say that subvocal speech is not useful for deaf readers. For some orally trained deaf or postlingually deaf readers, words may be mouthed or silently spoken on the lips during the reading process (Conrad, 1979; Litchenstein, 1998). This may aid in short-term memory, which underlies reading behaviors. The reader moves from recognizing letters to comprehending a word, sentence, or passage and holds this information in memory as he or she moves on to comprehending more print. But researchers are unclear on whether it is good reading that produces "inner speech" or whether it is the spoken language ability that facilitates good reading in deaf persons (Marschark, 1993; Marschark & Lukomski, 2001).

The *reading by eye* approach may be useful for deaf readers in identifying words, sentences, and the gist of the text. But the *reading by ear* approach may be useful for analyzing some words by breaking down the unit words into smaller parts—either dactylicly through finger-spelling or phonetically through subvocal speech or lip movements, or by using visual cues as in those used in cued speech (LaSasso & Metzger, 1998). More research is needed to determine how deaf readers from different backgrounds decode printed words and phrases.

Recognizing Words

Reading is getting the meaning or the gist of a text. Perceptually, this task may seem overwhelming. Children must recognize 52 upper- and lower-case letters, 10 numerals and their combinations, punctuation and spaces between words, and that is just the beginning of it. Children must learn the meanings of the words (semantics) as well as how the words are arranged together (grammar).

But deaf children easily learn the letters of the alphabet. In a study of deaf children in kindergarten and first grade, it was found that letter recognition and sight word recognition were part of the children's prereading skills. As emergent readers, they learn that finger-spelling can be linked to letters on the page and that a word's meaning can be matched to a familiar sign and concept (Andrews, 1986).

Deaf children's early attempts at using finger-spelling is not for spelling words though. They use finger-spelling like they use signs—to represent whole meanings. For instance, a deaf boy may make the B finger-spelled handshape on his cheek to represent his friend Bob, and then finger-spell B-O-B as a whole sign. Later, with letter awareness, the children break words down to the finger-spelled equivalent. For young deaf readers, the sign-to-print connections signal the beginning of an emerging sight-word vocabulary. For example, signing deaf children will use the sign CAT when they see the printed letters *c-a-t* in a story. In contrast, many hearing children connect the sounds and syllables to meaning through spoken words that correspond to written English equivalents. (Some hearing readers do not learn sound-out strategies and rely on sight words.) They will use phonological awareness of syllables, rhyming, and phonemes. Rhyming helps children form auditory categories of words. It facilitates connections of similar-sounding words to new words when children come across them in print. Rhyming also helps with phonemic awareness and segmentation skills. Hearing children's early writing errors indicate that they are developing phonological awareness and using it to segment words. Many deaf children will use finger-spelling to segment words and develop a kind of visual and motor memory for words. Deaf children's spelling errors reveal that they are developing awareness of orthography and visual patterns of letter combinations (Andrews, 1986).

Results of studies are mixed as to whether deaf readers use phonological information to a great extent while reading. Some studies indicated that they use phonological information and rhyming awareness. Yet other researchers have noted that deaf children develop visual orthographic rhyming and speech-reading rhyming skills that are qualitatively different from hearing children's auditory rhyming skills (see reviews by LaSasso & Metzger, 1998).

Researchers have established links between phonological coding, awareness and short-term memory, and the reading processes as mentioned earlier. However, the research on phonological awareness is not conclusive regarding to *what extent* these skills support the reading process for deaf students or if they are useful only when used in combination with other visual codes (e.g., signing, finger-spelling). Lichtenstein (1998) reports that the phonological skills of oral deaf readers contribute to better grammatical skills and better reading comprehension in skilled deaf readers, because having a phonological representation is more efficient than a signing or visual code for the memory demands of reading. More research is needed about the interaction between visual and acoustic data in the phonological representations in deaf readers

For the young, deaf, signing reader, the sign-meaning-print matching may begin with a one-to-one correspondence between a sign and a word (i.e., CAT, *cat*). It eventually progresses to more than one sign or sign phase. As in any translation from one language to another, there is not always a one-to-one correspondence (Andrews, 1986).

The sign-meaning-print connection later will progress to a word-to-word association as deaf readers use context to figure out words they do not know. For example, a deaf reader might come across a new word, such as *acorn,* in a story. He or she might may understand from the story context that an acorn is a nut. Mentally, the deaf reader visualizes the sign NUT and transfers its meaning to the new word, *acorn*. The child signs the word NUT, then finger-spells the word A-C-O-R-N to keep it in memory. Deaf students acquire large vocabularies using this strategy. The sign plus finger-spelling is an easy way to acquire English vocabulary, especially for English words for which there is no sign equivalent, such as brand names for cars, grammatical features of English, and so on (Padden & Ramsey, 2000).

There is also some evidence indicating that deaf readers use visual hand-shapes such as those used in the cued speech system to recognize and read words. The advantage to using cued speech, according to its proponents, is that it provides visual phonological information about English that neither signed systems of English or ASL provide (LaSasso & Metzger, 1998) (see Chapter 7).

Researchers and educators have tried a variety of ways of visually representing sign language and matching it to English print graphically in order to mediate print for deaf students. These techniques have been used to teach hearing people sign language. This is particularly noticeable in any sign-language text where you can see many graphic pictures of signs.

Figuring out ways to map a visual sign language onto print has motivated educators in many creative directions. Reading materials have been developed that graphically illustrate the sign and printed word, which match invented signs to English print words.*

Research on the effects of the use of graphic illustrations of signs on deaf children's reading comprehension is not conclusive. Wilson and Hyde (1997) report gains in reading comprehension from the use of these sign materials. Drasgow and Paul (1995), in a review of Manually Coded English (MCE) studies, report that even though some deaf children have benefited from learning to read and write using these systems, many deaf children still do not achieve the literacy skills at the levels they should be capable of achieving. In other words, these techniques may be useful in helping deaf children develop a sight-word vocabulary, but not the understanding of stories and other connected texts.

Other researchers have devised strategies for deaf readers that involve decoding or analyzing a graphic picture of a sign according to its sign parts (Supalla, Wix, McKee, 2001) (see Chapter 4). The rationale is that just as hearing students decode a word based on its sounds, Supalla and colleagues hypothesize that young deaf readers can build a substantial sign-word vocabulary by analyzing print words according to their sign parts or formational parameters of handshape, location, and movement. These investigators have created dictionaries that organize the signs around their sign parts.

Supalla's group has also created a sign-writing system based on what they call *ASL graphemes*. These ASL graphemes represent signs, much like alphabetic writing does for spoken words. Supalla and colleagues developed and adapted their sign-writing system from the SignFont system (1989). Efforts to devise sign-writing systems began with Stokoe, Casterline, and Croneberg (1965) when they wrote the first ASL dictionary. These various systems differ in the number of graphemes they use.

There are also examples of graphic representations of ASL signs, phrases, and sentences. For instance, the "Bilingual Corner" is a regular feature in the *Silent*

---

*See our textbook webpage and companion DVD for graphic representations of these examples: http://hal.lamar.edu/~andrewssjf/bookindex.htm.

News, a popular newspaper for deaf readers. For example, a drawing will be made of a person making an ASL sign. Underneath the picture will be a caption with the English equivalent to the ASL sign.

The examples demonstrate the creative attempts by educators to provide a bridge from signs to print in order to build sight-word vocabulary. A large, quickly accessible vocabulary is critical to fluent reading. Poor readers are impeded by weak vocabularies, and this happens frequently to deaf readers (Kelly, 1996). In fact, compared to hearing readers, deaf readers have smaller vocabularies, acquire words at a slower rate, and have a narrower range of context in word learning (Lederberg & Spencer, 2001). This can be explained in part by deaf students' lack of access to the English language, in multiple ways that are meaningful and comprehensible to them.

Reading, Writing, and Spelling Development

Like hearing students, deaf readers learn reading, writing, and spelling rules. However, deaf readers will also add finger-spelling to their letter awareness, letter naming, and word-spelling skills; and sign language to their word identification (Padden & Ramsey, 2000); and comprehension skills using visual reading strategies (Grushkin, 1998; Wilbur, 2000).

Deaf children progress similarly to hearing children in acquiring spelling skills. However, when hearing children produce spellings that sound like English words (e.g., *der ant Geen* for Dear Aunt Jean), deaf children produce spellings that are based on graphic and visual characteristics of words (Romig, 1985). Some deaf students will draw pictures of signs in their writing. The grammar of ASL also affects deaf children's writing. The following writing sample of a 10-year-old deaf student illustrates spelling and writing errors.

> **KNIGHT AND THE DAGON**
> Once upon a time a big castle with lonley boy name is Knight and other is a stone stuck at hat where dagon live. One day dagon rad book about "How fight Knight." Knight think and get book about cook and he finish it with it so he go to made a stone sivler body. he fix a round with sivler hammer and he strew on it and he pow it up so it can be stay hard and he made everything ready so he put it on and he get his horse and his knife and dagon has no supply to fight but his nose have fire and then Knight say 1...2...3...go both of us run toward than to back and both fell down and Knight only go to library and read.

Researchers have characterized deaf students' writing as being repetitive; using more simple syntactic structures, run-on sentences, and restricted vocabulary; and lacking complex syntactic forms (DeVilliers, 1991). Students have difficulty with the mechanics of writing (e.g., punctuation, capitalization) and frequently misspell words based on graphic similarities rather than sound, as the sample writing demonstrates. This may be explained in part by the lack of practice in English compositional skills.

Reading Comprehension

Reading involves more that letter naming, spelling, and word reading. It involves getting the meaning or the gist of a text. A good literacy program involves giving children opportunities to sample quality children's literature, including those with multicultural themes, a variety of text genres, writing activities, read-aloud, guided reading, and independent reading sessions, as well as basic skill work in word and grammar analyses. Such a balanced approach to literacy is supported for deaf students (Gallimore, 1999; Smith, 1999).

Researchers have shown that deaf readers and writers have difficulties with the vocabulary and grammar of English (DeVilliers, 1991; Quigley et al., 1977). They have difficulty writing coherent stories (Yoshinaga-Itano & Snyder, 1985), but their memories for story items increase when they practice signing the stories (Andrews, 1986).

One of the authors composed the following story to illustrate these story, word, and grammar difficulties deaf readers face.

> THE CAT, THE DOG, AND THE ANT
> One crisp fall day in a sunny spot in the woods a cat was chased around a tree by a dog. When the dog barked, the cat was bit by an ant. Full of fear and pain, the cat ran up the tree like lightning. Up in the tree, he pulled an acorn from a branch and dropped it on the dog. The dog barked and the ant crawled up the dog's leg. The cat laughed when the ant was carried away with the dog. He knew the dog would get his just desserts and he felt happy. What goes around comes around, he thought to himself.

The vocabulary words—*day, cat, dog, tree, ant, chase*—are easy to read in a list. But when the words are combined into the sentences, and the sentences are combined into a story, the text becomes a minefield of comprehension problems. For instance, deaf readers may have difficulty with passive constructions. They may read the first sentence as *the cat chased the dog* instead of *the dog chased the cat*. Deaf readers impose a subject-verb-object word order on sentences (Quigley et al., 1977).

If asked the question, "Where was the dog when he was hit by the acorn?" the deaf reader may go to the text and use a visual matching strategy. The reader will try to find similar phrases and copy the answer. But the dog's location is not explicitly stated in the story, so the reader must read the first few sentences to infer the ant's location. Visual matching strategies may work for some questions but not for those questions that require inferences from story ideas. Deaf readers often overly rely on visual or verbatim matching on text-based tests (LaSasso, 1999). Deaf students may also guess at answers rather than try to solve problems by relying on their limited reading skills and background knowledge (Marschark & Everhart, 1999).

Deaf readers can often bypass the grammar level if they understand the meaning of the story (Ewoldt, 1981). However, there are certain constructions in English that are problematic for deaf readers even if they understand the story. In our story, the word particles *ran up* and *carried away* may be difficult to understand (Payne & Quigley, 1987). Multiple-meaning words such as *bark, head, bit,* and *run* change meaning depending on the context. To be *carried away* by a dog is different from to be *carried away* by an idea.

Deaf readers may also have difficulty understanding figurative language, as in *to run like lightning* (Girorcelli, 1982), and pronouns (Quigley et al., 1977). Young readers who have been stung by a red ant can feel the cat's pain. But those who have not had these emotional experiences may not be able to empathize with the characters (Gray & Hosie, 1996). Deaf students may have difficulty with the meaning of the moral of the story—*what goes around comes around*. In terms of a story grammar, this story has a beginning, a middle, and an end, which unfolds according to a plot with a moral. These concepts aid in comprehension only if the student has a sense of the parts of a story.

We have only scratched the surface in our analysis of reading comprehension, but it highlights the challenges deaf readers face. The crux of the comprehension problems is that many deaf students are learning the English language at the same time they are learning to read. Unlike hearing students who bring a level of English language competency to the reading process, deaf readers often do not have this English language competence. This makes reading English even more difficult for deaf students.

Language-Teaching Approaches and Bridges to Literacy

The research is divided on which language-teaching approach leads to higher reading scores. Researchers studying children who are enrolled in monolingual oral/aural programs report that some oral deaf children have high literacy scores and that this is a function of their overall English language development. Factors that predicted this achievement include early intervention, attendance in an oral/aural program and a high level of family motivation (see reviews in Marschark, 2000).

There is another view. Researchers have examined the relationship between deaf children's language abilities using ASL and their literacy achievement. This work has been partly an outgrowth of studies done in the 1960s and 1970s that showed the beneficial effects of sign language on English language learning in deaf children (see reviews in Vernon & Andrews, 1990). Researchers have tested deaf students on different measures of ASL grammar and have compared these ASL scores with reading achievement scores and writing measures. They have found that deaf students who have higher ASL competence also have higher English reading scores compared to children who had lower ASL skills (see studies in Butler & Prinz, 1998; Chamberlain, Morford, & Mayberry, 2000).

Researchers have also summarized visual teaching techniques (Grushkin, 1998; Wilbur, 2000) that highlight how teachers use ASL as a bridge to English. This work is based on the notion that if students have competence in one language, they can transfer it to a second language. Cummins (2000) calls this the Linguistic Inter-dependence model. This model theorizes that there is a common proficiency under-lying all languages, and that literacy skills in one language can transfer to literacy skills in the second language. Mayer and Wells (1996) argue that this cannot be applied to deaf education because certain assumptions for the Cummins model are not met. Specifically, ASL has no written form. Likewise, Mayer and Akamatsu (1999) argue that there is little linguistic interdependence between a native sign lan-guage and the written form of a spoken language. These authors contend that English-based signing may be useful to mediate sign to print. Others argue that bilingual approaches to language teaching and language learning should include only ASL and English and not include the invented sign systems (see reviews by Nover & Andrews, 2000).

Whether one supports the monolingual, language-mixing (invented sys-tems), or bilingual approaches to language teaching and language learning (Chap-ter 7), it remains that the field lacks a coherent theory of teaching English literacy to deaf children. Given that there are alternative pathways for language acquisition using vision, it may be that deaf children would benefit from new paradigms of English literacy instruction that capitalize on visual pathways. This does not mean abandoning all auditory strategies, but it would mean focusing primarily on visual pathways using auditory pathways as secondary.

Many teachers use visual strategies to link signs with print, but there is no the-ory of reading that pulls these strategies together. Such a model might build on the approaches deaf adults use in reading to their young deaf children. Perhaps the model could also be built on how deaf adults read to deaf children (Schleper, 1997).

The work of Gallimore (1999) represents a beginning in the conceptualization of such a framework. Gallimore modified techniques such as read-alouds, guided reading, word analyses, and mini-grammar lessons found to be successful with hearing children. She applied a balanced approach to teaching reading (Lyons & Pinnell, 2001) in her work with deaf students.

Figure 5.2 represents a graphic of what Gallimore (1999) and Bailes (2001) pro-pose that reading lessons should look like for deaf students. These researchers incorporate comprehension skills as well as word and grammar skills within a reading lesson using a balanced (top-down and bottom-up) approach with interac-tive activities.

In the guided reading approach, first the teacher signs the whole story to the students (ASL *storytelling*) (Gallimore, 1999). Second, the teacher takes one page of text, and provides translation of the meaning of the page (*storyreading*). The teacher does not sign the text word for word but signs the meaning of whole phrases and sentences (Gallimore, 1999). In the *guided reading* portion, the teacher thinks of a particular reading skill to teach (e.g., finding the main idea or multiple meaning words, etc.) then discusses how students can use this skill to understand the words and the whole story. In the *mini-grammar* lesson, the teacher again takes a piece of the text and emphasizes a particular skill in grammar (e.g., past tense, passive sen-tences, etc.). The teacher then repeats these steps going back to the full text. This kind of interactive approach to teaching reading to deaf children by using signs,

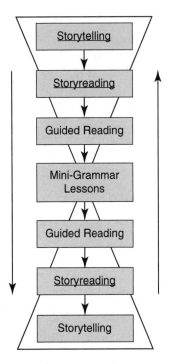

FIGURE 5.2   Teaching Reading to Deaf Students

finger-spelling, print, and bridging strategies from English to sign has been used in several classroom ethnographic studies of reading teachers working with deaf students (Bailes, 2001; Gallimore, 1999).

Literacy and Content Subjects

Another void in the field is the lack of research on literacy in the content subjects (Chapter 6). Very little research has been done on the ways deaf readers use reading and writing in content subject areas such as math, science, and social studies. To become science literate, the reader must not only understand the concepts of science and the technical science vocabulary but also know how to use reading and writing in the science laboratory and classroom. Science literacy is not simply learning new science vocabulary. Science literacy means learning how to use reading and writing to learn science concepts as well as science methods of investigation (McIntosh, Sulzen, Reeder, & Kidd, 1994).

The subject of math is also difficult for deaf students because of the reading of math word or story problems. The math vocabulary is difficult and the math operations may be hidden, as illustrated in the following math word problem:

> Natalie has 5 toy cars. She has 8 fewer than Cole. How many toy cars does Cole have?

The grammar of this sentence is simple—but the vocabulary is tricky. The math student could read the word *fewer* and think that he or she needs to use the subtraction operation, when, in fact, this word problem calls for addition.

Miscue (Error) Analysis and Eye Movements

Researchers have examined how deaf readers process print by examining the errors they make while reading. In one of the first studies to examine reading errors, it was found that deaf readers relied too much on graphic information, such as signing CAT for *cart* and FROG for *fog*. The readers used finger-spelling as a placeholder while reading sentences (e.g., finger-spelling unfamiliar words). But when the deaf readers figured out the meaning in the story, they went back and signed the word (Ewoldt, 1981). In another study examining metacognitive strategies of deaf readers in high school, one deaf reader fingerspelled T-H-E for the word *there* and signed FATHER for the word *farther*. In other words, the deaf readers were guessing based on the graphic similarities between words rather than reading the words for meaning (Andrews & Mason, 1991).

Eye movements of captioned deaf viewers have also shed light on the ways deaf persons comprehend print. Jensema and colleagues (2000) studied six deaf adults who watched video segments with and without captions. The additions of captions to a video resulted in a major change in eye movement patterns, with the viewing process becoming more of a reading process. For adult readers, caption reading dominated eye movements, while viewing the screen action was secondary. The data indicate that adult readers who depend on speech-reading for communicating focus more on the actor's lips than on the captions. Those who do not have strong English skills may spend all or most of the time reading the captions. The authors found that the higher the captioning speeds, the more time was spent on reading captions. In a follow-up study, Jensema and colleagues (2000) studied the eye movements of 23 deaf people ages 14 to 61. It was found that those people being studied gazed at the captions 84 percent of the time, at the video picture 14 percent of the time, and off the video 2 percent of the time. Age, sex, and education level had little influence on the time spent viewing captions. The researchers conclude that the large amount of time viewing captions (84 percent) suggests that viewing captions is primarily a reading task. Given that people normally watch 30 hours of television per week, deaf persons are spending about 25 hours a week viewing printed material. The conclusion has implications for the teaching of reading to deaf children and youth (Jensema et al., 2000).

SOCIOCULTURAL PROCESSES

Language and literacy learning have broad cultural implications, as these involve home and school communities (Heath, 1983). Children will learn different styles of asking and answering questions, listening, and telling stories, depending on their culture.

Deaf adults and Deaf teachers also have culturally different ways of presenting conversations and reading lessons to young Deaf children. In a study of four Deaf parents of hearing toddlers in Puerto Rico, Rodriguez (2001) found that Deaf parents created a dynamic triangle between themselves, their young toddler, and objects (e.g., food, toys, or a book). Deaf parents signed within the triangle, pointing to the object or making the signs on the child's body or on the book, toy, or food item. The triangle was expanded or reduced in size as the parent moved toward or leaned away to let the child respond (Rodriguez, 2001).

In a study with three African American families reading to their preschool deaf children, Smith (1999) found that by teaching parents basic sign language communication skills, introducing children's books with African American themes, and providing modeling, guidance, support, and feedback to reading, she could increase the home literacy behaviors. Smith, who herself is African American, attributed the program's success to the fact that she shared the parents' cultural heritage. She established trust and rapport, and she taught directly to the parents' level and needs. Smith also introduced the parents to an African American deaf adult who read to the deaf children, thus providing this role modeling for parents.

Research on other Deaf parents and teachers reading to deaf children shows that they use a variety of strategies such as moving the location of the sign to pictures in a book or on the child's body. Deaf adults elaborate on the child's background experience tied to the story, expand on concepts in the book in sign language, finger-spell names of characters and places, ask questions to check the child's comprehension while reading, and use eye gaze and visual attention-getting strategies to obtain, maintain, and keep the child's attention during the conversation or book reading lesson (Mather, 1997).

There are few studies that have examined how oral deaf adults or hearing parents who do not use a sign language read to their children. Anecdotal evidence from deaf graduate students suggests that oral deaf mothers and hearing mothers use picture clues, mouth words, and pantomime to mediate print. More home studies are needed to document such behaviors.

Bilingualism and Reading English as a Second Language

The field of bilingualism and English as a second language offers educators in deaf education many insights and intriguing parallels into the reading-acquisition process. For instance, children from China, Japan, Korea, and Saudi Arabia must learn different orthographies compared to their spoken language. Similarly, deaf children who use sign language will associate pictures of signs and finger-spelling with print. Oral deaf children will use mouth movements, lip-reading, or what they hear via amplification, and match these to print. Like other second language learners, many deaf readers are not necessarily proficient in using a first language and mapping it onto a written language (Cummins, 2000).

Like other second language learners, when signing deaf children begin to write English, they often mix the two languages (ASL and English) and create what second language researchers call an *interlanguage*. This provides a fascinating inside view of their language-processing strategies. An interlanguage grammar is established when the student's writing is influenced by both the first and the second language. Take, for example, the following language sample by a Deaf writer:

> HOW DO I FIND EARTH
> I not know much about Earth. I have no feel about Earth, but I finish learn about Earth. People need care for home. People need respect. People are nice to earth. Animals can live long if animals eat healthy food, drink clean water and breathe clean air. Animals live free. Each help people and animals live. Each is very pretty because blue water, colors many different. Earth need nicely. Earth not need mess.

The underlined phrases highlight our key points. This deaf writer is struggling with articles and verb tenses—a common developmental error for people learning English as a second language. One can also note interference or transfer in which the child's dominant ASL has influenced the writing of English. For instance, the child used the ASL sign FINISH to show past tense with the verb phrase *learned about Earth*. In the next to last sentence, the child also used another ASL grammatical feature. In ASL word order, the adjective can follow the noun, as in the phrase *colors many different* (Nover & Andrews, 2000).

The deaf writer has transferred his or her knowledge of past tense in ASL and incorporated it into his or her English sentence. Deaf writers also make other kinds of errors that young children make in learning a first language. For example, when deaf children learn the *-ed* rule for past tense, they often overgeneralize this rule as they write English. These overgeneralizations persist even into high school or adulthood for many deaf students (Wilbur, 2000).

There are countless factors that affect the child who is learning to read and write a second language. These factors include age, affective factors, cognitive factors, and the kind of second language instruction the student receives (Baker, 2001). The second language literature may provide potentially new ways of understanding and instructing the deaf reader and writer (Nover & Andrews, 2000).

Technology in the Classroom

The microchip has resulted in many new gadgets and electronic devices for the classroom teacher. Technology, however, as the saying goes, is only as good as the teacher who is using it. Numerous technologies are available to assist the teacher in the literacy classroom. There are communication technologies such as cochlear implants, hearing aids (analog, digital), and FM systems and phone amplifiers. These auditory technologies provide sound awareness and, with training, some understanding of speech. This can enhance phonological awareness for reading, spelling, and writing.

Deaf people use text telephones (TTYs), email, and wireless pagers to communicate. Using these devices is essentially engaging in reading and writing. Today, with high-speed lines at most universities and agencies, videoconferencing is becoming a common practice. Video relay systems are being established in the United States. More and more deaf and hearing people are using desktop videoconferencing software to conduct business.

There are also steno-based systems that use the stenographic machine—the court reporter's machine. A trained stenographer uses a 24-key machine to encode spoken English phonetically into a computer. It is then converted to English text and displayed on a computer screen or television monitor in real time. The text is generally produced verbatim. This system is called CART (Communication Access Real-Time Translation) when used in the schools. It is also used in courtrooms and at professional conferences.

In addition, there are computer-assisted note-taking (CAN) systems. For these systems, a typist with special training uses a standard QWERTY keyboard and types words onto a laptop computer as they are being spoken. These can take the form of summary notes or verbatim text. Some CAN systems include the use of computerized word abbreviation software that has been developed for extensive abbreviation of words and phrases being entered into the computer.

The C-Print system was developed by Dr. Michael Stinson and his colleagues at the National Technical Institute for the Deaf in Rochester, New York. The C-Print system includes training and specialized software. The specialized software produces real-time text through automatic speech recognition and a computerized keyboard-based abbreviation system. An intermediary operator (or "captionist") in the classroom with the deaf or hard of hearing students dictates into a microphone linked to a laptop computer containing automatic speech recognition software and often along with abbreviation software. The software also has computer network capabilities and displays for the captionist (host) and student (client) computers. This software enables students to participate in class discussion, highlight text produced by the captionist, and easily take their own notes.

Studies by Stinson and colleagues have shown that speech-to-text transcription systems such as C-Print are effective in increasing accessibility in the mainstream class for deaf students (Elliot, Stinson, McKee, Everhart, & Francis, 2001). Deaf students who were raised orally when they enter high school or college use these note-taking systems widely.

Today, decoders for translating closed-captioned signals into words that appear on the screen are built into all TV screens at least 13 inches in diameter. In larger cities, such as Houston, first-run movies are captioned for deaf audiences. The National Center for Accessible Media (NCAM) has developed virtual vision glasses. The system includes an oversized pair of eyeglasses and a small liquid crystal display that sits at the very top of the glasses and faces straight down. Captions are created by a computer and sent to displays through cables that hold the glasses to the seat. Through lenses and a mirror, the captions on the display are reflected onto the eyeglasses. As the wearer looks at the screen, the captions appear to float in midair. Reactions have been mixed. The glasses are expensive ($700 each), can be fatiguing to wear throughout a movie, and have cables that can be annoying (Clark, 1994). Other movie captioning systems include a seatback display or a rearview display of the movie captions (Clark, 1994).

There is also computer software that can be used by teachers, such as multimedia CD-ROMs. These materials present ASL movies, graphics, animation, text, and audio. Some are interactive, meaning the student can interact with the materials in game or question-and-answer formats. Numerous desktop software is available for teachers and students to create language lessons. The Internet has many tools that teachers can use for literacy teaching, such as web-based courses, web-casting, videostreaming, encyclopedias, and so on.

Other technologies that can be used in the reading classroom are document projectors that allow the teacher to place a book under a camera and have it projected on a screen. There are also SmartBoards, which are electronic screens that function as a computer. In addition, digital cameras allow the reading teacher to take pictures of language experiences for preparing writing lessons. Digtal camcorders can be used to take movies of children and adults using sign language. Digital still shots as well as movies can be imported into software programs such as PowerPoint to develop creative language and literacy lessons that demonstrate both languages—ASL and English—to deaf students.

Web-based courses with videostreaming are also available for deaf students. The Internet does not yet support clear and fast transmission of sign. Future developments with Internet II may open up more opportunities for teachers and students to transmit sign language.

Videoconferencing allows students in a distant geographic place to take courses on a variety of subjects. Deaf teenagers in a Dallas Regional Day school are now taking an algebra class via distance learning from the Texas School for the Deaf (TSD), several hours away. These deaf mainstream students can benefit from having a deaf instructor teaching them algebraic equations. Likewise, teachers from the Texas School for the Deaf can teach sign language to hearing high schools from around the state. Another use of videoconferencing that benefits students is the virtual field trip. Deaf students from TSD can have a videoconference with education specialists from the Cincinnati Zoo or other museums and parks around the country.

Of course, in setting up a totally visual environment with videoconferencing and young deaf students, there are challenges. For example, with interpreters, there will be a lag time, especially if the education specialist wants to involve the children in hands-on activities. Also, how does one set up a slide show as well as include the interpreter as the education specialist is talking? As videoconferencing is being set up in more state schools for the deaf and more programs offered to deaf students, these issues will no doubt be addressed.

There are also computer programs that use virtual reality (VR). Virtual reality is an interactive multimedia environment based on the computer during which the user is assimilated into and becomes an active participant in the virtual world. This technology can present information in a three-dimensional (3-D) format in real time, thus enabling the user to become an active participant in an environment that communicates interactively without the use of words.*

Signing avatars are three-dimensional computer characters that communicate in sign language and include the use of facial expressions (www.signingavatar.com). Until recently, much of the technology has focused on hearing systems to

---

*See our textbook webpage and companion DVD for pictures of these technologies.

access information using text or captions. Today, companies are developing signing avatars or cartoon characters using animation technologies that allow the characters to communicate in sign language. This technology has the potential use for teaching parents sign language as well as teaching literacy to young deaf children.

In England, researchers are experimenting with digital avatars as signing translators at the post office. A computer program takes spoken English and converts it to real-time text. The digital avatar then takes this English text and signs its meaning on a display screen. With a computer screen displaying the signing avatar, a deaf or hard-of-hearing person can communicate with a postal worker and complete his or her business. Of course, this post office avatar is not a fluent translator, but it can be programmed with a set of predictable phrases (e.g., Want to buy some stamps?). Avatars cannot translate oral conversations into real-time text, but perhaps with improvements in technology, such a device may be possible. Future signing avatars may someday appear on mobile phones or hand-held computers to translate real-time between English and sign language. Such technologies could change the communication and literacy experiences of the Deaf community (*BBC News,* March 2, 2002).

So far, little research has been done on the effectiveness of the use of technology to teach literacy. Most of the research on technology and reading has centered on television captioning These studies have pointed to the positive effects of presenting captioning to deaf students to aid their reading comprehension. But the captioning speed and reading level of the captioning must be regulated if the child is to benefit (Jensema, McCann, & Ramsey, 1996).

Multimedia combines text, graphics, photographs, movies, and animation. There are many multimedia programs with ASL movies that are available to reading teachers. In a study on the use of multimedia with deaf students, Gentry (1999) compared deaf elementary school children's performance in each of four treatments: print plus picture, print plus ASL movies, print without pictures, and print with ASL movies and pictures. Gentry reports that deaf students' retelling and comprehension score increased when they were allowed to view the pictures and the movies, rather then just view the print alone. She suggests that these kinds of materials have potential for building reading comprehension in deaf children. She also reports that many deaf students initially did not know how to focus on the signer in the movies. The students had to be trained to get information from the movies.

Unique Populations with Literacy Needs Using Sign Language

About 30 to 40 percent of deaf children have disabilities that are educationally significant. Deaf children with cognitive and learning disabilities typically use sign language for communication and learn literacy for functional purposes (Vernon & Andrews, 1990). A communication and literacy curriculum for children with special needs includes communication/language, functional math, social/emotional aspects, domestic, community living, health, and human sexuality with sign language. They can learn social or pragmatic skills using sign language, such as greeting a person, meeting strangers, carrying on conversations, and so on. Although deaf children with specific disabilities may not be able to read a textbook, they can benefit from teachers who focus on vocabulary skills related to reading medicine bottles, safety signs, menus, job applications, newspapers, phone books, and recipes. Math literacy skills include budgeting, making grocery lists, having a bank account, and carrying out similar function-related activities.

Sign language and finger-spelling have potential for use with hearing children who have language learning disabilities as well as with children who have communication disorder associated speech impairments, vision impairments, mental retardation, aphasia, dyslexia, autism, and auditory processing. Children with these communication and literacy disorders are not able to use phonological information and segment sounds in order to develop a phonologically structured lexicon (Vernon & Andrews, 1990).

Signs and finger-spelling have also been used with hearing children who have reading, writing, and spelling disorders for the same reason—the inability to use phonological information in the literacy process (Daniels, 2001). Because signs and finger-spelling do not require auditory processing and auditory memory, they allow the teacher to use a multisensory approach and to capitalize on the visual learning strengths of the student (Daniels, 2001; Greenberg, Vernon, DuBois, & McKnight, 1982).

Daniels (2001) has conducted numerous studies on using sign language with hearing children. In several studies conducted over a 10-year span, Daniels compared children who had no signing with the treatment group of hearing bimodal students who used sign in the reading classroom. The treatment group performed higher on the Peabody Picture Vocabulary Test.

Researchers know very little about the literacy development of children with diminishing vision and hearing problems, particularly those who are deaf-blind. There are gifted children in the public schools with vision and hearing problems who need special services. Persons with impaired vision and hearing will use a variety of communication strategies: speech, speech-reading, finger-spelling into the hand, signing in the hand or in close proximity to the face, reading, and writing. The literacy research on these populations is virtually nonexistent. There are only a few case studies of deaf-blind adults who have good reading vision and the ability to read and write English. One deaf-blind individual with Usher syndrome (Chapter 3) said that after he lost his vision, he began reading more because other avenues of recreation were no longer open to him. Many deaf persons with Usher syndrome will learn braille, a tactile form of communication based on raised dots on a page. Using braille allows the deaf-blind person to use other communication technologies, such as Teletouch and TeleBraille, as well as writing for communication (Duncan, Prickett, Finkelstein, Vernon, & Hollingsworth, 1988). The Teletouch is a portable communication device that has one braille cell on which the deaf-blind person places his or her finger while the speaker uses a typewriter-like keyboard on the other side. The TeleBraille is an electronic device that provides a braille keyboard on one side and a typewriter keyboard and print display on the other side, so that a deaf-blind person and another person can type messages to each other. However, since braille is based on English, the deaf-blind person must have English skills. Many deaf children who lose their vision may not have the English skills to learn braille. Deaf-blind children and youth with residual vision and hearing may use enlarged print and amplifiers on their computers. They may also use tactile books and sign language to learn about reading (Miles, 2000). How deaf-blind children, youth, and adults acquire, develop, and retain their reading and writing skills is an unexplored area of research.*

CONCLUSION

The average reading achievement of deaf high school students is around the fourth-grade level (Traxler, 2000). Standardized reading tests, however, cannot tell the whole story. Most deaf adults use reading and writing every day. In using the TTY, email, and television captioning, deaf persons are essentially reading and writing. New auditory technologies, such as cochlear implants, may provide further information on how deaf readers using audition can access the phonological code to assist them in reading, given that some researchers highlight the importance of phonological awareness in learning to read. New visual technologies can present both ASL and English to the student in the classroom. The field of deaf education currently lacks a coherent theory of literacy instruction that could guide classroom teachers in utilizing the best literacy practices. Further, there is a need for more research on the prevalence of reading disabilities, including dyslexia in the deaf population. As Superintendent Tucker noted in the opening of this chapter, deaf children must be given plenty of practice in reading and writing. But this must occur in an environment where children are guided by teachers who can help them bridge their communication system to English print. Note-taking systems such as CAN (computer-assisted note-taking), CART (Communication Access Real-Time Translation) and C-Print hold promise in providing deaf students with full access to English. However, to use these systems, deaf students must have English reading ability.

SUGGESTED READINGS

Ashton-Warner, S. (1963). *Teacher.* New York: Simon & Shuster.
> In this classic book, Sylvia Ashton-Warner tells how she taught reading to Maori Indians in New Zealand. After she found out they were not learning to read using British methods, she created literacy methods by incorporating the language and culture of the Maori Indians in her classroom instruction. Her findings are strikingly relevant to the teaching of literacy to deaf students.

Bryson, B. (1990). *Mother Tongue: English and How It Got That Way.* New York: Avon Books.
> This highly readable book written by the humorous author Bill Bryson provides a wealth of information about the English language. It would be useful for reading teachers, as it could contribute to their understanding of the complexities of the English language.

* See our textbook webpage and companion DVD for case studies of deaf readers.

CHAPTER SIX

EDUCATIONAL ASPECTS

Deaf people can do anything hearing people can do—except hear!
—I. King Jordan, Gallaudet University President

We can—if given a chance. That chance has to begin with a good education.
—Bowe, 1991, p. x

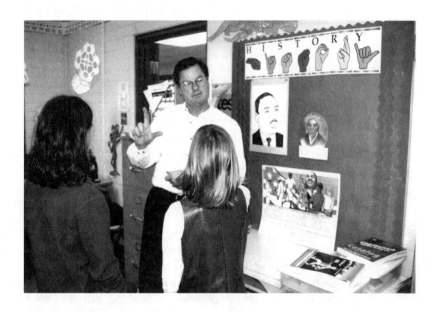

Education involves the transmission of academic information and culturally tinged values deemed important by society. For deaf children, education must also reinforce basic language acquisition to a greater extent than it does for hearing children. Educators have a monumental task. They have to take into account the diversity in all children, including individual learning styles, when deciding what and how to teach. In educating deaf children, a number of approaches have been developed to counteract long-standing academic achievement problems. This complicates decisions about how best to educate deaf children, since no one approach provides "the final answer." The bottom line is that one must be sensitive to exactly what the educational needs of these children are, whether these needs are being met, and how educational laws influence the educational process.

CHAPTER OBJECTIVES

This chapter focuses on deaf education aspects, including the laws that are currently influencing educational decisions, the types of educational programs and services that are available, the factors that determine the most appropriate educational placement of deaf children, and the pros and cons of each. Discussion will also center on the role of teachers and educational interpreters in various deaf education programs, multicultural issues in the classroom, and deaf education in other countries.

PLACEMENT ISSUES

With so many educational options available, the decision regarding the educational placement of deaf children is very complex. There are state residential schools for the deaf, day schools for deaf students, public schools with self-contained classrooms, regular public education, and programs that educate deaf children using oral communication, cued speech, or combinations of various communication philosophies and methods. Also available are programs that promote bilingual education, incorporating ASL and English. Charter schools for deaf students have been established in recent years.

Further complicating matters, these programs vary in academic quality, availability, and affordability. Also, the needs of deaf children vary, including how they communicate, where they are in terms of language and cognitive development, and how they use their residual hearing. Deaf children also differ in their ability to use sign language, speech, hearing aids, and cochlear implants. In addition, some children have to contend with additional disabilities, such as visual impairment, mental retardation, and learning disabilities (Stewart & Kluwin, 2001).

Sometimes the placement decision comes easily, such as when a deaf child's needs are clearly indicated and the educational program best suited to meet those needs is available where the child lives. Unfortunately, most deaf children live in areas where the best educational placement may not be available; however, by law, public schools are instructed to meet those children's needs. In reality, these schools may be ill prepared for deaf students and provide inadequate educational services (Lane, Hoffmeister, & Bahan, 1996; Ramsey, 1997; Siegel, 2000).

Each deaf and hard-of-hearing child deserves a quality, communication-driven program that facilitates the development of age-level language skills, whether in spoken English, ASL, or some combination of both. Such a program should provide a critical mass of communication, cognitive peers, teachers and staff able to communicate directly with deaf and hard-of-hearing students, administrators who understand the unique needs of these students, deaf and hard-of-hearing role models, and access to extracurricular and other important school activities. The child's communication needs should be a prime determinant for his or her educational placement (Siegel, 2000).

Due to the long-standing documentation of academic underachievement at the time of school completion for the majority of deaf students, it is important to consider the type of academic environment in which deaf children can flourish and maximize their academic skills. The reasons for underachievement are complex, involving etiology, level of hearing loss, parent hearing status, the nature of early environmental stimulation, and social factors, among others (Marschark, 1993). If children enter the educational system with linguistic deficits as well as limited factual knowledge of the world, schools are expected to make up the lag (Moores, 2001a). This is a daunting task. Schools need to integrate both communication aspects and academics optimally in order to minimize academic underachievement.

The fact of the matter is that achievement results among deaf children do vary. Deaf students can attain good to exceptional academic achievement. It is not unrealistic to expect that deaf children's academic achievement should match that of their hearing peers. This expectation, however, demands effective curriculum planning for classes with deaf children that are in line with the general curriculum (Moores, 2001a).

Before considering the different educational programs for deaf children, it is important to understand the role of the Individuals with Disabilities Education Act.

INDIVIDUALS WITH DISABILITIES EDUCATION ACT (IDEA)

The Education of All Handicapped Children Act of 1975 (PL 94-142), which preceded IDEA, was enacted in 1975 by the United States Congress. This law was strongly supported by parents who wanted their mentally retarded children integrated into public school settings and exposed to normal classrooms rather than kept in segregated settings (Kauffman, 2001). The efforts of professionals working with mentally retarded children as well as advocacy groups for people with disabilities facilitated the passage of PL 94-142. Additionally, the 1963–65 rubella epidemic generated a large group of deaf children that existing residential programs could not absorb. New local programs were needed to accommodate this bulge of students. PL 94-142 was seen as a way of ensuring program standards (Moores, 2001a).

The act mandated a free, appropriate public education (FAPE) for all children with disabilities, and listed several procedural safeguards to protect the rights of these children and their parents. It called for nondiscriminatory testing and an annual required individualized education plan (IEP) appropriate to each child's needs. The process of developing the IEP for each child included parental involvement, with the ultimate goal of placing the child in the least restrictive environment (LRE) that best meets the child's needs.

Although the Individuals with Disabilities Education Act has been viewed as the "mainstreaming law," it actually only mandates both an appropriate education and an education in the least restrictive environment, whether in residential schools, day schools, day classes, resource rooms, and itinerant programs. This continuum of alternative services also includes instruction in regular classes supported by additional services such as interpreting, special classes, special schools, home instruction, and instruction in hospitals and institutions.

The goal of LRE was to provide an environment without barriers. Unfortunately, the individual needs of many deaf children have been subsumed to the greater goal of inclusion, with the LRE being defined to mean the typical hearing classroom. This is based on the assumption that deaf students need hearing children to model appropriate behavior as well as standard language and conventional communication. In reality, access to language and communication may be limited since the dialogue swirling around these deaf students tends to be auditory (Ramsey, 1997). Being mainstreamed is often viewed as legally inclusive when in reality it is exclusion for too many deaf children (Siegel, 2000). The ramifications of full inclusion for deaf children can range from easy integration into the mainstream to total exclusion with feelings of isolation, rejection, and negative self-worth (Stinson & Leigh, 1995). There are many success stories, but one also needs to scrutinize the implications of receiving information secondhand through interpreters rather than directly from teachers and having limited access to peer communication due to difficulties in understanding.

Section 504 is another law that facilitates communication access, including assistive technology in schools, particularly those of higher learning. It mandates that any institution receiving federal assistance or indirectly benefiting from such assistance provide access to individuals with disabilities (National Association of the Deaf, 2000a).

The goal of the National Deaf Education Project (Siegel, 2000)—a collaborative project of the American Society for Deaf Children (ASDC), the Conference of Educational Administrators of Schools and Programs for the Deaf (CEASD), the Convention of American Instructors of the Deaf (CAID), Gallaudet University, the National Association of the Deaf (NAD), and the National Technical Institute for the Deaf (NTID)—is to clarify the education and communication needs of deaf and hard-of-hearing children (Siegel, 2000). It aims to define the necessary fundamental systemic educational changes needed to support IDEA, based on the principle that all deaf and hard-of-hearing children are entitled to a language-rich educational system that is communication-rich and communication-driven, and to ensure equal access to education. Under IDEA, a rich language environment is not required, but without this language-rich environment, deaf children cannot develop. It is critical to understand the types of educational programs and their services for deaf children in order to get some insight into the ways various settings influence communication accessibility.

SCHOOL PLACEMENTS

Early Intervention Programs

IDEA requires that deaf children age 3 and older be enrolled in early intervention programs. The impetus for these programs was the increased awareness of the influence the early years had on later functioning (Moores, 2001a). The linguistic deficits often noted in deaf children may be reduced or eliminated if they receive appropriate early language training (Marschark, 1993, Moores, 2001a). This training can be signed or spoken, and provided by deaf and hearing parents, early intervention program staff, and peers. These children usually fare better in the social domain than do those without the benefit of such experience (Marschark, 1993).

However, to be truly effective, early intervention needs to take place at the time hearing loss is identified and prior to age 3 to enhance the potential for language and psychosocial development (Calderon & Greenberg, 1997). More recent federal legislation (PL 99-457 and PL 101-476) mandates individualized family service plans. The programs that develop the family service plans are generally housed within public school districts and day/residential schools for deaf children (Lane, Hoffmeister, & Bahan, 1996; Marschark, 1997; Moores, 2001a). Recommendations for services are made after thorough evaluation, preferably involving a team of professionals and parents or caregivers (Calderon & Greenberg, 1997; Moores, 2001b).

Necessary program services include providing general information about deafness and the implications (short term and long term) for the child and other family members. Counseling and support are available as family members work through their own adjustment to the presence of deafness in their child. The training component focuses on helping family members develop skills related to the proper fitting and care of amplification, the provision of socially accessible and intellectually stimulating environments, and effective communication techniques, often through parent child tutorials. Assistive technology devices and services are also provided (Calderon & Greenberg, 1997; Moores, 2001a).

Excellent early intervention programs exist. However, they cannot always totally overcome all the linguistic, social, and academic difficulties that may emerge (Marschark, 1997; Moores, 2001a; Calderon & Greenberg, 1997). No specific program design can provide all the various levels of services required to match the diverse needs of deaf children and their families, largely due to cost. Specifying a standard model program is also complicated due to the paucity of methodologically sound research on the effectiveness of early intervention programs. The low incidence and heterogeneous nature of the deaf population, the ongoing controversies regarding language and teaching approaches, as well as the lack of appropriate outcome measures for intervention strategies and family functioning compounds the difficulties in doing neutral, scientific investigation (Calderon & Greenberg, 1997). Chapter 8 provides additional details on early intervention programs.

Residential Schools

Residential schools for the deaf supported by states were the first schools that provided formal deaf education (Van Cleve & Crouch, 1989). It all started with Reverend Thomas Gallaudet, a pastor whose encounter with a deaf young girl, Alice Cosgwell, fueled his desire to educate her. Her father, Dr. Mason Cogswell, was determined to start a school, and so he financially supported Gallaudet's endeavors to learn about European teaching methods. Gallaudet visited a school in Great Britain that used the oral method to teach deaf children. Since the school administrators refused to train him, Gallaudet traveled to another school in Paris, France. There, he met several educated deaf people using sign language, and was successful in convincing a deaf teacher, Laurent Clerc, to come to America and collaborate with him and Dr. Cogswell. The three men were instrumental in establishing the first residential school for the deaf in America, now known as the American School for the Deaf, in Hartford, Connecticut. Soon thereafter, other states established their own public state school for the deaf. For more information on the history of residential schools, see Van Cleve and Crouch (1989).

Before PL 94-142, state residential schools were one of two main options for educating most deaf children, the other being day schools. The residential schools generally were large complexes of buildings designed to accommodate children between the ages of 4 and 20, grouped by age, gender, and sometimes the severity of additional disabilities, if any. Today, physical size has decreased. Classes consist only of deaf children, therefore eliminating any need for educational interpreters. Students are offered a full range of extracurricular activities such as athletic opportunities, social clubs, drama, and Jr. NAD (explained in Chapter 10) activities to facilitate leadership development. Deaf adults often work at these schools as teachers, administrators, and staff. They become role models for appropriate social behavior, sex roles, moral reasoning, and interactions with hearing individuals.

I never had to be so conscious about my own deafness because everybody was deaf. It was not a big deal. It was so nice to have complete access to communication at all times. Everybody signed and also I felt a sense of belonging. It was not a problem socializing with my peers. When I went home where nobody was deaf and did not know sign language, I struggled with the inaccessibility of information and the isolation. I would demand to know what was going on, but was told that I had to accept my limitation since I lived in a hearing world. Boy, did that make me mad! —Graduate of a residential school for the deaf

Support services—such as speech therapy, residual hearing training, and physical therapy—are usually provided by trained full-time professional deafness specialists. In addition, these schools work with state vocational rehabilitation agencies to plan for the students' transition to postsecondary education or to the working world (Marschark, 1997).

Additional advantages are that residential schools provide in-depth socialization with children creating their own family of friends that last for life. They learn to be comfortable with their deafness. If the schools use sign language, the children are in an environment where they can understand what staff, teachers, and peers are saying and what is going on at all times, unlike back at home where they may be less attuned to what is going on in a hearing environment. Deaf children who attend residential schools tend to be better adjusted and more emotionally mature than deaf children enrolled in public school programs (Lane, Hoffmeister, & Bahan, 1996; Marschark, 1997). However, quality public school placement together with appropriate quality services can be positive factors that facilitate adjustment.

Traditionally, residential school children went home only for summers and holidays, basically because of distance factors, transportation problems, and costs. Consequently, children were not with their families sufficiently enough to maintain close relationships or for parents to learn sign language to communicate with their deaf children. Since families are now recognized as critical socializing agents who can facilitate the developing academic potential of their child, children are encouraged to go home as much as possible, generally every weekend (Marschark, 1993; Bodner-Johnson & Sass-Lehrer, 1999). Residential schools now welcome day pupils.

In one sense, residential schools are artificial environments, not a true reflection of the real world. As a result, residential school children are said to have missed out on various life experiences to which most children their ages are exposed, including the opportunity to socialize with their hearing peers. This has encouraged a perception that residential schools are the most restrictive place to which a state or public school district could choose to send a child with special needs. The current preference is to provide supplementary support services in general education classrooms for students with special needs (Reschly, 2000). However, residential schools for deaf children may in actuality be the LRE, providing full communication access and deaf role models to facilitate the exchange of ideas and thoughts, which encourages educational growth (Lane, Hoffmeister, & Bahan, 1996).

One of the disadvantages of being at a residential school for the deaf was that I did not get to go home that often. School was hours away from home. I was often homesick and so envious of my hearing siblings who did not have to go to a boarding school. My family never could maintain their sign language skills. What was the point of learning sign language if I was never around. —Graduate of a residential school for the deaf

■ ■ ■ ■ ■

I did write home that school was like prison. My parents thought that was funny. In reality, school was so structured that we were not able to be independent. They were so concerned about liability which was understandable, but at what cost? I heard stories of graduates who went wild because they were not used to such freedom. For me, it was an incredible experience to be able to do anything I wanted without having to ask for permission. I was nineteen when I graduated from school!
—Graduate of a residential school for the deaf

Day Schools

Day schools for deaf children are usually found in larger metropolitan areas. They are similar to residential schools except for the lack of dormitories. In comparison to most mainstream settings (discussed later in this chapter), day schools provide a more accessible communication environment in that teaching is directed specifically at deaf students. Also, there is a concentrated body of deaf peers with whom to socialize (Moores, 2001a).

According to Lane, Hoffmeister, and Bahan (1996), disadvantages include the fact that the number of deaf staff available to students tends to be small. Since students often do not live in close proximity to the school or classmates, there are fewer opportunities to socialize with older deaf students after school, in contrast to residential schools. Most of the teaching staff is hearing, and communication access will vary depending on how well these teachers communicate with their deaf students.

Charter Schools

Charter schools—such as the Magnet School for the Deaf in Jefferson County, Colorado; the Jean Massieu Academy in Duncanville, Texas; and the Ohio Valley Oral School in Montgomery, Ohio—represent a new trend in day school programs that educate deaf children using either bilingual or oral educational approaches. They are usually operated by a group of parents, teachers, and/or Deaf community members as a semi-autonomous school of choice within a school district, operating under a "charter" contract between the members of the charter school community and the local board of education (www.colorado.edu/CDSS/MSD/9/22/00).

The Magnet School for the Deaf aims to provide deaf children from early childhood to 12th grade with an education that is Deaf-friendly, supportive of the child's home, and managed by the parents, the Deaf Community, and the school personnel. The educational approach is based on the premise that deaf children are visually oriented and therefore need to be in an environment that provides access to a visual language, (e.g., ASL) to facilitate thinking skills, learning, and playing. American Sign Language is considered a stepping-stone to learning English, seen as a necessary part of a deaf child's education. There are multiage classrooms along with a family education program that provides support in learning ASL. It is also a

■ ■ ■ ■ ■

Day schools was the best option for me because I had deaf family at home and communications was not an issue. I had best of both worlds, going to a school for the deaf and then go home after I was finished with classes and activities for the day. I did not have to tolerate the structured group living arrangement that is usually the norm for residential school for the deaf. I had freedom to go anywhere and the freedom to discuss most things with my family. I did not realize how lucky I was until I brought home a friend from school for one night and he told me this was the first time he understood and enjoyed the family conversation during dinner and it was about what I learned at school. —Day school graduate

licensed childcare and educational center with additional services such as auditory and speech training (www.colorado.edu/CDSS/MSD).

The Jean Massieu Academy in Irving, Texas, encourages innovative teaching methods, utilizing ASL as the instructional language with emphasis on mastery of English in reading and writing, while following the Texas Essential Knowledge and Skills curriculum (www.jeanmassieu.com). Parents believe that American Sign Language will facilitate the learning of English, which the school mission considers a necessary part of the education of deaf children. Students participate in the statewide testing program in reading, writing, and mathematics. The Jean Massieu Academy first began on August 11, 1999, with 23 students. Currently there are over 100 students. What is unique about this charter school is that approximately one-third of the students are hearing. Most of them know sign language as result of having deaf parents or a deaf relative.

The Ohio Valley Oral School, one of about 35 oral-deaf education schools in the country (www.oraldeafed.org), was founded by parents whose children had been enrolled in early intervention programs within local school districts. These parents wanted more oral education for their children than what was offered, as they felt this would give their deaf children better opportunities in the hearing world. This school offers accelerated speech and language skills development, along with regular curriculum offerings. The goal is to prepare students for mainstreaming in regular traditional classrooms by the third grade.

Public School Placement Alternatives

The number of deaf students in public school has grown rapidly. With it comes considerable discussion about whether an inclusive approach can work successfully in educating deaf students. Much of the discussion concerns the caution that must be taken when placing deaf students in public schools with hearing peers because of the communicative, developmental, educational, and social implications, including the lack of sufficient deaf peers for increased positive exposure to communication and social experiences (Siegel, 2000; Stinson & Antia, 1999).

The terms *inclusion, mainstreaming,* and *integration* are often used interchangeably, thereby creating confusion regarding the public school placement of deaf students. *Inclusion* and *mainstreaming* are educational practices, whereas *integration* is an outcome of these practices (Hardy & Kachman, 1995).

Inclusion.   The inclusion philosophy as derived from the Regular Education Initiative (REI) means that the regular classroom will change to accommodate different learners, with special services being offered as needed within the regular classroom (Stinson & Antia, 1999). In practice, it reflects the placement of all students who have disabilities in their neighborhood schools with same-age peers without disabilities—that is, in the regular classroom (Hardy & Kachman, 1995). These students are theoretically provided with all the support services, such as sign-language interpreters or itinerant teachers, which they may need to succeed in the regular classroom. However, there is no assurance that the environment will be accessible, particularly for deaf students, who may be the only deaf pupils in the school. Consequently, this tendency to consider an inclusion environment as the LRE is in direct violation of the Individuals with Disabilities Education Act (IDEA), when it should be seen as one of several placement options for the LRE. For this reason, the National Association of the Deaf (see Chapter 10) has come out against the "one shoe fits all" inclusion concept, because it disregards the unique abilities and needs of each child and runs counter to the provision of a free, appropriate public education (FAPE) in the LRE (National Association of the Deaf, 2002). The NAD advocates that the IEP ensures that each child's individual needs are considered in deciding educational placement. In this vein, inclusion is appropriate for children when their needs are addressed.

Mainstreaming.   Although the philosophy of mainstreaming implies that a child will adapt to the regular classroom (Stinson & Antia, 1999), mainstreaming broadly covers educating deaf children within the regular public school, but not necessarily all day in the regular classroom. Mainstreaming within the public school environment refers to a broader and more realistic range of placement options—including total inclusion, self-contained classrooms only for deaf students within local public schools, resource rooms, itinerant programs, and team teaching classrooms—than does inclusion (Stinson & Antia, 1999). For example, deaf children in a resource room or a self-contained classroom with other deaf students may be mainstreamed only for specific classes such as mathematics or physical education (Hardy & Kachman, 1995).

Resource Rooms.   Mainstreamed deaf students can receive services individually or in small groups from specialized teachers available in resource rooms (Stewart & Kluwin, 2001). These teachers are trained to work with students varying in age, hearing loss, presence of additional disabilities, and academic achievement. Their services cover consultation and collaboration with teaching staff, who may request assistance with specific students who demonstrate academic need, resource room teaching and tutoring, and general education classroom support (Stewart & Kluwin, 2001). A greater percentage of resource room classes exist at the high school level, although resource room teachers work at all levels of schooling (Stewart & Kluwin, 2001).

I was mainstreamed for a lot of my classes during my middle school years. I was allowed to take Spanish in high school with an interpreter, but English was forbidden regardless of how much I begged to take it. Finally, by my sophomore year in high school, the program finally relented and allowed me to take mainstreamed English with a warning that if I earned at least one bad grade, I would be pulled out. I was later recommended by my teacher in that class to take Honors English, and was completely mainstreamed in 10th grade. —Graduate of a mainstream program

Itinerant Teachers.   Itinerant teachers are special education teachers who travel from school to school to serve mainstreamed students when there are insufficient students in any one school to justify a resource room teacher on site. Their numbers have grown due to the increase in deaf and hard-of-hearing students attending local neighborhood schools. As do resource teachers, they provide two major categories of service: consultation and direct service, which Smith (1997) covers in detail. In brief, consultation services tend to be "advice and guidance" usually provided to students who are doing well in the classroom, school staff, and parents. "Direct service" students are those who need scheduled instruction or tutoring daily or weekly, depending on individual needs. The itinerant teacher can either assist the teacher in the classroom or take the student out for individual work that supports the regular teacher's instruction through various reinforcement strategies.

Additional services may range from providing supplemental materials for a specific topic, to giving a lesson on hearing loss to the other children, and/or teaching sign language to all of the students (Smith, 1997). Itinerant teachers need to be able to interact positively with staff and students, use effective communication skills, be flexible due to frequent schedule and instructional strategy changes, and provide emotional and social support as needed. They must focus on student needs and assess academic, speech, audiological, and social needs in order to write goals, objectives, and necessary accommodations for the student's annual IEP and three-year evaluations within a multidisciplinary format that includes teachers, school psychologists, audiologists, and other school personnel. They also may play a role in transition planning when students are preparing for the next stage, whether school or work.

Certification requirements for itinerant teachers vary from state to state. Some states do not require these teachers to have regular classroom experience first, even though such experience enables them to understand regular classroom procedures and needs and thereby better integrate service to students within the scope of the teacher's total classroom operations (Smith, 1997).

Participants in a qualitative research study conducted by Yarger and Luckner (1999) to investigate itinerant teachers' perceptions of their responsibilities, job satisfaction, and effectiveness reported that they spent approximately 60 percent of their time working directly with students. The rest of their time was spent traveling between schools and consulting with general education teachers and families. Satisfactory aspects of the job included variety, autonomy, time for reflection, and the diversity of students with whom they worked. Participants recognized the importance of being able to use a variety of signed communication methods such as sign language and signed English, but acknowledged their inability to do so. They were concerned about isolation, time and budget constraints, and travel distances between schools. The researchers recommend that future research focus on what constitutes effective teacher training for itinerant positions, developing profiles of deaf and hard-of-hearing students who are likely to succeed with itinerant services, and investigating the efficacy of the itinerant model of service delivery.

Team Teaching.   A team teaching classroom involves a general education teacher and a teacher of the deaf teaching a group of hearing and deaf children (Stewart & Kluwin, 2001). Roughly 5 deaf students are combined with approximately 15 hearing students. While both teachers develop daily activities, the teacher of the deaf usually has the responsibility of developing IEPs for the deaf students.

Additional Services.   Additional services include various personnel such as speech pathologists, multicultural specialists, and school psychologists. They should have expertise in working with deaf students to provide effective services, but that is not always the case.

Collaboration Issues.   In order for inclusion to work for deaf children, the regular education teacher must work in partnership with a teacher of the deaf or a special educator to adapt the curriculum and to develop classroom strategies that promote social and academic integration of all pupils. Antia (1999) interviewed classroom and special education teachers in order to examine one school's attempts to integrate deaf children. She found that special educators did some direct teaching and assisted classroom teachers in making curricular adaptations. To do this, they had to know the general classroom curriculum and methods as well as details about the classroom in which the deaf child was included (which they usually lacked). All too often, they had unrealistic expectations of regular teachers in that they would make suggestions that did not fit the classroom culture or the classroom teacher's style. At times, they perceived their expertise as undervalued by the classroom teachers who took on major responsibility for educating the deaf children in their classrooms. In turn, the need for classroom teachers to maintain ownership of their deaf students tended to limit effective collaboration with the special educators, whose suggestions were seen as threatening. Another interesting finding of that study was that both the classroom teachers and the special education teachers communicated more with the sign language interpreters than with each other in order to obtain crucial information about the students with whom the interpreters worked closely. The problems noted in this study hindered the full integration of deaf children into the academic life of the classroom.

Educational Interpreting.   The Registry of Interpreters for the Deaf (RID), a membership association that certifies interpreters, views interpreting as a highly specialized professional field (RID, 2000). Knowing sign language or taking a couple of sign-language classes does not qualify a person to be an educational interpreter. It takes extensive training and experience over a long period of time to understand interpreting issues. Oral transliteration (mouthing words) also requires specialized training. Those who are rewarded RID certification must successfully pass national tests that assess language knowledge, communication skills, ethics, cultural issues, and professionalism—all critical for quality interpreting.

The Registry of Interpreters for the Deaf's standard practice paper on interpreting in educational settings (K–12) states that educational interpreters facilitate communication between deaf students and others, including teachers, service providers, and peers. Schick (2001) explains the roles and functions of educational interpreters, who may interpret classroom activities, field trips, club meetings, assemblies, counseling sessions, and athletic competitions. The types of interpreting they may do include sign-language interpreting, oral transliteration, simultaneous interpreting (signing every English word), and reverse/voice interpreting for those who are signing (Schick, 2001; RID, 2000).

Educational interpreter duties depend on a number of factors, such as the number of deaf students in the school or district, the distribution across grade levels and school buildings, the type of employment (full time, part time, or hourly basis), and the interpreter's background, knowledge, and skill (Schick, 2001; RID, 2000). Jones (1999) describes the multiple duties performed by educational interpreters. They are part of the educational team, attend meetings concerning deaf students for

---

I had to convince my program to provide me with interpreters for physical education class because I hated the feeling of being lost and confused. The program would attempt to change my mind, but I was really stubborn. I always liked to have complete access to information and feel comfortable, and the program finally gave me an interpreter for P.E. classes. —Graduate of a mainstream program.

I was an active participant in my regular IEP meetings. What I hated the most was that my interpreters evaluated my class performance. I felt my privacy and independence as a student were being trampled on. I repeatedly requested that interpreter evaluations be left out of my IEP, to no avail. —Graduate of a mainstream program

When I was in 6th grade, I had an oral interpreter come to my class. It was great since I could look at one person to follow everything that was said. At my public high school, I requested oral interpreters, but was forced to use the sign language interpreters already on staff. This was pretty ridiculous since at this point I knew no sign language. I asked the interpreters to mouth for me, but they kept signing, so I eventually enrolled in a sign language class so I could know what they were saying. I also did not have the same access to my own teachers. These sign language interpreters instituted silly rules that I needed to talk to them first, rather than going to my own teacher. It became a battle between me and the interpreters. I fought not only for access to my education, but also for the sense of independence that I'd worked my entire life for. I felt the interpreters weren't doing their job, which was helping me understand what was happening in the classroom, but were trying to make me communicate through sign language. —Graduate of an inclusion setting

whom they interpret, and provide input to parents. They also function as language models for deaf children. In addition, educational interpreters prepare for the interpreting task and work with teachers to develop ways of increasing interaction between deaf students and their peers (RID, 2000). In some schools, the interpreter may also interpret for deaf parents, deaf teachers, and other deaf employees. They may tutor deaf students or teach sign language and explain "deafness" to hearing school staff and children if qualified to do so. Nonetheless, they often are viewed as paraprofessionals despite the demands of their job. Since some schools assign responsibilities such as copying and filing work, playground supervision, and monitor duties, it is critical to have a clearly detailed job description prior to hiring in order to minimize confusion.

Even with the presence of educational interpreters, there are barriers to accessibility. Some, not all, states have certification process for educational interpreting that will ensure quality interpreting. In this relatively new profession, quality interpreters are unfortunately not the norm. It is difficult to find interpreters with broad basic knowledge of subject areas such as mathematics, social studies, and language arts, and who can interpret technical concepts and terminology accurately and meaningfully, much less ones who understand child development as well. Importantly, educational interpreters must have signing skills just above the signing level of the deaf child in order to facilitate language development. Many teachers do not know how to integrate their work with that of the educational interpreter (Jones, 1999), thereby limiting the effectiveness of the interpreter. Interpreter training programs tend not to focus on educational interpreting roles, which is problematic considering the complex nature of the job (Jones, 1999).

In addition, many deaf children enter the public school system with insufficient skills in English or ASL to benefit from interpreting, and academic and social goals cannot be achieved via interpreting alone (Winston, 2001). The English that is interpreted is not always understood clearly by the recipient, as confirmed by preliminary findings from a small-scale ethnographic study that examined the patterns of communication of deaf students, educational interpreters, teachers, and hearing classmates in a high school setting (Nover, 1995). The linguistic signals that deaf students perceived were not the spoken or written English words, but fingerspelled English words and ASL signs. The use of Manually Coded English, a "pidginized" form of English and ASL often used by interpreters, did not allow deaf students to see a complete representation of English unless they could lip-read well, thereby limiting their access to an English language model. Manualy Coded English appears to be ineffective for deaf children unless they possess adequate

■ ■ ■ ■ ■ ▬▬▬▬▬▬▬▬▬▬▬▬▬▬▬▬▬▬▬▬▬▬▬▬▬▬▬▬▬▬▬▬▬▬▬▬▬▬

I used to have this horrendous interpreter who absolutely had no receptive skills and kept asking me to teach her some sign language for certain words often throughout the class period. It infuriated me tremendously to a point that I complained furiously to my mother. —A mainstreamed graduate knowledge of English (Nover, 1995). Furthermore, when lectures are transliterated, deaf students miss many English words, because they receive both English and ASL representations (Nover, 1995).

Children go through developmental changes that affect their ability to understand and use interpreters. If their understanding of language is limited, this will have an impact on their ability to benefit from interpreters (Schick, 2001). It is common for children learning any language to make mistakes in understanding and expressing the language. When the child receives messages from the interpreter that do not make sense, and responds accordingly, mistakes are reinforced, the child appears less "bright," and the child is less willing to communicate in response to negative feedback. It is critical that interpreters match the child's level in order to accurately conceptualize the message and reflect the child's comments (Schick, 2001). Attunement to the evolving nature of the child's language is necessary. Too few educational interpreters "have it."

School should be a place for children to reinforce the use of language that will help them absorb new information and build their thinking skills. Activities that are not understood deprive children of this opportunity. For example, when the teacher writes something on the board and simultaneously describes how to do it, or instructs students to look at an object while explaining what it means, most hearing children can integrate both auditory and visual information simultaneously (Schick, 2001). Deaf children usually are watching the interpreter rather than the object. In that case, interpreting creates a barrier to visual access. The educational interpreter can educate the teacher and students about the uninterpretability of such situations and assist in developing teaching strategies to facilitate visual accessibility. It is critical that one understands the implications of deaf children learning through interpreters in order to increase their effectiveness, particularly since children do not automatically know how interpreters are supposed to work (Schick, 2001; Winston, 2001).

Such barriers may seem tremendous, but there is hope. The public school classroom can be communicatively accessible for deaf children with the collaboration of teachers, interpreters, and parents. Interpreters do facilitate classroom accessibility for children with a good language foundation. The scarcity of research in the area of educational interpreting needs to be remedied, and educational interpreters must be recognized as professionals (Stewart & Kluwin, 2001). Teachers, parents, and students must weigh the advantages and disadvantages of choosing an interpreted education. Once an interpreted education is chosen for the deaf

■ ■ ■ ■ ■

I often refrained from participating in classroom discussions because I knew my interpreters did not have good reception skills and the process of voicing would be painstakingly slow. The students would wait and watch. Often the interpreters would relay incorrect information and I ended up feeling even more stupid. As an adolescent, this was damaging to my self-esteem. —Student in mainstream program

■ ■ ■ ■ ■

I am thankful that I had the opportunity to be mainstreamed with interpreters, because I honestly know that I would not have come far in education if mainstreaming was not a possibility for me. It certainly was an uphill battle for me, but I received good education. As result, I succeed. —Mainstreamed graduate

child, its accessibility should be evaluated continually, along with classroom adaptations, to ensure that the deaf child has access to a large portion of the learning experience (Winston, 2001).

Placement Changes and Consequences

Often, deaf children experience different educational placements, including placement in residential schools, depending on their needs at any point during their education. Historically, only children with the most residual hearing and the best oral communication skills were placed in resource rooms and itinerant settings (Moores, 2001a). With growing acceptance of the use of educational interpreters in regular classrooms, there are more profoundly deaf children in regular classrooms. Such placements allow deaf children to remain with their families, learn strategies for interacting with hearing peers, and have (theoretically) the same education as their hearing peers. Interestingly, Holden-Pitt (1997) notes an increase in residential school placement during the high school years.

Statistics for local program placement indicate that 52 percent of the schools with deaf and hard-of-hearing children had one deaf or hard-of-hearing child, whereas 24 percent had two to three deaf or hard-of-hearing children, with the number of programs in which there was one deaf or hard-of-hearing student increasing from 1,797 in 1979 to 4,412 programs in 1986 (Siegel, 2000, p. 16). Many of these pupils are placed in inappropriate or inadequately supported mainstreaming programs as a result of their IEP, which may not list all the services each child needs for success (Siegel, 2000). Fiscal factors often make it difficult to provide the most appropriate education for deaf children, including necessary one-to-one services such as sign language or oral interpreting, speech therapy, and psychological evaluation by a school psychologist familiar with deafness.

■ ■ ■ ■ ■

My city had a mainstream program in elementary, middle, and high school. There were approximately 50 students, but the numbers have now declined. One of the reasons was the city's difficult financial situation. The program no longer exists. The city now places deaf and hard-of-hearing students alongside students who have learning disabilities and/or multiple disabilities. I am relieved to say that I did not have to experience what the children are now experiencing. —Graduate of a mainstream program

However, deaf children do flourish in the public school setting when provided with the services they need. Public school placement alternatives can offer routine, positive communication between deaf and hearing students and pave the way for psychosocial growth, but there is no standard formula for success. Some key factors that should be considered in placement decisions are the student's communication abilities, educational achievement, personality, social and emotional adjustment, and family support.

Since parents do have responsibility for decisions concerning their child, they may have to invest enormous time and energy to acquire the services needed for their deaf child (Christiansen & Leigh, 2002). Parents have the right to ask any questions regarding whether the educational placement they are considering for their child provides an environment conducive to learning. They should be familiar with the school's philosophy, administrative structure, instructional program, faculty/staff qualifications, support services available for the child and parents, extracurricular activities, and interpreter quality if their child is placed in a mainstreaming setting, and know how their child will be evaluated. The National Information Center on Deafness mainstreaming booklet (NICD, 1991) lists questions about communication abilities; educational achievement; and personality, psychosocial adjustment, and family support that will facilitate placement decisions and IEP planning.

Parents dissatisfied with IEP recommendations have had to resort to litigation, not always with results in their favor (Siegel, 2000). Issues center on communication issues, the provision of support services, and the definition of LRE as applied to specific cases. The outcome of court cases tends to rest on how well school districts comply with IDEA procedures and document their efforts. In one case, the court ruled in favor of the parent that a deaf student should be admitted to the state school because the school district did not provide a FAPE (*Barbour County Bd. of Educ.* v. *Parent, 1999*). Required services were not provided and there was no demonstrable educational progress. In another case, the court ruled for the school district, which argued that the proposed IEP was reasonably calculated to provide an educational benefit to the student and therefore was appropriate under IDEA, even though the parent preferred a different educational methodology (*Brougham* v. *Town of Yarmouth*, 1993).

USE OF TESTING IN EDUCATION

Currently, many states advocate the use of standardized tests as a way of assessing what students have learned. The No Child Left Behind Act of 2001 mandates that education agencies, specifically schools and educators, be held accountable for improving performance of all student groups (www.whitehouse.gov). This law was enacted in part because of widespread belief that schools were not effective enough in training all students. Consequently, the expectation is that schools will meet established standards for both academic content and academic achievement. Student progress and achievement will be measured annually for every child. The goal is to ensure that schools identify what needs to be done to facilitate student progress toward these established standards.

What this means is that states are now required to use standardized tests as critical criteria for tracking, promotion, and graduation. In other words, statewide testing is now viewed as high-stakes testing. If certain standards are not achieved (in other words, if certain tests are not passed), the student will not receive a high school diploma, no matter how much the student may have learned in non tested areas. The implications for deaf students, many of whom historically have had difficulty achieving reading comprehension scores higher than a fourth-grade level, will be devastating (Johnson, 2001). The possibility of higher drop-out rates, worsening employment potential, and increased reliance on Social Security Insurance (SSI; see Chapter 10) for financial support is very real. Standardized tests tend to be low on contextual redundancy and use grammatical constructions that are difficult for nonnative users of English to understand. Even bright deaf students sometimes struggle to discern what the test items are asking because of language constructions.

Educators of deaf and hard-of-hearing students have joined forces with organizations such as the National Education Association, the National Parent Teacher Association, the National Conference of School Superintendents, and the American Educational Research Association to protest high-stakes testing because they believe such testing is unfair and discriminatory to many students (Johnson, 2001). At the same time, these educators do not want to avoid accountability; therefore, they are analyzing ways to ensure that deaf students obtain the necessary tools to succeed in this competitive world. Educators of deaf students are now increasingly grappling with major issues such as test construction, standards appropriate for different levels as the child progresses through the education system, appropriate types of test accommodations (including the role of American Sign Language in conveying instructions and test items), and the development of effective curriculum approaches designed to facilitate annual student progress from the early years onward in alignment with the assessment demands for high school diplomas. An alternative to high-stakes testing would be to use a multiple measure approach, including portfolios in addition to tests and other evaluative components, as the basis for educational decisions (Randall, McAnally, Rittenhouse, Russell, & Sorensen, 2000). The National Task Force on Equity in Testing Deaf and Hard-of-Hearing Individuals—a cooperative effort involving deaf, hard-of-hearing, and hearing professionals that was established to promote full access to learning and equity in testing deaf and hard-of-hearing students—is a major factor in the movement to ensure that these students are not left behind (www.gri.gallaudet.edu/TestEquity).

MULTICULTURAL ISSUES

A significant issue facing deaf educators in the United States today is that of deaf children whose families belong to diverse ethnic groups and use a language other than English or ASL as their primary mode of communication (Christensen, 2000).

Deaf and hearing professionals representing all ethnic and racial backgrounds must consider ways to work together for the benefit of all deaf children. The long-standing practices of discrimination, unequal treatment, low expectations, and unacceptable achievement patterns of multicultural deaf and hearing children need to be addressed by these professionals (Fischgrund & Akamatsu, 1993).

As part of the long-standing patterns of discrimination, multicultural students have found their racial or ethnic affiliation, either by itself or in addition to their deafness, being devalued (Christensen, 1993). African American and Hispanic deaf students, for example, may be pressured by both hearing people and deaf people to be "Deaf first," to be part of the "Deaf culture" (Christensen, 1993). The cultural ways that they share with their families of origin may be rejected in the schools for deaf children. In order to succeed, they may feel they need to affirm Deaf culture and become raceless. As will be discussed in Chapter 9, this is not psychologically healthy for identity development.

To increase sensitivity, professionals need to understand the interactive effects of students who not only belong to diverse racial, linguistic, and ethnic groups but who are also exploring Deaf culture. These students are connected to more than one culture, each with a different center (Humphries, 1993). Children from diverse ethnic origins will have to balance their home culture, the dominant culture of America, and the culture of the Deaf community (Corbett, 1999).

Researchers have stated that equity and quality in the education of multicultural deaf students can be achieved within the current educational framework, with curricula being adapted to increase student awareness and knowledge of all ethnic, racial, and cultural groups, including their own, and Deaf culture. This process will enhance each student's identity development, promote the positive values of cultural differences within an egalitarian framework, and prepare the students to cope with and function in a multicultural society (Christensen, 2000).

To do this effectively, one approach that educators can use is the trilingual and tricultural perspective, which encompasses the home language and culture, the school language and the culture, and the visual language and culture of Deaf people (Christensen, 2000). Other countries—such as China, where the language of the dominant culture coexists with local languages—have much to teach the United States. Chinese deaf children may grow up bilingual, and more often multilingual, as they encounter the languages of their families, their neighborhoods, and the educational and political arenas, though the degree of competency in each language will vary (Callaway, 2000). These children generally have the ability to learn to communicate effectively in more than one language and adjust comfortably to unfamiliar cultural environments.

When a deaf child's family incorporates an additional language, such as English or sign language, all family members need appropriate intervention to help them achieve comprehensible communication. Christensen (2000) claims that trilingual education research supports the use of signed language as a bridge between two different spoken languages. She notes that Spanish-speaking parents have reported an increase in communication with their deaf child and greater mutual understanding when they were able to utilize ASL skills in conjunction with spoken Spanish. Sussman and Lopez-Holzman (2001) describe techniques used to facilitate language development within all curricular content using an interactive/experiential model in the context of an oral program. They feel students are empowered, with less chance for failure, when the home language and culture are incorporated into the school's program, even if the program is based on English.

The important process of understanding and respecting the personal cultures of their students is facilitated when educators themselves examine their own attitudes regarding ethnicity and race, and how these attitudes influence the power relationships within the classroom and school setting that favor one ethnic group over another (Welch, 2000). The probability that they are overwhelmingly white and less identifiable as role models makes this process more difficult. To enhance their ability to promote healthy multiculturalism within schools, in-depth treatment of diversity issues should be incorporated within teacher-training programs, textbooks, educational media, and computer programs, to create good learning atmospheres (Christensen, 2000). This goal has been endorsed by professional organizations such as the National Conference of Educational Administrators Serving the Deaf (CEASD), which regularly addresses the needs of deaf children from diverse ethnic, racial, and linguistic backgrounds in their symposiums. The Council on Education of the Deaf (CED) requires the inclusion of multicultural coursework in teacher training programs for the deaf (http://deafed.educ.kent.edu/cedman1.html). The Convention of American Instructors of the Deaf (CAID) has a special-interest group on multicultural issues in education of the deaf. The Teachers of English to Speakers of Other Languages (TESOL) has a section for educators of deaf students who are developing a growing body of information on ASL/English bilingual biculturalism. Unfortunately, the field still lacks practical, research-based information on how to teach deaf children from diverse backgrounds (Sussman & Lopez-Holzman, 2001). Educators must work collaboratively to rectify this situation in order to help deaf and hard-of-hearing children from multicultural backgrounds achieve their fullest potential.

TEACHER TRAINING ISSUES

Teacher-training programs strive to help teachers effectively maximize their ability to help all children achieve their potential and develop emotionally, socially, and intellectually into productive adults. Teacher certification is essential to ensure the quality of teachers, and each state has its own certification requirements that students in deaf education-training programs are expected to complete. Additionally, the Council on Education of the Deaf (CED) has its own national certification standards that teacher training programs must meet (http://deafed.net). The CED lists 173 standards required of all special education teachers and 66 specialized standards in the area of deaf and hard-of-hearing education within the following areas of competence: philosophical, historical, and legal foundations; learner characteristics; assessment, diagnosis, and evaluation; instructional content and evaluation; planning and managing the teaching and learning environment; managing student behavior and social interaction; communication and collaborative partnerships; and professionalism and ethical practices. (See http://deafed.net for further information on those standards.) Training in the basic academic areas—mathematics, science, social studies, and English—is also necessary.

Interestingly, the most common topics for national certification requirements for teachers of the deaf continue to be aural habilitation, audiology, speech pathology, audiometry, and hearing aids. There is a need for more training in the content areas for deaf children (Lytle & Rovins, 1997), considering that the gap between deaf and hearing students' academic achievement scores remains unacceptably large. The expectation that the curriculum for deaf children should be the same as that for hearing children may help to increase teacher training in academic contents.

The settings in which teachers of deaf and hard-of-hearing students may work also need to be considered within the spectrum of training. Miller (2000) reports that most training programs emphasize preparation for teaching in residential schools and self-contained settings rather than mainstream settings, where most deaf education takes place today. To facilitate successful mainstream education, training should include methods of collaboration with general education teachers and parents, information on effective individualized education programs, and defined specialized roles of itinerant teachers, resource room teachers, and teachers who team teach (Miller, 2000).

Obviously, training teachers to work with deaf and hard-of-hearing children from various ethnic and racial backgrounds is increasingly crucial, as is training to teach deaf and hard-of-hearing children with special needs. This includes understanding their cognitive capacities and knowing appropriate learning strategies when considering how additional disabilities such as mental retardation interact with deafness. All these variables are in addition to the regular teacher certification requirements, which impose time constraints on those training programs (Moores, 2001a).

What teacher training emphasizes depends on its philosophy regarding the education of deaf children. For example, if the focus is that of oral communication based on the premise that deaf children are capable of achieving understandable spoken language, as much time as possible would be devoted to the training of strategies for enhancing spoken language within the classroom (Moores, 2001a). Teachers have to balance this with the need to provide content material. In recent years, more programs have begun to incorporate training in the expression and reception of ASL, in addition to the teaching of speech reading and the use of residual hearing, English grammar, and literacy (reading and writing). Programs must also address how to maintain higher academic standards—no easy task. Additionally, training programs need to cover the potential benefits that both improved technology for speech reception and production as well as sign-language learning and academics offer when properly used in instructional programs (Moores, 2001a). Bilingual-bicultural instruction is now being offered in many teacher-training programs in the United States (Nover & Andrews, 2000).

Teacher-training programs should also encourage innovative cognitive strategies to enhance learning. For example, the Lexington School for the Deaf (LSD) has

■ ■ ■ ■ ■

The time came to register for 12th grade English; however, the person responsible for approving class registration (to make sure enough interpreters were available) discouraged me. The deaf education teacher specifically told me that because most of the material was Shakespearean, I would not be able to keep up with the classes. It was, to quote, "too hard." I was stubborn and asked the teacher of that class if I could register, and the teacher was very supportive. I enjoyed that class immensely and had no problem keeping up. —Mainstreamed graduate

successfully used a cognitive strategy approach called the *mediated learning experience.* Students learn to reason, draw inferences, and analyze experiences that are carefully planned by teachers for optimal learning. This approach has been used at LSD for several years, and academic achievement scores have improved (Johnson, 2001).

Equally important is the expectation that teachers have of their students. New teachers need to be aware of the danger of stereotyping deaf students. They may have been told about deaf students who have low reading levels and difficulty in mastering English. In spite of those facts, they should believe that deaf students are capable of learning and expect more from them.

Another area of training involves transition points enroute to productive and satisfying lives, which can counteract the employment problems that have been a bane for deaf adults (see Chapters 2 and 10). Relative to education, this requires teaching specific knowledge and critical skills that will help students navigate the move from high school to postsecondary education or vocational training and work, including interpersonal, decision-making, and coping skills, in addition to learning about and trying out careers (LeNard, 2001). To be effective, schools need to implement transition programs that incorporate outcome-oriented interdisciplinary curriculum offerings and utilize deaf peers and mentors as positive role models for motivating student involvement in planning for their future (LeNard, 2001).

Training Deaf Teachers

There is an urgent need to train deaf teachers and administrators. One significant hurdle has been the difficulties in obtaining professional certification in many states (Lane, Hoffmeister, & Bahan, 1996). Moores (2001b) reports that none of the deaf teachers in one residential school passed the state teacher's competency test at the first try. This test had a vocal component, which is an invalid representation of these deaf teachers' communication abilities.

Part of the mission of the National Task Force on Equity in Testing Deaf and Hard-of-Hearing Individuals is to increase the pool of deaf and hard-of-hearing professionals (www.gri.gallaudet.edu/TestEquity). Its members advocate the use of multiple measures for all college and graduate school admissions and professional licensure and certification. For teacher certification, one such measure could involve a job analysis of teaching performance, which would be in accordance with the Americans with Disabilities Act (Moores, 2001b).

Training Minority Teachers

The scarcity of minority and minority deaf professionals in deaf education is well documented (Andrews & Jordan, 1993; LaSasso & Wilson, 2000). Current training program admission standards designed for white, hearing populations need to be modified, not lowered, in ways that reflect the strengths of minority and minority deaf teachers. Providing support services and leadership training, becoming multiculturally sensitive, and revising old curricula to reflect current multicultural reality will facilitate the training and retention of these unique individuals. This process will address the lack of ethnically diverse hearing and deaf professionals in education, who represent the type of role models sorely lacking today.

INTERNATIONAL DEAF EDUCATION

Deaf educators in countries outside the United States are grappling with issues concerning the best approaches to educating deaf children—issues that are also germane to what is going on in American deaf education, as indicated by a review of *American Annals of the Deaf* articles published between 1996 and 2000 (Moores, Jatho, & Creech, 2001). Different countries have developed various educational approaches to meet the needs of their deaf children, as reported by Brelje (1999). This comprehensive report includes descriptions of the historical evolution of deaf education and background information covering the extent and type of educational services for deaf children.

Model educational programs for deaf children have emerged in developing nations such as the Holy Land Institute for the Deaf in Salt, Jordan; the Lakeside School for the Deaf in Jocotepec, Mexico; the Atafaluna School in Gaza; and the programs of the Society for the Care of the Handicapped in the Gaza Strip (Moulton, Andrews, & Smith, 1996; Silverman & Moulton, 2002). Basically, these programs started with small numbers of deaf children and grew over time, adding academic, vocational, and residential programs as needed. The Holy Land Institute for the Deaf in Jordan has one unit for deaf students and another one for deaf children with multiple challenges. Their teachers use the Jordanian Sign Language (JSL) for communication and instruction. Deaf adults also serve as teachers and teaching assistants to reinforce the bilingual curriculum (Brelje, 1999).

The Atafaluna School for Deaf Children in Gaza was established by Jeri Shawa, an American fluent in Arabic. Under the guidance of Japanese and U. S. educators of deaf children, Shawa trained a cohort of local teachers and recruited Arab audiological technicians. In addition, the Society for the Care of the Handicapped (SCH) in the Gaza Strip, a nonprofit Palestinian Rehabilitation agency managed by Dr. Hatem Abu Ghazaleh, provides services to deaf children and adults with the help of a comprehensive training program begun in 1991 by SCH and Lamar University in Beaumont, Texas, as a joint collaborative effort. In Jocotepec, Mexico, the Lakeside School for the Deaf originated in a chicken coop and now is located in a large physical plant. It was established by Ms. Gwen Chan, who sought input from deaf education experts and adapted their suggestions to fit local cultural and economic reality (Moulton, Andrews, & Smith, 1996). These efforts are a small sampling of worldwide efforts to help deaf children take their places in the societies in which they live, thereby enhancing their potential to become contributing members in their countries (Brelje, 1999).

BILL OF RIGHTS FOR DEAF AND HARD-OF-HEARING CHILDREN

The National Association of the Deaf (NAD) saw the development of a Bill of Rights for deaf and hard-of-hearing children as necessary to emphasize their need for quality education and draw attention to the plight of those children who were not flourishing in local educational systems (www.nad.org). The Bill of Rights, as currently conceptualized, states that such children have the right to appropriate communication access with the help of qualified and certified personnel who will adhere to educational standards in educational settings with a sufficient number of similarly aged, same-language mode peers at similar ability levels. Some states have enacted their own Bill of Rights, including Louisiana, South Dakota, California, Rhode Island, Colorado, and Montana (www.nad.org). The NAD recommends that other states follow suit.

CONCLUSION

The education of deaf and hard-of-hearing children involves a spectrum of educational options for children whose needs vary in a multitude of ways. In any placement, each child deserves a quality, communication-driven program that will facilitate the development of age-level language skills and provide a critical mass of communication as well as age and cognitive peers (Siegel, 2000). Schools need to face this responsibility. Research is needed on determining the best educational practice for deaf children in a variety of domains, including multiculturalism, special needs, language, and content areas, to name a few. Teacher and interpreter training programs must adapt to current needs. The training of deaf teachers and administrators, including those from diverse ethnic backgrounds, needs to be a priority.

SUGGESTED READINGS

Connor, L. (1992). *The History of the Lexington School for the Deaf (1864–1985)*. New York: Lexington School for the Deaf.
   The world-famous Lexington School for the Deaf had its roots in the oral education movement. This book chronicles how Lexington served thousands of deaf children and evolved to address the needs of today's deaf children.

Langdon, H., & Cheng, L. (2002). *Collaborating with Interpreters and Translators: A Guide for Communication Disorders Professionals*. Eau Claire, WI: Thinking Publications.

This book was written for speech pathologists and audiologists but could be used by teachers of deaf children who work with families who are non-English speaking. The authors explain how to use interpreters in clinical and educational settings. They also give examples of potential conflicts in interpersonal communication between people who use different languages and who are from different cultures. A handy resource of tests and case histories of students are given in the book's appendix.

Reed, R. (2000). *Historic MSD: The Story of the Missouri School for the Deaf*. Fulton, MO: Ovid Bell Press.

This is a fascinating history of one of the oldest residential schools for the deaf, established in 1835. It is filled with interesting details of the people, places, and events that shaped the deaf students who attended MSD. The book contains photographs of students, newpaper clippings, architecture, and historical documents related to the school. The history of MSD gives readers a full picture of the thoughts, feelings, and beliefs deaf people have about their schools.

Winzer, M., & Mazurek, K. (Eds.) (2000). *Special Education in the 21st Century: Issues of Inclusion and Reform*. Washington, DC: Gallaudet University Press.

In order to support educational reform, this book scrutinizes classroom practices for different groups, including deaf students. It also tackles issues that confront teacher-training programs, which have to accommodate a greater variety of practices in order to enhance the learning of an increasingly diverse group of learners.

CHAPTER SEVEN

LANGUAGE LEARNING AND LANGUAGE TEACHING APPROACHES

A Sociocultural View

*The teacher is no longer merely the-one-who-teaches, but one who is himself
taught in dialogue with the students, who in turn while being taught also teach.*

—Friere, 1970, p. 2

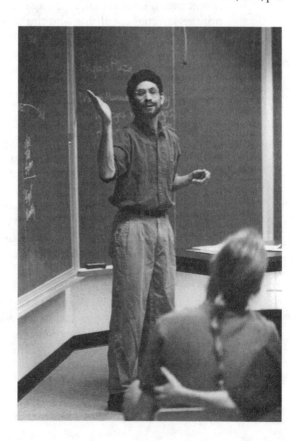

Words amuse, inspire, endear us to others, mask and uncover truths, lift us up and put us down. By its nature, language is creative, playful, humorous, loving, full of feeling, and much more. Used as a tool for thinking, a system for communicating, and a means for literacy expression, language enables people to relate to each other in creative and meaningful ways. Educators have debated for centuries about how deaf students learn language and what are the best approaches to teach them. However, research on the most effective language learning and language teaching for deaf students is far from conclusive (Marschark, 2000b). To understand the impact of deafness on language in the lives of deaf persons, it is necessary to explore the different languages and modes of communication they use with each other. How the community uses the languages can inform educators on what instructional strategies can best be used in the schools.

CHAPTER OBJECTIVES

This chapter examines how teachers use one language (monolingual) or two language (language-mixing or bilingual) approaches for instruction.* Using a sociocultural framework, language teaching approaches can be classified into three categories: monolingual, language-mixing, and bilingual approaches. Each incorporates language, culture, and the community. Each also has specific pedagogical techniques, support services, assessment strategies, and technology applications. Technology is included because the auditory and visual digital technologies available today can enhance language teaching and learning goals.

COMMUNICATION COMPETENCE

Deaf adults are monolingual, bilingual or multilingual, bicultural or multicultural individuals who use diverse languages and modes of communication (Grosjean, 1998). Deaf adults and children develop bridging strategies using more than one language to maintain family, work, and peer relationships. For instance, they may learn some spoken English, Navaho, or Spanish, depending on the family heritage. They may learn a sign language such as ASL, or Mexican Sign Language, or Puerto Rican Sign Language, or any other indigenous sign language, or they may use a contact sign language along with the written language of their society. They may combine, mix, or change (code switch) languages depending on their communication partners (Grosjean, 1998).

Variables such as the extent and type of hearing loss, age of onset, the home language, and reliance on vision and/or audition affect language learning (Quigley & Kretchmer, 1982). Many prelingually deaf children typically depend on vision for communication, and use a visual-gestural sign language incorporating eye gazes, head tilts, facial expressions, and the use of space, handshapes, signs, and

---

*See our textbook webpage and companion DVD for websites and photographs of technology used in the three language approaches: http://hal.lamar.edu/~andrewsjf/bookindex.htm.

movement. A number of them will also benefit to varying degrees from early amplification. Many hard-of-hearing children and children with progressive hearing losses who first acquire spoken English may learn ASL later in life as a second language to support their learning in academic content areas (e.g., concepts in a social studies class) (Grushkin, 1998).

The average age of identification of children with hearing loss in the United States ranges from 12 to 36 months (Chapter 3). But with newborn hearing screening, identification of hearing loss can happen shortly after birth (Joint Committee on Infant Hearing, 2000). Whether newborn screening does in fact improve long-term language outcomes remains to be seen due to various complex factors (see Chapter 8 for details). However, in general, deaf children who receive early language training through the many parent/infant programs located in speech and hearing clinics and residential schools for the deaf through the United States do better in language development than children who do not receive these services (Yoshinaga-Itano, 2000).

From their caregivers, children learn about conversational turn taking and how to express an idea clearly. They develop social and cognitive skills as they participate in and observe communication events, actively figuring out the many ways that language is used in different social situations. Slowly, children build a complex system called *communication competence.* Family activities such as informal conversations, storytelling, and responding to child questions allow the child to freely express feelings and opinions, all of which contribute to the child's communication competence. The impact of deafness on family communication competence is well documented (see Marschark, 2000b, for reviews). Typically, but not always, many hearing families of deaf children have difficulty establishing communication with their deaf children. There is much variability to this issue.

Many prelingually deaf children who are initially exposed to sign language as their first language function much like second language English learners. They use their first language to think and communicate, and build English literacy skills on this base. For many deaf children, though, the first language to which they are exposed does not necessarily become their dominant language. These children may learn ASL in later childhood. Because it is fully accessible to them, it may become their dominant or "first fully acquired" language. These children then learn English like other second language learners do (Mounty, 1986).

For the most part, deaf children depend primarily on visual pathways to access language and secondarily on audition through amplification. The use of hearing aids and cochlear implants to utilize residual hearing does not always mean the child will fully understand spoken language sufficiently to learn its linguistic rules. These devices may at the very least function only to alert deaf children to the fact that a communication event is occurring (Marschark, 2000b; Spencer, 2002). Nonetheless, many deaf children find these auditory devices very helpful in supporting their overall communication with hearing persons.

Children learn language in communities. Within these communities, they show much flexibility in how they use language. For instance, the language learned on the playground may be informal, unstructured, and made up of gestures, speech, and signs. In the classroom, deaf children freely mix speech, ASL, English-based signing, finger-spelling, writing, and drawing, depending on what languages their teachers are using (Maxwell & Doyle, 1996). Deaf children taught with a signed system of English may include more ASL-like signing on the playground (Supalla, 1991). The children will often mix ASL grammar with English grammar in their writing. Such language-mixing is a natural sociolinguistic process for persons learning a second language. That is, second language learners fall back on what language they know best and mix it with the new language they are learning (Baker, 2001; Cummins, 2000).

Deaf adults also mix English and ASL (contact signing) when communicating with each other or with hearing people (Lucas & Valli, 1992). Although language-mixing is a natural sociolinguistic phenomenon, few second language theorists advocate it as a teaching method because it does not provide children with an accurate model of either language. Nonetheless, most second language learners at some stage of their language learning will mix the languages.

Families, schools, and clinics provide language programming organized around their language teaching belief systems (Nover & Moll, 1997). Oftentimes, deaf children change what language they are taught to fit their conversational needs. They may mix languages. However, if they are regularly exposed to more than one language in the early years, and receive adequate exposure in each, they are usually able to separate the languages. This does takes time, however.

MONOLINGUAL APPROACHES

Teachers who use monolingual approaches focus on one language—English—based on the assumption that deaf children can acquire spoken language following the same developmental language milestones as hearing children do (Chapter 4). Deaf children will require in-depth training to acquire spoken language that hearing children acquire effortlessly and naturally. Key components include early identification and early intervention (Yoshinaga-Itano, 2000), the use of residual hearing to learn spoken language, intensive auditory and speech training, and audiological management (Eastabrooks, 2000). Strong parent involvement, amplification technology, developmentally appropriate language instruction, and a range of classroom options (self-contained, mainstreamed, or inclusion settings) are used (Chapter 6).

The goal of the *auditory-verbal approach* is that deaf and hard-of-hearing children will grow up to be children who function much like children with normal hearing do (Eastabrooks, 2000). This approach focuses exclusively on using audition to facilitate language development. The use of visual strategies such as speech-reading is minimized. Children attend private clinics at auditory-verbal centers. The *auditory-oral approach* differs somewhat in that it more frequently incorporates a variety of visual strategies, primarily speech-reading, along with consistent auditory reinforcement, to facilitate language learning. Sign language is not taught in oral/aural or auditory-verbal programs.

The sounds that a prelingually deaf child "hears" or "senses" (with amplification) are qualitatively different from the sounds a hearing person hears (as described later in this section). Intensive auditory training is needed to recognize these sounds and to learn what they mean in order to facilitate the development of language and speech. Nowadays, auditory training can be enjoyable with competent clinicians playing sound games with younger children or using contemporary music lyrics with high school students.

In the auditory-oral approach, training in speech-reading may be done in conjunction with auditory training. Some clinicians will use cued speech to minimize the ambiguity of speech-reading (Cornett, 1967). (Cued speech is described later in this chapter.)

Speech training includes the development of speech production skills (duration, loudness, pitch, and articulation) developed at the phonetic level (isolated syllables) and the phonological level (words, phrases, and sentences) (Ling, 1976). Techniques have been devised to make speech training a positive and fun learning experience. Speech training also benefits from the use of technology, such as computer-based visual displays of speech production.

The process of learning to listen and speak depends in large part on the effectiveness of the child's response to amplification (hearing aids, cochlear implants, and auditory assistive listening devices). Parents and teachers typically check amplification systems to make sure these are working. The following list (Waltzman & Cohen, 2000) illustrates what teachers need to know about cochlear implants.

- Up-to-date information about cochlear implants
- The difference between cochlear implants and hearing aids
- The expectations for cochlear implants
- The fundamentals of an implant system
- The basics of the tuning process
- How to monitor the system's functions
- How to troubleshoot the system

In classes, some oral-deaf students may use oral interpreters to assist them in following spoken dialogue. They may also use a computerized note-taking system such as Communication Access Real-Time Translation (CART), C-Print, or other captioning and speech-to-text software. Teachers, too, may use captioning software to develop language lessons using graphics and movies. Students will use email, wireless laptop labs, and a variety of other digital communication technologies for English instruction. They may also enroll in web-based courses. Such technologies, when used properly, can provide added exposure to the English language to supplement the use of amplification (see Table 7.1).

The goal of the monolingual approach is to fully assimilate the deaf child into the hearing, mainstream culture, attend school along side hearing peers, and use the standard school curriculum. Deaf culture and ASL are not introduced into the curriculum. Instead, cultural values, such as talking and listening and behaving

TABLE 7.1   Monolingual Approaches to Language Teaching of Deaf Children

APPROACH	DESCRIPTION	ADVANTAGES/ DISADVANTAGES	USE OF TECHNOLOGY
Auditory-Oral	Develops spoken language and listening skills at all ages, incorporating visual methods including lip-reading	*Advantages:* Uses home language; strong parent involvement *Disadvantages:* Not all deaf children benefit; speech training can be tedious; auditory functioning, even with amplification implants, is highly variable among deaf students	*Auditory technology:* Hearing aids, cochlear implants, and auditory assistive listening devices, such as amplifiers and FM systems *Visual technology:* TTYs, relay services, alerting devices, captioning, computers, email, wireless pagers, fax, Communication Access Real-Time Translation (CART), C-Print
Auditory-Verbal	Develops listening skills and verbal communication: early identification, audiologic and medical involvement, parents as models; helps child use sounds; follows normal hearing child development milestones developing speech/language, observing and evaluating child's progress; participates with normal hearing children in regular education classes	*Advantages:* Uses home language; strong parent involvement *Disadvantages:* Not all children benefit; does not use visual cues such as speech reading in instruction	Same as above

like a "hearing person," are emphasized. Many deaf children instructed in monolingual classes may switch to language-mixing or bilingual programs during their school careers depending on individual needs (Spencer, 2002).

Support services for the monolingual approaches include intensive speech and auditory therapy at home and at school. Audiological services include hearing aid repair as well as cochlear implant mapping (described later in this chapter) and maintenance. Family support groups include organizations such as the Cochlear Implant Association (CIA), the Alexander Graham Bell Association for the Deaf and Hard of Hearing (AGB), and the Auditory-Verbal International, Inc. (AVI). These organizations provide opportunities for families to meet oral deaf adults who use hearing aids or cochlear implants. *Volta Voices* is a periodical published by AGB that also contains information on family experiences, camps, workshops, and parent-teacher conventions. See the appendix at the end of Chapter 10 for websites.

Issues with Monolingual Approaches

At the center of the debate on monolingual versus bilingual teaching approaches lies the issue: How effective is speech and auditory training in developing communication with prelingually deaf children? For monolingual proponents, auditory management is crucial. For bilingual proponents, language is learned and most effectively taught using vision. This very issue has been the crux of a historically heated debate called the *"oral-manual" controversy* (Winefield, 1987; Vernon & Andrews, 1990).

In practice, how deaf children use their eyes and ears for language learning is highly variable. Depending on their communication partners, family background, and physical characteristics (extent and type of hearing loss, age of onset, etiology, etc.), they will use various communication modes to a greater or lesser extent.

Speech, speech-reading, and auditory training can enhance the speech and listening skills of deaf children, but there are limitations. Studies have indicated that intensive speech therapy has led to improvements in various aspects of speech production, but prelingually and profoundly deaf children have thus far rarely developed intelligible speech (Marschark, 2000b). What may happen is that for some deaf students, there occurs a leveling off of progress. Many factors may influence this process, including innate abilities and skills in deciphering sounds that differ qualitatively from the normal sound, the nature of the audiogram, and environmental support. Ongoing instruction may be needed to maintain existing skills. It is counterproductive to continue extensive speech training when children are not understood or when there is no evidence of improvement. Professionals may then recommend sign language training.

It is a mistaken assumption that those who lose their hearing can replace listening with speech-reading. Speech-reading is not easy because almost two-thirds of the 42 sounds of English either are invisible or look like some other sounds formed on the lips (Hardy, 1970). All of this creates ambiguity for the lip-reader. Beards and moustaches, protruding teeth, different accents, hands or newpapers covering the mouth, and so on are obstacles. In group situations, by the time the deaf speech-reader notices one person has stopped talking, the next conversationalist may be halfway through his or her statement. Teachers who talk while facing the wall or who have lights glaring in their faces compound these difficulties. Dimly lit rooms make speech-reading practically impossible (Vernon & Andrews, 1990).

For these reasons, speech-reading is difficult even for deaf adults who already know English. It is also virtually impossible for a child born deaf to learn language using speech-reading alone without amplification, although there are rare exceptions. The average deaf child understands about 5 percent of what is said through speech-reading (Mindel & Vernon, 1971). Speech-reading is of some use when the deaf person knows the context and when the conversation is simple. For example, in a school program, deaf children will anticipate questions from visitors, such as "What is your name?" "How old are you?" and "Where are you from?" The speech-reading task becomes one of guessing or distinguishing which question was asked before responding. When communication moves beyond simple exchanges to more complex communication, speech-reading becomes relatively inadequate (Vernon & Andrews, 1990).

Through the years, hearing aid, FM (frequency modulation), and cochlear implant technology has improved significantly and benefited many persons with hearing losses. Today, more than 35,000 people have received cochlear implants worldwide (Christiansen & Leigh, 2002). Currently, 1 out of 10 deaf children receive the implant, and it is predicted that 1 out of every 3 deaf children will receive a cochlear implant in the future, especially with the age for candidacy being lowered to 18 months and even younger (Christiansen & Leigh, 2002).

Contrary to popular assumptions, hearing aids and cochlear implants do not make spoken language fully accessible to prelingually deaf children. For example, hearing aids are not tuned to speech sounds the way normal hearing is (Vernon & Andrews, 1990). Background noise and reverberation may be loud and are amplified disproportionately. An air conditioner may sound like a roaring ocean. Wearing a hearing aid is not like wearing glasses. Glasses can correct imperfections in the lens of the eye and often deliver a perfect image to the retina. Amplification devices make sounds louder, but not necessarily clearer. Thus, the brain gets an unclear message. As a result, for many deaf people, amplification devices by themselves are not helpful for understanding language without training in identifying sounds. The public is sometimes confused at this point; they assume that the presence of the aid means that the wearer can, with some effort, understand speech or can automatically learn to understand speech with training. Some deaf children may find that the discomfort and trouble with amplification devices far outweigh any benefits they get by wearing them.

When deaf people do not benefit from hearing aids, they may be referred to a surgeon for cochlear implant surgery. The cochlear implant prosthesis is a device that includes an external package made up of a microphone and a speech processor. The implant also has an internal package, an array of electrodes that are surgically implanted into the cochlea in the inner ear. The external and internal components of the implant are connected through magnetic coupling. The implant is designed to create "hearing sensation" through direct electrical stimulation of the auditory nerve (Waltzman & Cohen, 2000).

Cochlear implants are different from hearing aids. Hearing aids amplify sounds and rely on the responsiveness of hair cells. Cochlear implants bypass the damaged hair cells and stimulate the auditory nerve directly. For some children, cochlear implants provide more benefits than both tactile aids and conventional hearing aids for developing speech perception and language (Geers & Moog, 1994).

Cochlear implant users do not hear the same sounds that people with normal hearing are able to hear. The sensation is not like amplified sound. Rather, it involves a different type of processing (Waltzman & Cohen, 2000). The implant user must learn how to use this new information. "Hearing as a sensation of sound" is not the same as hearing with the ability to understand conversational or academic language in the classroom. Few experts dispute that implants help postlingually deaf adults comprehend spoken language, but most currently agree that the effectiveness of cochlear implants for prelingually deaf children varies widely

(Spencer, 2002; Waltzman & Cohen, 2000). Prelingually deaf adults have generally shown little improvement in speech perception scores after cochlear implantation (Waltzman & Cohen, 2000; Spencer, 2002).

How does one define *effectiveness*? Success means different things to different people. If children recognize environmental sounds, parents may view this as success. Professionals in cochlear implant centers prepare parents and deaf adults for the possibility that environmental sounds may be the sole benefit (Christiansen & Leigh, 2002). Others may define success as being able to process language, use the telephone, or listen to music. Professionals do agree that even with an implant, deaf children do not process speech and proceed with spoken language development in the same automatic manner that hearing children do, at least not without intensive training (Spencer, 2002). Noisy environments remain a problem for all implant users, significantly detracting from their speech-perception abilities.

Researchers have identified factors such as age of onset of deafness, age of implantation, the child's language and listening skills before the implant, the nature and intensity of therapy, the kind of therapy provided after the implant, intactness of the child's neurological system, and resources and involvement of the family as reasons for the variability in results that researchers have noted (Spencer, 2002; Waltzman & Cohen, 2000). Many of the assessment measures have been speech perception and speech production tests as well as some language measures. However, there is little research on the use of the implant in a noisy classroom, at the dinner table, on the playground, or in other real-life listening situations. More research is needed about the implant's effectiveness in enabling the child to understand and comprehend language in real-life situations involving groups of conversational partners.

Spencer (2002) indicates that performance of children with implants rarely reaches the average range in speech and language expected for hearing children of the same age. But she notes that the range of benefits is significant—some children make great progress in speech production, whereas others get little benefit (Spencer, 2002). Most children with cochlear implants still require support services in the school setting, such as interpreter services, itinerant teacher services, and so on. However, what experts know today about speech perception and language development results may change as younger children are implanted and the technology improves (Christiansen & Leigh, 2002).

Each child is fit individually for the cochlear implant. The speech processor must be carefully "mapped" by an audiologist with special training. The audiologist determines the appropriate electrode stimulation based on the child's audiogram. There must be close communication between the cochlear implant client and the audiologist in order to find the appropriate setting for the speech processor in the implant. Audiologists refer to this as finding the hearing *threshold level (T level)* and the *comfort level (C level).* In other words, with cooperation with the implant user, they must discuss how the client can best hear sounds comfortably using the speech processor. For the pediatric audiologist, programming the speech processor for the infant and young child requires care and patience because of the child's limited communication skills (Waltzman & Cohen, 2000).

Many implant centers that provide the mapping for the speech processor are often located many miles away from the schools where the implanted children are enrolled. If the speech processor needs re-programming or adjustment, the children will be without their implant for some time. They may have to make multiple visits to the implant center and lose instructional time at school (Waltzman & Cohen, 2000). Improvements have led to reductions in surgical risks and device failure. Approximately 6 percent of the 439 cases reported in the Gallaudet Research Institute survey of parents with children who had cochlear implants needed reimplantation (Christiansen & Leigh, 2002). Today, a good insurance plan will often pick up surgical costs (Christiansen & Leigh, 2002).

Many children with implants will simultaneously sign and speak, or just speak while their parents speak and sign to them. Many will occasionally sign with deaf friends while primarily using speech in daily life. Thus, children with cochlear implants do not necessarily stop the use of sign language. Recent statistics reported in Christiansen and Leigh (2002) indicate that children with cochlear implants are placed in educational settings ranging from residential schools for the deaf to full mainstreaming (See Chapter 6 for explanations of educational settings.) In mainstream settings, 40 percent of the children currently receive sign-language interpreting and 13 percent receive oral interpreting. They require the same kind of support services provided to other deaf and hard-of-hearing students in the school system.

Since residential schools are now admitting students with cochlear implants, researchers need to investigate whether and how ASL and the various sign systems currently being used are compatible with cochlear implant usage. Educational and family service centers are currently working on developing various strategies to explore the best practices for integrating ASL and cochlear implant usage.

Goldberg and Flexer (2001) report on consumer surveys covering the outcomes of aural rehabilitation approaches. All of the respondents in the 2001 survey were graduates from aural rehabilitation programs. They had attended local schools and were employed in a variety of jobs, professions, and careers. A majority of the subjects used hearing aids. Almost all respondents mentioned that their mothers dedicated much time to their development. About 62 percent used text telephones and 72 percent reported they had some use of voice telephones. About two-thirds of the group reported that they had a learning disability. Regarding socialization, 76 percent said they functioned in the hearing world and 21 percent said they functioned in both deaf and hearing worlds (Goldberg & Flexer, 2001).

LANGUAGE-MIXING

Since schools for the deaf were established, signs have been used in most schools. In 1880, signs were banned after an international conference in Milan (Van Cleve & Crouch, 1989). With research on the benefits of early use of manual communication among deaf children of deaf parents, signing was reintroduced into the schools using language-mixing or combined use of sign and English codes in the 1970s. The purpose of these combined approaches was to give deaf children a communication system as early as possible that was visually accessible through sign language while mirroring the form of their parents' English language. Thus, manual codes of English were invented to achieve this goal.

Today, the majority of deaf children are taught using some form of sign language and speech. We define *language-mixing approaches* as techniques that mix ASL with English in the form of an invented manual code of English and speech. Cued speech differs from the standard manual use of language in that it uses handshapes that are not intended to be signs.

Orin Cornett developed cued speech for use as a supplement to speech reading. It is a sound-based system composed of eight handshapes representing the groups of consonants, which are placed in four positions around the face that indicate groups of vowel sounds. Combined with the natural lip movements of speech, the cues make spoken language visible (Cornett, 1967).

Cued speech has been adapted to more than 56 languages and dialects. LaSasso and Metzger (1998) provide a comprehensive review of case studies of deaf children cuers. They find mixed results for the effectiveness of cueing for expressive language, indicating its weakness for meeting all communication needs. More positive results were shown for studies on the use of cueing for written word recognition and reading comprehension. The researchers conclude that deaf children who use cueing at home and at school are able to use phonological processing to read and write more effectively than children who use only cueing at school. Specifically, cueing helps make phonological information visible for reading and writing. The authors suggest that cueing be incorporated into language approaches such as the bilingual/bicultural approach as a tool to provide the deaf child with access to phonological information, including rhyming, alliteration, onomatopoeia, accents, and dialects (LaSasso & Metzger, 1998).

Using both signs and speech is referred to as *total communication*. This term incorporates a philosophy that supports the use of all modes—visual, gestural, auditory, and written. It is also referred to as *bimodal* or *simultaneous communication (SimCom), Sign Supported Speech (SSS)*, or *Siglish* or *Ameslish* (Andrews & Vernon, 1990). English-based signing can also be labeled as *pidgin*. Linguists have recently rejected the term *pidgin* in favor of the term *contact signing* (Lucas & Valli, 1992). Contact signing refers to communication that blends features of ASL and English.

Such language-mixing approaches most typically combine ASL lexicon signs with a variety of English invented signs and invented signs for morphemes (e.g., *-ing, -ed, -s*). These systems also use speech and put the ASL and invented signs in English word order. Today, most deaf children enrolled in special education programs use some kind of signing. Language-mixing approach proponents assume that signed English provides a visual representation of English on the hands, and consequently deaf students will acquire English skills.

There are several manual codes of English, commonly referred to as *MCE*. Individuals' knowledge of ASL and English will influence how they use these manual codes. Some will use more ASL features and others will use more English features depending on their language background. A historical perspective and current uses of these systems are provided by Stedt and Moores (1990).

Additional types of English-based signing include systems called Signed English (SE; Bornstein, 1982), Signing Essential English (SEE 1; Anthony, 1971), Signing Exact English (SEE 2; Gustason, Pfetzing, & Zawolkow, 1978), Linguistics of Visual English (LOVE; Wampler, 1971), and other forms such as Conceptually Accurate Signed English (CASE). The Rochester Method, which started at the Rochester School for the Deaf, combines finger-spelling with speech (Vernon & Andrews, 1990).

Language-mixing approaches also take advantage of various technologies including amplification and cochlear implants. Teachers may utilize multimedia and videotapes in ASL and Signed English, TV captioning, and captioning software for creating language lessons. They may use multimedia and other software programs to enable deaf children to create their own stories using sign language movies, animation, graphics, photographs, and English print. Deaf persons who use language-mixing approaches may use video relay services as well. Table 7.2 summarizes the various language-mixing approaches.

The goals of the language-mixing approaches are to develop proficiency in English and to assimilate the deaf child into the hearing world. Signs are used to support the development of speech and written English. Both modalities are used—the visual-gestural and the auditory-oral—but speech is considered to be the primary signal with signs playing a supportive role.

Early intervention using signs and speech is emphasized, together with visually oriented attention-getting strategies (Meadow-Orlans, Mertens, Sass-Lehrer, & Olson, 1997). Deaf mothers are seen as models, since they naturally use these visual strategies and their communication with their deaf infants has been characterized as less intrusive, more communicative, and more cognitively and socially stimulating (Mohay, 2000). (Details are provided in Chapter 8.)

Although children in language-mixing programs are introduced to Deaf culture through interaction with other deaf children and deaf adults, English may be given more status and prestige because of the focus on the child learning English—spoken, signed, and written—in contrast to ASL.

Both deaf and hearing members participate in language-mixing approaches. Parents and professionals who are hearing may feel more comfortable learning and using language-mixing approaches because of their native competence in English. Language-mixing approaches have received support from adult deaf people because it allows signing in the classroom, but few deaf adults use these signed systems. When communicating with hearing people, deaf adults prefer to use contact signing, which blends features of ASL and English and does not use invented signs.

With language-mixing approaches came an awareness that sign-language competence is a part of the deaf child's language proficiency. Educators have added directions in sign language to tests used for hearing children. There are also some tests that have been designed specifically for sign-language vocabulary development such as the Carolina Picture Vocabulary Test. Syntax tests, such as the Grammatical Analyses of Elicited Language (GAEL) and the Rhode Test of Syntax, allows the child to use speech and signs. In their book, *Psychoeducational Assessment of Hearing-Impaired Students: Infancy through High School*, Bradley-Johnson and

TABLE 7.2   Language-Mixing Approaches

APPROACH	DESCRIPTION	ADVANTAGES/ DISADVANTAGES	USE OF TECHNOLOGY
Signed English (SE; Bornstein, 1982)	Uses ASL signs as base; consists of more than 3,000 signs, 14 sign markers to represent English morphemes; finger-spelling may be used, follows English word order	*Advantages:* Provides a visual representation of English; easier for parents to learn compared to ASL; many instruction materials and videotapes have been developed for teachers and parents; of all the manual codes of English, probably the least complex to learn for parents *Disadvantages:* Lacks affect; does not follow linguistic rules of language formation	*Auditory technology:* Hearing aids, cochlear implants, assistive listening devices, and FM systems *Visual technology:* Captioning, email, TTYs, video relay services, computers, visual listening devices, instant message, Communication Access Real-Time Translation (CART), C-Print, Smartboards, LCD projectors, document projectors, ASL/English videotapes and CD-ROMs, digital cameras, digital camcorders, multimedia CD-ROMs, DVDs that present the two languages
Signing Essential English (SEE 1; Anthony, 1971)	Categorizes signs into basic compounds and complex words; uses two-out-of-three rule involving sound, spelling, and meaning; words with multiple meanings are signed the same (e.g., *run, can, tie*) because criteria sound and spelling are used; contains more than 50 invented signs for English morphemes	*Advantages:* Provides visual representation of English; parents may have easier time learning it because of its English word order *Disadvantages:* Lacks affect; system is slow, cumbersome, and awkward to learn by many; multiple meaning words are signed the same, which often confuses deaf children (e.g., *ball* for *dance* and *ball* for *toy* are signed the same)	Same as above

(continued)

TABLE 7.2   Continued

APPROACH	DESCRIPTION	ADVANTAGES/ DISADVANTAGES	USE OF TECHNOLOGY
Signing Exact English (SEE 2; Gustason, Pfetzing, & Zwalkow, 1978)	Uses basic words from ASL lexicon; invents signs for English morphemes; English is signed as it is spoken; is translatable to only one English equivalent; three-point criterion (sound, meaning, spelling) rule is applied; complex words are basic words with addition of an affix or inflection (e.g., *-ing, -ed, -ly*); uses initialized signs; compared to SEE 1, SEE 2 has less invented morpheme signs	Same as above	
Rochester Method (Vernon & Andrews, 1990)	Is an alphabetic system that incorporates finger-spelling and speech; uses the 26 letters of the manual alphabet that correspond to the English alphabet	*Advantages:* User can spell words for which there is no sign; spellings of words can be acquired manually; can assist in early reading instruction for letter awareness and spelling *Disadvantages:* Lacks affect; person must know English to understand it	
Cued Speech (Cornett, 1967)	A manual system that uses hand cues to make English sounds or the phonemes visible; uses 8 handshapes and four hand locations near the face to supplement the lip, teeth, and tongue movements to eliminate ambiguity of speech-reading	*Advantages:* Provides visual representation of speech sounds in speech and reading *Disadvantages:* Cues have no meaning in themselves; group discussions are difficult; must be face to face with the speaker; user must make complex associations and interpret them; difficult for young children developing language	

TABLE 7.2   Continued

APPROACH	DESCRIPTION	ADVANTAGES/ DISADVANTAGES	USE OF TECHNOLOGY
Conceptually Accurate Signed English (CASE)	Resembles SEE 2 as described above; used in day programs in Texas	Same as above	Same as above
Linguistics of Visual English (LOVE; Wampler, 1972)	System is based on hand positions that represent morphemes; LOVE distinguishes morphemes on the basis of similarity in sound, spelling, or meaning; LOVE signs are also designed to represent speech rhythms; used by preschool and kindergarden children	Same as above	Same as above

Evans (1991) provide a comprehensive review of cognitive and academic achievement, speech, reading, writing, and sign-language tests.

The Stanford Achievement Test–9th edition, a multiple-choice standardized tests normed on deaf students, is used in most language-mixing programs. The directions are given in sign language. The Stanford–9 assesses reading, language, science, math, and social studies.

A recent development in language-mixing schools is the use of ASL checklists that are based on psycholinguistic research into the developmental milestones of deaf children of Deaf parents (French, 1999). These checklists provide the teacher with information on what ASL signs and structures the deaf child has learned. Most schools still do not collect data on the signing proficiency of deaf children and focus only on English proficiency (Nover & Andrews, 2000).

Numerous journal articles describe ideas for teachers who use language-mixing approaches in the classroom to teach speech, language, reading, and writing. There are also published teaching materials using manual codes of English, such as the Signed English story series and sign-language instructional books and videotapes published by Gallaudet University Press and Modern Signs Press. Publications such as *Odyssey Magazine* (Gallaudet University) contain language teaching ideas for parents and teachers as well as information on camps, workshops, and conferences for parents and teachers. There are also parent groups, such as the American Society for Deaf Children.

Issues with Language-Mixing Approaches

Linguists have criticized language-mixing approaches on the grounds that English-based signing does not represent authentic sign languages. Sign languages are natural languages, have developed over time in a community of users, are acquired naturally if children are exposed to them, and are organized according to linguistic principles found in other human languages (Valli & Lucas, 2000). In contrast, manual codes have been invented by committees, not communities, are taught rather than acquired, and lack the phonological, semantic, and grammatical structure of ASL (Valli & Lucas, 2000).

Critics have noted that it is impossible to accurately model two languages when they are mixed. For instance, when ASL, a visual-spatial grammar, is combined with English, an auditory-vocal-linear sequential language, speech can be slurred and slowed. The quality of ASL is altered as the facial grammar features, essential to ASL, can be omitted and the linguistic principle of sign formation are violated. The quality of English is also changed. Morphemes and grammatical endings essential to English syntax can be dropped (Drasgow & Paul, 1995).

Critics of English-based signing claim that a child must be competent in English morphology and syntax to comprehend and learn from these codes. But many deaf children—even after years of intervention and speech and auditory training—arrive at school with little competence in English. Therefore, English-based signing may not be the appropriate language for instruction (Wilbur, 2000). Some researchers have questioned the learning of English literacy through English-based sign codes (see reviews by Drasgow & Paul, 1995)

But proponents of English-based signing disagree. They say the systems make English visible to students. They assume that deaf children will acquire English naturally through seeing it, and that this will lead to English written competence. They also argue that parents find it easier to learn signed systems. Some studies show that deaf children who use language-mixing approaches do achieve proficiency in English (Vernon & Andrews, 1990). Other researchers see language-mixing approaches as providing bridges from ASL to written English and as facilitating English grammar if the codes are appropriately used after the child has demonstrated understanding of the concept (Mayer & Wells, 1996; Mayer & Akamatsu, 1999).

BILINGUAL APPROACHES

Bilingual bicultural approaches are used in programs in North and South America, Australia, Europe, and China (Callaway, 2000; Metzger, 2000; Nover & Andrews, 2000). Specifically, teachers using bilingual-bicultural approaches utilize the sign language of the Deaf community as the language of instruction (e.g., ASL in the United States) and they teach the majority hearing community's language as a second language (e.g., English in the United States) (see Table 7.3).

Like most hearing bilinguals, deaf bilinguals are rarely equally fluent in both languages (unless they are balanced bilinguals). They are considered bilingual

TABLE 7.3   **Bilingual Approach, Description, Advantages/Disadvantages, and Use of Technology**

APPROACH	DESCRIPTION	ADVANTAGES/ DISADVANTAGES	USE OF TECHNOLOGY
Bilingual-Bicultural	Uses two languages (ASL and English) and promotes understanding of two cultures (Deaf and hearing)	*Advantages:* Visual access to a complete grammar and lexicon through ASL; learning English as a second language, Deaf bilingual persons have economic (employment) benefits (can work within the Deaf community) *Disadvantages:* ASL proficiency for hearing persons is a challenge; hearing acquire ASL as a L2 and need a Deaf community to interact with; deaf persons are limited to using ASL only with the Deaf community	Captioning, email, computers, Instant message, Computer Assisted Real Time Notetaking (CART), C-Print, Smartboards, LCD projectors, document projectors, ASL/English videotapes and CD-ROMs, digital cameras, digital camcorders, multimedia CD-ROMs, DVDs that present the two languages

because they use both languages. American Sign Language is often marginalized and given less status by the majority culture, similar to minority languages and dialects (e.g., Spanish, Black English Venacular, Gaelic, Welsh). Deaf bilinguals, like hearing bilinguals, are often educated in remedial English classes rather than enrichment programs. Unlike most hearing bilinguals, deaf bilinguals never learn to write their first language, as ASL does not have a written form. Attempts, though, have been made with ASL written systems (e.g., signed illustrations, ASL graphemes, and glossing), but they are not widely used (Stokoe, 1960; Supalla, Wix, and McKee, 2001). Deaf bilinguals with hearing parents also differ from hearing bilinguals in that Deaf culture and ASL are not passed down within biological families but through other Deaf adults and children in the community (Grosjean, 1998). Knowledge of Deaf culture and ASL acquisition are often delayed until early childhood or early adolescence, and in some cases even in adulthood (Nover & Moll, 1997).

By convention, the language learned first is called *L1* and the language learned second is *L2*. This is not perfect nomenclature, however, because sometimes L1 and L2 are learned simultaneously, and sometimes the language that one is exposed to first in childhood turns out to be the secondary language in adolescence or adulthood. Such is the case for deaf children of hearing parents who are first exposed to English and later in childhood to ASL. For these deaf children, ASL later may become their dominant and most comfortable language because the grammar and lexicon of ASL is visually and fully accessible to them, whereas English is not (Mounty, 1986).

Many deaf adults learn ASL at different periods in their lives—at birth if their parents are Deaf (simultaneous bilingualism), or in early or late childhood (sequential bilingualism) depending on their education program and access to other deaf peers and adults. Some oral deaf adults and postlingually deaf adults learn spoken and written English in childhood but later learn ASL as a second language in adulthood. Deaf students use both languages—ASL and English—to promote their overall language learning. Deaf bilinguals, though, widely vary on how much they use ASL and English.

In Deaf families, the English language is "added" to the family household language as an L2. Additive bilingualism is a situation in which a second language adds to, rather than detracts from or replaces the first language. Deaf children of hearing parents will learn ASL sequentially after being exposed to English. Often, hearing parents will "add" ASL to the family language of English, thus creating an "additive" language home environment.

It is commonly assumed that it is more difficult for older children and adults to learn a second language. Recently, however, researchers have noted the fallacy of this assumption. Although children will have a pronunciation or phonological advantage if they learn a second language early in life, the cognitive advantages of older language learners assists in their learning of a second language at a faster rate than younger language learners (Bialystok & Hakuta, 1994). This holds true for deaf ASL learners. Age is a critical factor in the deaf child's acquisition of the complex morphological and syntactic systems of ASL (Newport, 1990) (i.e., the earlier the better for ASL acquisition). However, many older deaf children and youth learn ASL later in life and become competent ASL users.

Second language acquisition is both similar to and different from first language acquisition. Just as for L1, the L2 learner uses creative processes to internalize the language. In other words, the learner does not simply imitate the language that is seen. Rather, the learner will internalize the rules of the language he or she is exposed to and go through a series of psycholinguistic developmental stages that involves creative use of language while moving toward the adult model of that language (Pinker, 1994).

The difference for L2 learners are that they are generally older, further along in their cognitive development, and have experienced a previous language. Second language learners use different strategies than first language learners use (Baker, 2001; Cummins, 2000). Second language learners go through a period of "language interference" during which they combine their L1 and L2 in their conversations or writing (Cummins, 2000) (see Chapter 5).

Researchers in bilingualism have pointed to the cognitive benefits of learning two languages. Individuals can learn to think and analyze concepts using two symbol systems. There are also linguistic advantages in that bilinguals can learn two different rule systems and use each language to think and talk about the other language (metalinguistic skills) (see Chapter 4). There are also advantages related to greater cognitive and cognitive flexibility and creativity (see reviews in Baker, 2001).

Studies show that deaf children of Deaf parents who were raised bilingually, learning ASL from birth and English as second language, demonstrate cognitive and linguistic advantage (see reviews in Vernon & Andrews, 1990; Wilbur, 2000).

But there is also the disadvantage of the "bilingual" child learning neither of the languages very well. This is the plight of many hearing immigrant children who have impoverished first languages and struggle to learn English as a second language in school (Cummins, 2000). These children have been described as "semilingual," meaning they are weak in both languages. Many deaf children also come to school with a weak or nonexistent first language and struggle to learn a second language. For these deaf children, the language-learning process is slowed and delayed in both ASL and in English. Some of these children may have learning and cognitive disabilities that delay their language learning.

The bilingual approach gives equal status to both ASL and English, and to two cultures (Deaf and hearing). The bilingual approach, similar to the language-mixing approaches, uses the linguistic developmental milestones of deaf children of Deaf parents. For instance, psycholinguistic studies of deaf babies acquiring language show that they go through predictable stages of finger-babbling, one-sign and two-sign utterance stages, and so on, as they acquire a complex syntax and morphology (Chamberlain, Morford, & Mayberry, 2000).

Studies in the 1970s showing the achievement levels of deaf children of Deaf parents have been used to support bilingual approaches (see reviews in Vernon & Andrews, 1990). In the 1990s, a series of studies established links between ASL and English language abilities. One volume of *Topics in Language Disorders* was devoted to this topic: *"ASL Proficiency and English Literacy Acquisition: New Perspectives"* (Butler & Prinz, 1998). Researchers have reported that children who have high scores on measures of ASL also have higher scores on measures of English literacy (Hoffmeister, 2000; Strong & Prinz, 2000). Some researchers argue that the ASL-to-English relationship does not happen naturally but must be cultivated through code-switching activities using finger-spelling and signs (Padden & Ramsey, 2000).

The bilingual language teaching approach involves parents, Deaf aides, Deaf staff, Deaf and hearing peers, and Deaf and hearing adults as communication partners with deaf language learners. This approach is supported by organizations such as the National Association of the Deaf and the American Society of Deaf Children.

In order to further examine bilingual approaches for deaf students Dr. Stephen Nover and colleagues have developed an ASL/English bilingual framework for language teaching and language learning (Nover, Christensen, & Cheng, 1998). This framework hypothesizes that language can best be taught to deaf students using two languages (ASL and English) in a bilingual approach using code-switching strategies. The model also includes an ESL (English as a second language) component. When deaf students have already developed a foundation in ASL and in English, they can further obtain practice in English composition by using only English in the classroom, not ASL. An English-only classroom may include computers linked up together on a network that allows students and teachers to write back and forth to each other whereby deaf students can further practice their English writing skills. The ASL/English bilingual framework is now used in 14 residential schools and in five university teacher-training programs.

This framework has been expanded by teachers, administrators, and university professors who work in concert with the Center for American Sign Language and English Bilingual Education and Research (CAEBER) directed by Dr. Nover. This center was established in 2000 at the New Mexico School for the Deaf (www.starschools.org/nmsd). It coordinates research and education efforts around the country that involve experimenting with ASL/English bilingual approaches. Figure 7.1 shows CAEBER's research and education activities.

Issues with Bilingual Approaches

Critics of bilingual education have raised several issues. Many parents have difficulty learning ASL or any sign language, so how can such an approach be effective in the home? Another issue is related to ASL competencies in teachers. Many teachers of deaf students and teacher-trainers at universities have weak or nonexistent ASL skills. If such an approach is to be implemented, how can those teachers' ASL skills be increased?

Another issue relates to testing. Maller, Singleton, Supalla, and Wix (1999) have produced the only ASL test with published psychometric properties. This test for deaf children ages 6 to 12 measures only 23 specific ASL syntactic structures. It

FIGURE 7.1 Center for ASL/English Bilingual Education and Research (CAEBER)

CAEBER activities include the following:

- Staff development training for more than 150 teachers in 14 residential schools for the deaf on bilingual methodology; theories in first and second language acquisition and literacy learning.
- Training for administrators at schools for the deaf who wish to establish ASL/English bilingual staff development
- Summer mentor training in ASL/English bilingual approaches
- Training for teachers and mentors in digital technologies to enhance ASL/English bilingual instruction
- Research on teachers' "levels of change" and students' academic achievement as a result of the training
- A bilingual kindergarten with deaf and hearing children who are learning two languages: ASL and English
- Development of web-based online courses for preservice teachers on ASL/English bilingual methodologies
- Development of a website database on deaf children's English reading and language achievement scores

must be administered, scored, and interpreted by an ASL linguist or trained coder. Analysis also involves many hours of videotaping children's signing. Thus, this test is not practical or usable for classroom teachers. There is a need for a test that teachers can use to assess the ASL abilities of deaf children.

Although there have been studies that show strong links between ASL acquisition and print acquisition (Butler & Prinz, 1998; Chamberlain et al., 2000; reviews by Wilbur, 2000), practitioners still confront the question of how ASL can be used to teach English, given that the form and structure of the two languages are so different (Chapter 4). In other words, what bridging strategies or combination of bridging strategies from the child's communication system to English are most effective?

A new issue is that of combining signing with cochlear implantation. The Laurent Clerc National Education Center has established a Cochlear Implant Education Center (http://clerccenter.gallaudet.edu/CIEC/). The goal of the center is to investigate, evaluate, and share best educational practices with children with implants. The center emphasizes programming that addresses the development of spoken language skills as well as the development of the child's visual language development through sign language.

More research is needed to discuss if and how implant technology can be incorporated in bilingual instruction, or vice versa. As more residential schools and day programs are seeing implanted children, special programs need to be developed.

CONCLUSION

Good education policy is one that encourages innovation within schools that leads to effective language learning (Bialystok & Hakuta, 1994). However, as Bialystok and Hakuta caution, one must not just inject bilingual theory into teacher training. The teachers must be allowed to critically examine, apply, and change theoretical aspects when new information emerges.

Invariably, the answers to effective language learning approaches ultimately depend on deaf adults themselves. Educators need to understand how they use language at home, at the workplace, and among family and friends. Additionally, consumer surveys and ethnographic studies on how deaf children use their languages—speech, finger-spelling, signed systems of English, ASL, reading, and writing—may provide the answers to how deaf children best learn language and how teachers can most effectively teach language.

SUGGESTED READINGS

Baker, C. (2000). *Foundations of Bilingual Education* (3rd ed.). Clevedon, England: Multilingual Matters, LTD.
    This is an excellent and very readable text on bilingualism in U.S. schools today. Baker includes a section on bilingualism and deaf people contrasting the medical view and the cultural view.

Estabrooks, W. (2000). Auditory-verbal practice. In S. Waltzman & N. Cohen (Eds.), *Cochlear Implants* (pp. 225–246). New York: Thieme.

The article provides a clear description of the auditory-verbal approach with graphics and charts of a hierarchy of listening skills. The author discusses the purpose of the hand cue in emphasizing audition. Tips are given to parents. The article ends with a section on auditory-verbal therapy for adults with cochlear implants.

Freeman, Y., & Freeman, D. (1998). *ESL/EFL Teaching: Principles for Success* (2nd ed.). Portsmouth, NH: Heinemann.

This book, written by a husband and wife team who are bilingual educators, provides case studies and guidelines for optimum second language learning in the bilingual classroom. It is written for hearing students but the principles within the book can be applied to deaf children's learning. There is also a strong emphasis on multiculturalism.

PSYCHOLOGICAL ISSUES IN CHILDHOOD

No crystal ball can foretell which critical events and experiences that occur in childhood will direct our later thinking and decisions.
—Sheridan, 2001, p. 1

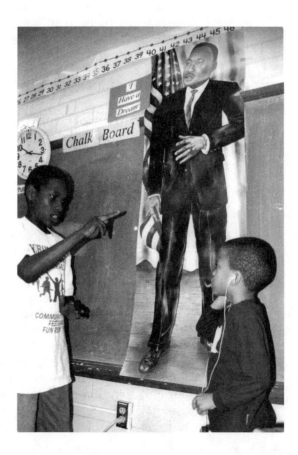

Developmental psychologists study the influence of multiple factors on development at every age and stage of life. These include biological, environmental, social, cultural, and behavioral influences. Some aspects of development, such as prenatal development and language development, are closely tied to critical periods, which are periods during which a child is maximally ready to process specific kinds of information, language being one. Interactions between the child and the environment, particularly during these critical periods, can profoundly influence how the child develops. With a deaf child, these interactions need to be shaped in ways that can maximize psychological development.

CHAPTER OBJECTIVES

This chapter discusses development issues with deaf children. It begins with the implications surrounding the parent/child relationship, and the importance of positive attachment. The text then looks at attachment between parents and their deaf children. Next, the role of early intervention programs is examined. Subsequently, the socioemotional development, self-esteem, and identity of deaf children and adolescents are addressed. The chapter then considers how childhood psychopathology may be manifested in deaf children, and ends with a discussion on psychological evaluations with deaf children.

THE PARENT/CHILD RELATIONSHIP

In more than 90 percent of families with deaf children, the parents are hearing and usually have no knowledge of or experience with deafness (Moores, 2001a). As indicated in Chapter 3, deafness has an impact on the family as well as on the deaf child (Koester & Meadow-Orlans, 1990). It is more than just the absence of hearing that families of newly diagnosed deaf children are addressing. Their world has changed. Hearing parents who are not familiar with deafness often view their deaf child with uncertainty (Christiansen & Leigh, 2002). They may not know what to expect in terms of goals and expectations for their deaf child's future. They also wonder about their roles and how to be effective parents in this new situation. They may experience feelings of guilt, confusion, and helplessness, all of which are understandable.

The phase covering the period of diagnosis is one of a series of major ecological transitions that families experience as they go through life (Harvey, 1989). The phases that encompass the other transitions include pregnancy, birth of a child, suspicion of hearing loss, entrance into school, postsecondary placement, marriage, having children, and the death of one's parents. Interestingly, the period covering suspicion of hearing loss may eventually be eliminated in part by the Newborn Infant Hearing Screening and Intervention Act of 1999 (PL 106-113). This law makes funding possible for states that are willing to establish hearing screening procedures for infants at birth. This process can prevent months of unnecessary uncertainty and frustration for parents and other family members, and facilitate the early initiation of services, amplification, communication, and educational placement for the deaf child in cases where the deafness is present at birth. It can limit potential language delays (Sheridan, 2001) and influence the evolution of attachment between parent or caregiver and child.

ATTACHMENT

The emotional bond that forms between the infant and caregivers during the first year is called *attachment*. John Bowlby's attachment theory posits that the infant's ability to thrive physically and psychologically depends on the quality of attachment (Bowlby, 1958). When caregivers are consistently warm and responsive to their infant's needs, the infant develops a secure attachment. In contrast, insecure attachment may develop when the caregivers are neglectful, inconsistent, or insensitive to their infant's moods or behaviors. The quality of attachment during infancy is associated with a variety of long-term effects (Goldsmith & Harman, 1994). Studies have shown that hearing preschoolers with a history of secure attachment tend to be more prosocial, empathic, and socially competent than are preschoolers with a history of insecure attachment (Collins & Gunnar, 1990; Kestenbaum, Farber, & Stroufe, 1989). Hearing adolescents with secure attachment histories demonstrate fewer problems, do better in school, and have more successful relationships with peers than do adolescents with insecure attachment in infancy (Sroufe, 1995).

Attachment is often assessed using Ainsworth's Strange Situation (Ainsworth, Blehar, Waters, & Wall, 1978). This assessment procedure, used with infants between 1 and 2 years of age, involves a stranger entering a room where a mother and child are playing with a variety of toys. The mother briefly remains with the child and then departs, leaving the child alone with the stranger. Shortly thereafter, the mother returns and spends a few minutes in the room, before departing and returning again. Through a one-way window, observers record the child's behavior during this sequence of separations and reunions with the mother. Attachment quality is assessed based on observations of the child's behavior toward the mother during the entire procedure.

When the mother is present, the securely attached child will use her as a secure base from which to explore the new environment and periodically return to her side (Ainsworth, Blehar, Waters, & Wall, 1978). The child will show distress when the mother leaves the room and will greet her happily when she returns, or is easily soothed by her. An insecurely attached child is less likely to explore the environment, even when in the mother's presence. During the mother's absence, the insecurely attached child may appear either very anxious or completely indifferent. Such infants will either ignore or avoid their mothers' attempts to comfort them.

The child's linguistic development emerges out of the typical, almost universal interaction between mothers and their infants that forms the basis for attachment. During this socialization procedure, secure attachment is reinforced when, for example, the infant cries, the mother touches and caresses the child, talks to the child, or picks up the child. The infant will usually cease fussing and look at the mother, who is smiling or speaking. The infant will respond by vocalizing. Such interactions continue back and forth as the dyad give each other cues. Over time, this procedure increases in complexity.

Hearing newborns are exposed to auditory information. They recognize their mother's voice very early, and become familiar with noises. Vision and voice enter reciprocally into play and become part of the early communication swirling around the infants (Montanini Manfredi, 1993). When the mother leaves physically, infants can still hear her even if they cannot see her.

In the case of children whose diagnosis of deafness is delayed, hearing parents do not know that their deaf infant cannot hear. They unknowingly deprive the infant of their presence every time they exit the infant's visual field (Montanini Manfredi, 1993). Deaf infants depend on tactile sensations, direct contact, and visual input for communication. They are incapable of foreseeing an arrival via noise, the sound of approaching steps, or a voice calling from the other room. If lack of hearing is not compensated for by visual and tactile stimulation on an ongoing basis, the deaf child's sense of isolation can be exacerbated, though these children are actually quite resilient.

It is typically the mother who is the first to identify and react to the infant behaviors that attract attention (Vernon & Andrews, 1990). Thus, it is she who generally first notices that her child is not reacting "normally." Usually, it takes a year or more to confirm the deafness (Christiansen & Leigh, 2002). During that period, the child may attempt to use nonverbal techniques to communicate that are not precise and that confuse the parents, making them feel powerless. The parents also are not able to discipline their child via auditory avenues. These difficulties can continue until the family enters an intervention program after diagnosis and hopefully learns how to communicate with the deaf child. Such delays can affect the child's language, socialization, and education experiences (Marschark, 1997; Vernon & Andrews, 1990). However, a number of families do develop temporarily effective communicative strategies, such as gestures, that work until early intervention specialists provide them with the necessary communication tools.

Early researchers described deaf children with hearing parents as less likely to be securely attached to their mothers based on anecdotal or observational rather than empirical studies (Marschark, 1993). They reasoned that the apparent role of hearing and speech enables the development of normal, reciprocal, mother/child relationships. Without this communication, reciprocity cannot transfer from nonverbal to verbal processes. Researchers theorized that the stress of waiting to confirm a child's hearing loss may lead to the mothers making incorrect interpretations of infant or child behaviors during the attachment process, such as thinking the child may be mentally retarded. The hearing mother/deaf child dyad may develop reciprocal behavior patterns that differ from those typically seen in hearing mother/hearing child dyads.

In an effort to understand the interactions between mothers' communication effectiveness and attachment in hearing-deaf child dyads, Greenberg and Marvin (1979) and Lederberg and Mobley (1990) ran studies that compared the relationships of deaf toddlers and their hearing mothers with those of a matched group of hearing toddlers and their mothers. They found that deaf toddlers and their mothers did not communicate with each other as well as hearing toddlers and their mothers. Mothers would talk and gesture when their children were not looking at them, and this frequently led to termination of the interaction. The mothers had not yet learned to coordinate communication with the children's visual attention. Also, deaf toddlers and their hearing mothers spent less of the free-play session interacting with each other than hearing toddlers and their mothers, maybe in part because deaf children must divide their attention between mother and toys.

Hearing mothers appeared to be dealing with more stress related to their difficulties in interacting with their deaf children than were mothers of hearing children. They were more pessimistic about their deaf children's future, less satisfied with being parents, and more dissatisfied with their lives. Interestingly, the stress and communication issues did not affect the quality of the relationship between mother and child. The two groups of mothers did not differ on affect, sensitivity, dominance, or teaching behavior. The children of those groups, both deaf and hearing, also did not differ on initiative, compliance, affect, attention span, pride in mastery, or creativity. Overall, however, it seems that deaf toddlers and their hearing mothers are able to establish positive, secure attachment relationships, even under less than ideal conditions (Lederberg & Prezbindowski, 2000). New work by Pipp-Siegel, Sedey, and Yoshinaga-Itano (2002) (see Chapter 3) indicates that, at least after the diagnostic phase, maternal stress may not be as much of a factor as once thought, particularly for mothers in early intervention programs. Their stress levels vary similarly to those for hearing mothers with hearing children.

Based on recent research on the attachment behaviors of deaf children with deaf parents (e.g., Koester, Papousek, & Smith-Gray, 2000; Meadow-Orlans, 1997), deaf parents do have the skills to facilitate optimal attachment bonds with their deaf children. Contrary to what earlier researchers hypothesized (e.g., Galenson, Miller, Kaplan, & Rothstein, 1979), general findings confirmed that exhibited attachment patterns follow almost exactly those reported for hearing children of similar ages. For example, studies investigating deaf mother and infant behaviors during face-to-face interactions in the first year of life show that deaf mothers modify their sign language when communicating with an infant—an activity that parallels that of vocal "motherese" of hearing children (Erting, Prezioso, & Hynes, 1990). Signs are simplified, and highly repetitious, and closer to the mother's face rather than within the larger space used among adult signing partners so that the infants can see the signs when looking at the mother. When the infant looks away or at other objects, the deaf parent tends to sign near the object or within the infant's visual field for effective communication (Koester, Papousek, & Smith-Gray, 2000).

The deaf infants themselves typically respond by mirroring their parents' signs (Koester, Papousek, & Smith-Gray, 2000). Specifically, these infants frequently move their own hands and arms, with parental praise and encouragement reinforcing these movements. These responses represent the precursor to the early gestures and signed communications produced by deaf infants, and are part of the attachment process.

Both eye gaze and maintaining eye contact during interaction are of particular importance. Koester, Papousek, and Smith-Gray (2000) report findings that conclude that deaf infants alternate their gaze between their deaf mothers and the surroundings more frequently. The length of time the deaf infants look at their deaf mothers tends to be longer in comparison to deaf infants with hearing mothers who spend more time looking at the surroundings.

Infant self-regulatory behaviors help to modulate responses to distress, displeasure, or overstimulation (Terwilliger, Kamman, & Koester, 1997). In deaf infants, these self-regulatory behaviors are reinforced when caregivers use facial and body expressions that the infants can imitate. Deaf mothers tend to be highly active and animated with their infants. This tends to elicit positive responses from the infants. When parents of deaf infants omit the use of eye contact or facial expressions, deaf infants are more likely to respond with protestations (Terwilliger, Kamman, & Koester, 1997). Deaf infants do vocalize, but more for protesting or stimulation. Without amplification that conveys speech sounds, the ability to learn conversational skills like hearing infants do is not reinforced. Visual stimuli, such as exaggerated facial expressions and visual language, as well as increased use of tactile contact and auditory amplification, will facilitate interactive communication and set the foundation for language development.

Hearing parents need to remember that deafness is very much a visual experience, even when auditory amplification is provided. They may require special help in learning to respond to and foster their deaf child's understanding of visual stimuli and signals, since this is a different communicative style for them (Swisher, 2000). They need to be taught the importance of responding to the child's early gestures using visual-gestural modes in addition to auditory stimuli. This entails awareness of eye contact and shifts in eye gaze, which indicate the infant's interests, level of attention, and receptiveness to environmental input.

Early interventionists and hearing caregivers have much to learn from how deaf parents utilize visual strategies, such as those already described, for interactive communication and for reinforcing self-regulatory behaviors (Koester, Papousek, & Smith-Gray, 2000; Swisher, 2000). Koester, Papousek, and Smith-Gray (2000, p. 56) include these strategies as part of *intuitive parenting*, which is defined as "nonconscious behaviors that in fact are ideally suited to support the human infant's natural inclination to adapt to its social world."

To maximize the effectiveness of appropriate auditory amplification in communicating about the environment to the infant or toddler, caregivers must link sounds with meaningful, naturalistic contexts (Goldberg, 1996; Maxon & Brackett, 1992). Daily routines and play times are opportunities for providing auditory information. For example, caregivers can use facial expressions and point to the sound source to direct the infant or toddler's attention to specific sounds in the environment, such as toy noisemakers or whistling kettles. They then communicate what is going on, using either spoken language, signed English, or ASL. The environment needs to be quiet to maximize the focus on the sound.

Information on the nature of attachment in deaf parents with hearing children is lacking. Most research with this population focuses on language and speech acquisition. As Meadow-Orlans (1997) reports, studies of family relationships tend to focus on older hearing children of deaf parents. Results suggest that the variability in relationship qualities parallels that found in the general population. Her pioneering study of interactive patterns in hearing infants with deaf parents used data based on observations of play behavior between these infants and their mothers at two different time intervals, when the infants were 12 months, and then 18 months of age. The interactive behavior of deaf parents and hearing children at age 18 months was ranked more negatively in comparison to the 12-month phase. Meadow-Orlans suggests that the mismatch between maternal and child hearing status may have influenced the intuitive understanding of how to respond to the behavior of the infant, considering that hearing parent/hearing infant and deaf parent/deaf infant dyads received more positive ratings. She emphasizes that many of these mismatched dyads do exhibit positive interactive behaviors, but may benefit from intervention programs to maximize effective interactions. Such programs play a crucial role in helping parents facilitate their children's psychosocial development.

EARLY INTERVENTION PROGRAMS

Public Law 94-142 applied only to children with disabilities from age 3 onward. Public Law 99-77 was designed to increase support for early intervention programs by shifting the focus to individualized family service plans (IFSPs), thereby addressing the urgent need for services during the child's first three years (Bernstein & Morrison, 1992; Moores, 2001a).

The home needs to provide consistent access to a natural language for deaf children if they are to have the tools they need to use during play, summon help, and communicate with their families, become literate, develop in positive ways, and achieve their fullest potential (Marschark, 1997). It is becoming evident that early intervention programs for young deaf children and their families provide critical services that will encourage positive developmental and educational outcomes for children who are deaf (Marschark, 2001). Such programs have proved to play a major factor in improving the overall language abilities of deaf children over the last two decades, essentially by providing families with the tools to maximize the deaf child's integration into the family, the neighborhood, and the school.

The ideal early intervention program should serve deaf children and their families from the time the child's hearing loss is identified (Calderon & Greenberg, 1997). As indicated in Chapters 3 and 6, parents and other family members need guidance regarding communication approaches and education as quickly as possible. Parents should also receive counseling and support as they work through their own feelings about their child's deafness and increase their own sense of comfort. At the same time, parents should be developing skills in providing intellectually and socially stimulating environments for their deaf child. (Marschark, 1997) They may also learn a manual form of communication, or techniques to stimulate oral communication, depending on the program philosophy of the early intervention program.

■ ■ ■ ■ ■

The mother of a deaf girl diagnosed at 10 months had this to say about her early intervention program: "[They were] wonderful. I mean I walked in and I just . . . cried and [they] just listened to me and said there are options, you know, it's not terrible, she's going to be fine, we have lots of kids and . . . they are fine. So that was the next thing that happened, and I think that was my ray of hope that things were going to be all right" (Christiansen & Leigh, 2002, p. 79).

In order to get some understanding of the extent and offerings of early intervention programs, Bernstein and Morrison (1992) surveyed state departments of education concerning available programs for deaf infants and preschool children and the characteristics of the programs. Sixteen states and the District of Columbia responded, identifying a total of 340 programs, of which 134 responded to the questionnaire. Some 69 percent were school-based programs and 41 percent were home-based, with professionals going into the homes. The numbers add up to more than 100 percent because some programs had both school-based and home-based services.

The activities in the two types of settings varied. Most of the school-based programs emphasized oral or Signed English development and academic readiness, whereas the home-based programs emphasized language/English development, auditory training, sign-language acquisition, and experiential and cognitive enrichment. Only 10.5 percent of the programs provided ASL instruction. The greatest overall emphasis reported for home training was for speech and auditory activities. Fathers and siblings were seldom involved in home-based training. The results suggested that state agencies usually do not understand what is going on in the early intervention field. However, on the positive side, more states are seeing the value of early identification, and IFSPs within early intervention programs are now being provided in the hopes of alleviating the educational deficiencies long noted in deaf children (Bernstein & Morrison, 1992).

At this point, there is no validated ideal comprehensive curriculum for early intervention programs that will address all the needs of all deaf children and their families (see Chapter 6). A curriculum that incorporates a variety of competencies such as counseling, child development, linguistics, speech and hearing, and instruction becomes complex, indeed. Funding is also problematic. Even though Congress established a reimbursement formula stipulating that by 1982 the federal government would reimburse the states for educating children with disabilities 40 percent of the excess cost per year above that required to educate a child without a disability, Moores (2001a, p. 234) reports that in reality the government expects states to pick up these extra costs and federal funding has never approached that legislated by Congress.

Professionals should be aware of the importance of including fathers as well as mothers in discussions of and decisions about their deaf children within early intervention programs. The fathers' roles in their children's lives are usually underestimated (Crowley, Keane, & Needham, 1982). In a survey of factors contributing to oral communication ability, it was been reported that even though participating parents strongly agreed on the need for paternal involvement, the father is less likely to be involved and tends to receive information from the mother about issues involving the deaf child (McCartney, 1986). This lower level of involvement tends to be true for fathers of young children with special needs as indicated in a review of the literature (Essex, Seltzer, & Krauss, 2002). That may change due to the cultural shift toward fathers being more involved in child rearing as mothers increasingly return to work.

Fathers may be at risk for stress just as mothers are, depending on factors such as education, culture, and personal attributes. Support groups can facilitate paternal involvement with their deaf children (Crowley, Keane, & Needham, 1982), particularly when provided within culturally sensitive contexts.

CHILD DEVELOPMENT AND DEAFNESS

Foundations for Language Development

Enhancing the visual strategies that can maximize reciprocal communication and language development will diminish the problems associated with limited communication, including language delay, and will facilitate play behavior that can lead to enjoyable complex interactions as well as optimal cognitive development and, in turn, healthy psychosocial development (Lederberg & Prezbindowski, 2000). Following is a list of visual communication strategies that parents can employ (Mohay, 2000):

1. Nonverbal communication
2. Gaining and directing attention
3. Making language salient to context
4. Reducing need for divided attention
5. Linking language and meaning
6. Modifying signs

Chapters 4 and 5 addressed language development issues, but it is important to emphasize that parents need to understand how to use the child's perceptual field and minimize divided attention while simultaneously helping the child track stimuli that will facilitate language development (Calderon & Greenberg, 1997). In terms of divided attention, deaf infants tend to divide their attention sequentially between the communication itself and the subject of communication (Koester & Meadow-Orlans, 1990). They cannot simultaneously attend to the visual surroundings and receive linguistic communication, except when provided with meaningful auditory information via appropriate amplification that they potentially can build on (there is no guarantee of this). For that reason, the visual tracking techniques described earlier are important. These strategies may at first seem unnatural for new hearing parents, as they are not part of the behavior repertory hearing parents typically assume with hearing infants. However, these parents can eventually arrive at an interactive style that is effective and mutually satisfying, in which each party responds to and influences the other's behavior (Maxon & Brackett, 1992). As this synchronic interaction, so critical for the process of language development, becomes more apparent to the hearing parents, their confidence in their new-found communication skills and their ability to parent their deaf infants will increase (Koester & Meadow-Orlans, 1990; Mohay, 2000).

Successful language development in deaf children tends to be facilitated by effective mother/child communication, enrollment in early intervention programs, and early use of sign language, although sign language is not necessarily the appropriate mode of communication for all deaf children (Marschark, 2001). Marschark notes that deaf children who were exposed to sign language during the early years tend to have more effective communication experiences and do well linguistically, cognitively, and socially. They are linguistically more fluent in ASL and English as adults. Children with cochlear implants have been found to benefit significantly from exposure to both sign language and spoken language, as based on a review of the literature done by Spencer (2002). Therefore, they can benefit from both visual and auditory enhancement strategies.

The Role of Play in Early Cognitive Development

Cognitive development is enhanced when children are provided with opportunities to explore their environment in the guise of play (Spencer & Deyo, 1993). Vygotsky, a sociohistorical theorist, and Piaget, a cognitive-developmental theorist, see play as enhancing the ability of children to develop and practice adult-like behaviors (Vygotsky, 1978; Piaget, 1929). The process of play, incorporating as it does both reality and pretense behavior, constitutes a critical step in the development of thinking (Vygotosky, 1978). For example, using a box and pretending it is a car provides a way for children to distinguish between objects and their meanings, and facilitates thinking about the mental representations of boxes as other objects, which in turn leads to flexibility in cognitive processing and the ability to abstract. The communities and cultures in which children live have a significant influence on the ways in which play behavior evolves and shapes cognitive behavior.

The importance of play in general and symbolic play in particular in the cognitive and social development of deaf children cannot be overemphasized (Marschark, 2000a). It is not the deaf child's lack of hearing, but rather delays in language development and disruptions in social interaction patterns that may interfere with the deaf child's acquisition and demonstration of symbolic play (Brown, Rickards, & Bortoli, 2001; Spencer & Deyo, 1993). In other words, the level of sophistication in symbolic play exhibited by deaf children may be a function of their level of language development, social behavior characteristics, and cognitive abilities. Evidence from studies with preschool and early school-age children shows that hearing mothers of deaf children are more likely to be controlling in their verbal and nonverbal interactions, particularly when communication is constricted (Musselman & Churchill, 1991) and to be more controlling of deaf children's behavior (Greenberg, Calderon, & Kusche, 1984). Brown, Rickards, and Bortoli (2001) suggest that when family members learn pretend-play techniques, this will enhance mutually satisfying interactions with their deaf children and facilitate positive attachment.

Psychosocial Development

Parents and educators need to attend to the child's psychosocial development since its successful outcome will lead to the development of a sense of competence and self-assurance (Calderon & Greenberg, 1997). In addition, the development of personal identity that evolves during the developmental process should ideally allow the child to acquire a solid sense of self in order to develop emotionally and socially and gain a sense of inner security (Calderon & Greenberg, 1997).

What constitutes the process of healthy psychosocial development? Erik Erikson's theoretical model of this process provides a useful frame of reference (Erikson, 1972). In this model, Erikson postulates eight psychosocial stages that characterize the course of personal and emotional development in human beings. Those successive stages each have a potential crisis and are described in terms of successful and unsuccessful solutions. The usual outcome is a balance between those two extremes. The successful solution of each stage depends on its level of difficulty and the individual, parental, and social/community resources that are immediately available. The eight stages, beginning with infancy, are (1) basic trust versus mistrust, (2) autonomy versus shame and doubt, (3) initiative versus guilt, (4) industry versus inferiority, (5) identity versus identity diffusion, (6) intimacy versus isolation (7) generativity versus stagnation, and (8) integrity versus despair. The last three stages cover the adult phases of life.

Schlesinger (2000) uses Erikson's psychosocial stages as a framework for tracing the psychosocial development of deaf individuals throughout the life course. We incorporate her observations into our discussion.

The first stage, that of basic trust versus mistrust, encompasses the early attachment stage. Next comes the autonomy versus shame and doubt stage, which takes place between 18 months and 3 years of age. It encompasses the initial process of learning the behaviors and attitudes appropriate to family and culture. According to Schlesinger, if meaningful reciprocal communication is limited, deaf children show delays. Hearing parents may overprotect their deaf children despite the advice of numerous professionals, thus hindering autonomy. In turn, the children may also initiate power struggles for autonomy that can take the guise of rebelliousness, such as refusing to maintain eye contact or communicate when, for example, pushed to do something they do not want to. When parents allow their children some exploratory leeway, these children learn to master new skills in their environments, thereby developing autonomy. Interestingly, Schlesinger notes that deaf parents with deaf children appear to be more comfortable in allowing more exploration. Power struggles do not appear to be as intense, with these children experiencing fewer eating and toilet training problems.

During the next stage of initiative vs. guilt, the task of children (ages 3 to 6) is to develop a sense of initiative with a feeling of the purposefulness of life and one's own self. Children begin to know whether they are "good" or "not so good" based on feedback. Ideally at this stage, parents show the child by example what behavior is appropriate and acceptable. The child, in turn, needs to be able to take some initiative in testing the environment, such as riding bikes down the block and stopping at streets to wait for the parent to catch up before crossing.

Deaf children who experience verbal inhibitions because of limited communication will often erupt in physical actions, especially if they are unable to express their feelings in words or signs during a time when children typically have a stream of questions. To avoid diminishing initiative, parents need to provide adequate information, establish reasons for external events and for behavior, and establish safety limits that do not overly restrict their deaf children's explorations.

Education settings may also place a premium on immobility when the emphasis is on children sitting still and paying attention at times. This may serve to limit the various ways in which initiative may be reinforced. But this also provides learning opportunities for new initiatives that can be reinforced during free periods. It is difficult to determine what the optimal teaching situation is for active deaf children with less auditory contact with the environment. Directing visual attention and utilizing good auditory monitoring will facilitate opportunities to encourage initiative within appropriate situations.

Self-concept is evolving during this phase, and deaf children need to be exposed to deaf adults in order to minimize the development of potentially distorted expectations of what happens to deaf children when they grow up. As a matter of fact, some children will express the belief that there are no deaf adults because they have never seen any (Lane, 1999). Analogous to this, multicultural studies show that the self-esteem and school achievement of disadvantaged children rise dramatically when successful adults of their own color or linguistic competence are introduced into their social and learning environment (Ervin-Tripp, 1966, as cited in Schlesinger, 2000).

For children ages 6 to 11, the task during the school-age period is to develop a sense of industry and accompanying feelings of competency. Failing that, the child will feel inferior. When children are struggling in school, this may heighten feelings of inferiority. It can be difficult to overcome such feelings. This can have repercussions for the next stage, which involves internalizing a positive sense of identity, and self-concept may suffer. In order to feel competent, children need to be around people such as teachers who will work at reinforcing their strengths. If parents avoid taking over and do not always tell their children what to do, this will encourage the child's sense of competency. This works when there is sufficient language foundation to explain possibilities that children can choose, and what the limits are.

When deaf children are able to converse and socialize at ease with their families and peers, whether through speech or sign, and internalize social rules, this leads to social competency (Marschark, 1993, 2000a). Deaf children with hearing parents are not as able to "eavesdrop" or listen to interactions taking place in their environment as do hearing children, who are more aware of events swirling around them. If families develop strategies such as quickly explaining what is going on, or making sure that the deaf child can see everyone in the room, there is less chance for the deaf child to be left out of the loop. Sometimes, unfortunately, even in well-meaning families, it is difficult to remember such strategies in the heat of the moment during stressful situations.

Also, deaf children are not easily able to acquire information through television and radio, unless they are exposed to captioned television programs and can comprehend the captions. Deaf children will learn a great deal about the world through reading books, only if their language development and reading skills are up to par. When deaf children are provided with adequate input concerning their social environment, using all sources of information possible, they develop basic understanding of events, social conventions, and typical age-appropriate expectations about relationships (Lederberg, 1993).

Deaf children can and do develop social relationships with deaf peers much like hearing children do with hearing peers. If they are not provided with this opportunity, or if they are and still do not develop these social relationships, this can be cause for concern. Loneliness and other social problems are potential consequences (Leigh & Stinson, 1991). It has been suggested that the social relationships between deaf children differ from those between hearing children in a number of ways, in part because of missing information about the ways hearing children socialize, and in part because of the visual nature of interaction with deaf peers (Marschark, 1993). Whether observed differences in social relationships are deficiencies rather than differences needs to be carefully scrutinized, depending on the age-appropriate nature of the interactions.

Deaf children are capable of developing good social relationships with hearing peers, but the success of these relationships is very dependent on their social and communicative competence in interacting with hearing peers (Bat-Chava & Deignan, 2001; Stinson & Antia, 1999). Deaf students who are in public schools with no deaf peers have been found to have less positive social and emotional experience, although there is considerable variability. Specifically, deaf children in mainstream settings are likely to be "neglected" by hearing peers (Stinson & Antia, 1999). Postsecondary deaf students more often than not report feelings of loneliness, rejection, and social isolation related to their earlier mainstream experiences (Foster, 1989; Stinson & Foster, 2000). Overall enrollment in residential schools has decreased drastically; however, deaf children of deaf parents do not show the same decline in percentage of residential school placement in comparison to deaf children of hearing parents (Holden-Pitt, 1997). The message may be that many deaf parents see their deaf children as benefiting from not only the educational experiences available in these schools but also the socialization and extracurricular opportunities available for optimal psychosocial development.

Due to the presence of more deaf children in the mainstream, professionals need to work with parents in helping these children establish social network connections within their home and school communities that will facilitate healthy psychosocial development (Calderon & Greenberg, 1997; Stinson & Antia, 1999). Every

■ ■ ■ ■ ■

Because of the large number of deaf people in my school, I was able to socialize with my deaf peers. I mainly interacted with two students who were fully mainstreamed. I did not socialize much (if at all) with my hearing peers. I also participated in different organizations and activities over the years, but always shifted to something new each semester or year in hopes of finding a place I could fit in and be accepted by my hearing peers. —Graduate of a large mainstream program

I did not socialize a lot during my middle and high school years, especially with hearing peers. I did participate in clubs and extracurricular activities, but I never felt comfortable in socializing with my hearing peers. I usually preferred to socialize with the deaf and hard-of-hearing students from the program. —Student who was fully mainstreamed at a school where her deaf and hard-of-hearing peers were in self-contained classrooms

I often feel that I have a firm grounding in the hearing side, with a few toes dipping into the deaf side like the hot water from a hot tub—touching it enough to get a feel of the heat, but not needing to immerse myself in the hot water. . . . I spent most of my time with my hearing friends. —Graduate of an inclusion setting

school setting with a deaf child should develop prevention-oriented strategies and programs that decrease high-risk student outcomes such as low academic achievement, social difficulties, and psychological distress (Greenberg, 2000; Greenberg & Kusche, 1998; Marschark, 1993; Stinson & Antia, 1999).

One example is a comprehensive school-based program known as Promoting Alternative Thinking Strategies (PATHS), developed by Kusche and Greenberg (1994), designed to improve deaf children's self-control, emotional understanding, and problem-solving skills through teaching social problem-solving behaviors. Its effectiveness was investigated in 11 Total Communication self-contained classrooms. Teachers were trained in the intervention model and provided PATHS lessons for one school year. Results of the study showed significant overall improvement in the deaf children's social problem-solving skills, emotional recognition skills, social competence, and even reading skills (Greenberg & Kusche, 1998).

The National Deaf Children's Society (NDCS), a leading national charity in the United Kingdom, did a three-year project involving PATHS in seven pilot schools with deaf children. Deaf children emerged with more positive social skills (NDCS, 1999). Early intervention programs can also benefit from the PATHS programs in terms of providing parents with strategies to develop their children's emotional vocabulary, facilitate peer relationships, discuss deaf issues, and set up informal social networks for their deaf children.

According to Greenberg (2000), the PATHS program has the potential to foster healthy deaf identities. This is the focus of the next stage in Erikson's (1972) psychosocial theory, which takes place during adolescence—a time when issues of independence and identity come into the picture. During this stage, the task is that of integrating earlier experiences into a true sense of identity as a separate individual. Adolescents seek to find out who they are. If the earlier crises of previous stages are resolved, the adolescent is then ready to work on identity explorations (Erikson, 1972).

Identity reflects how people define themselves, what they find important, and what goals they want to accomplish in life. Membership in groups often plays a key role in fostering adolescents' identities. Groups can also endorse values and goals that teenagers may adopt. Before adolescents achieve a true sense of their adult identity, most need considerable time to explore their various options for the different affiliations in their lives.

Deaf adolescents also need time to explore various options, particularly deaf identity issues. The extent of exposure to deaf adult role models and the perceptions of selves as deaf or Deaf can influence identity development. A deaf person who has attended hearing schools may absorb the standard view of deafness as a disability, while, in contrast, the culture within the school for the deaf may facilitate the construction of identity as a culturally Deaf person (Bat-Chava, 2000). Bat-Chava indicates that her research findings (see Chapter 9 for further explanation of these and identity issues in general) appear to support Tajfel's (1981) Social Identity Theory. This theory states that members of minority groups will achieve positive social identity via two avenues: (1) by attempting to gain access to the mainstream through individual mobility or (2) by working with other group members to bring about social change. Deaf persons may access the mainstream through being "culturally hearing" and assimilating into hearing groups. However, assuming a bicultural identity (comfort with both hearing and Deaf cultures) does not necessarily preclude involvement with hearing groups. The second avenue is represented by deaf individuals getting involved with Deaf culture and working for changes related to Deaf culture interactions with the majority hearing society. Deaf adolescents will join either group insofar as they benefit from the group in terms of positive self-esteem or self-image. Without this, they will leave the group physically or psychologically (Bat-Chava, 2000).

I always compare my identity to a line, with the deaf world on one side and the hearing world on the other. . . . My family falls on the hearing side. My friends are mostly on the hearing side. . . . Yet, I can't deny my deaf identity. It has shaped too much of who I am and what I am. My deaf friends are like myself: oral, wear hearing aids or cochlear implants, attend hearing colleges, and work in the hearing world. What we have in common is our deafness, and also our lives in the hearing world. I pass in the hearing world. My deaf identity is equal with my other identities, that of a female, a Jewish person, a resident of the Midwest. My deaf identity has shaped my everyday experiences and the way I see the world. I would not be successful in the hearing world without the support of my deaf friends. I will always remain in the middle. I need both worlds, both sets of friendships to thrive. I will never cross the line completely, since I know I need both sides to be a successful and happy person. —Graduate of an inclusion setting

Crocker and Major (1989, as cited in Bat-Chava, 2000) "propose that members of stigmatized groups who have stronger group identity will have higher self-esteem than those with weaker group identity" (p. 421). What this implies is that deaf persons who espouse deaf identities will have higher self-esteem. Bat-Chava's (1993, 1994) and Maxwell-McCaw's (2001) research supports the presence of a relationship between self-esteem and having either deaf or bicultural identities. Observations of deaf children of deaf parents indicate that they tend to feel more self-confident, have higher self-esteem, and are able to maintain self-confidence in school (Marschark, 1993). One explanation for such positive self-esteem is that deaf parents are able to successfully navigate lives as deaf people and thus can model successful patterns of adjustment with both hearing and deaf people for their deaf children (Lane, Hoffmeister, & Bahan, 1996). We note that although these deaf children may not necessarily struggle with deaf identity issues per se, they may confront other general types of identity issues germane to adolescence.

What about deaf adolescents with hearing parents? If they have not had significant exposure to other deaf peers, they may start to express more interest in exploring connections with deaf peers (not all do). This can be difficult if their hearing parents convey the message that socializing with hearing peers is a desirable goal, preferable to intermingling with deaf adults (Bat-Chava, 2000; Leigh & Stinson, 1991). It becomes even more frustrating if socialization with hearing peers is shallow. When these adolescents start to express preferences for socializing with other deaf peers, exploring Deaf culture, and distancing from the family because of communication difficulties, parents do not always have an easy time "letting go" (Leigh, 1987; Schlesinger, 2000). Parents will handle this phase much better if they are truly comfortable with having deaf children; allow socialization experiences with deaf peers, including the use of sign language, that can lead to comfort and identification with Deaf culture; and frame this stage as a rite of passage (Lane, Hoffmeister, & Bahan, 1996; Leigh, 1987; Leigh & Stinson, 1991). Parents need to understand that such exploration does not necessarily lead to ultimate rejection of connections with hearing individuals. Maintaining open communication with their adolescents during this stage is critical.

Lytle (1987) provides empirical support indicating that deaf college women do successfully resolve the same Eriksonian psychosocial stages of development as their hearing peers, deal with the same set of identity issues, and are similarly classified into four identity status categories (Marcia, 1993). These categories reflect identity status as influenced by Erikson's (1972) criteria of the presence or absence of crisis (period of time spent in exploring alternatives) and commitment.

Specifically, *identity achievement* is characterized by commitment to choices made after exploring alternatives in different areas. *Foreclosure* is commitment without crisis. Those achieving this status tend not to spend time considering alternatives and depend on their parents or significant others to develop life plans for them. *Moratorium* is defined as a status in which a person is currently experiencing crisis and has not made a commitment in resolving this crisis. If there is no commitment and no crisis, the result is *identity diffusion*. Such individuals have superficial relationships and are often lonely and unhappy. Individuals in the identity achievement category have been found to be more mature and competent in relationships than people in the other three categories (Marcia, 1993). During adolescence, identity categorizations can change. From late adolescence onward, more people are in moratorium or achievement status in terms of identity. The others may remain in foreclosure or diffusion (Kroger, 1993).

Identity status is influenced by factors such as the degree of encouragement that parents allow for autonomy and exploration of differences (Kroger, 1993). Other factors include one's levels of ego development, moral reasoning, self-certainty, self-esteem, performance under stress, and intimacy. More research on these factors in young deaf people can facilitate the development of effective programs to strengthen their psychosocial adaptation and identities.

The Role of Deaf Professionals in Psychosocial Development

Deaf professionals who can facilitate the process of self-esteem usually do not have a major role in providing learning models for hearing parents and their deaf children (see Chapter 6). Early intervention specialists tend to be hearing. Regardless, these professionals should be trained to meet with parents in their home and share with them what it means to be a deaf person in today's world. Hearing specialists can emphasize the use of deaf role models with whom they can model accessible language and language acquisition strategies for the deaf child from birth onward. If parents also hire deaf babysitters and invite deaf people, either signing or oral, to meet their child, the child will have additional exposure to language and social models throughout the developing years. Being exposed to the successful lives of deaf people can only enhance the deaf child's and adolescent's sense of self as a psychologically healthy person.

CHILDHOOD PSYCHOPATHOLOGY

Formal studies of the psychological adjustment of deaf children date back to the late 1800s and early 1900s, about the time psychological tests first came into use (Pollard, 1992–93). Caution needs to be taken when investigating childhood psychopathology where deaf children are concerned, since many test instruments used for diagnostic purposes are verbally loaded and lack deaf norms. Also, they are often inappropriately administered to children, thus changing the meaning of the questions and hence the responses. (See Chapter 9 for a discussion of psychometric issues.) There have been many cases where gross misdiagnoses have resulted in irreversible psychological and educational damage. As reported in Lane (1999), Matti Hodge and Alberto Valdez spent most of their lives in institutions after having been misdiagnosed as mentally retarded based on low IQ scores. These scores were revealed to have been sadly incorrect, as later retesting indicated normal intellectual functioning. Lack of awareness by psychologists of appropriate testing procedures with deaf individuals is at the heart of the problem (Leigh, Corbett, Gutman, & Morere, 1996).

Studies assessing the prevalence and to some extent the nature of psychological maladjustment among deaf children were conducted back in the 1970s. Most of them report higher rates of psychological maladjustment problems among deaf children compared to hearing peers (e.g., Chess & Fernandez, 1980; Freeman, Malkin, & Hastings, 1975). Based on a review of the literature up to 1980, Meadow (1980) observes that the prevalence of emotional and behavioral pathology among deaf children ranges from 8 to 22 percent, compared with rates of from 2 to 10 percent for the general child population.

Rehkemper (1996) identifies a significant drop in the percentages of deaf children diagnosed with emotional and neurological behavioral problems in studies conducted after the 1970s. She attributes the previous higher prevalence rate to the presence of children affected by the rubella epidemic of the 1960s, which resulted in a significant increase of multiple disabilities in addition to hearing loss. The subsequent improvement in rates after the 1970s may have been due to improved educational intervention practices as well as changes in diagnostic criteria.

More recent information on prevalence rates were provided by Karchmer and Allen (1999) through a set of questions that were added to the 1997–98 Annual Survey of Deaf and Hard of Hearing Children and Youth. These questions, which teachers answered, were designed to assess the functioning of children in their classrooms. Findings extrapolated from information on 30,198 students suggest a broader range and higher prevalence of functional limitations than would be assumed by analyzing categories of additional disabilities alone. Within this large sample, 74 percent reported no specific condition in addition to deafness; 22.6 percent had one additional condition; and 3.2 percent had more than one specific condition. The specific conditions reported in addition to deafness were learning disability and mental retardation (most prevalent), followed by attention deficit disorder, cerebral palsy, and legal blindness. Conditions that included emotional or behavior disorders, autism, and asthma, among others, made up 3.8 percent of students with specific conditions in addition to deafness. About a quarter of the students had one or more of the specific conditions checked. Since the information was provided by teachers, not trained diagnosticians, Karchmer and Allen acknowledge that some of these teachers may have had difficulty communicating with their students and, as result, judge their students as exhibiting inappropriate social behavior when in fact this may not necessarily be the case.

The methodology for estimating emotional or behavioral disorders has not been well developed even for hearing children (Anderson & Werry, 1994). The methodological problems are similar to those in conducting a poll or making a projection during an election. Different numbers will emerge depending on how the sample is selected, what questions are asked, and how those questions are asked. For deaf children scattered in different school settings, obtaining accurate figures becomes even more problematic. The prevalence rates reported thus far are open to question because of problems related to diagnostic criteria, the expertise of the evaluators regarding deafness and child psychopathology, and whether the sampling studied was truly representative of the general population of deaf children (Anderson & Werry, 1994). (See Chapter 9 for further discussion.)

In addition to the problem of determining criteria for various diagnoses, diagnosticians face the complexity of separating the impact of deafness from the disorder itself, such as in the case of learning disability (LD). There is almost no research on how learning disabilities are manifested in deaf children, or on how to separate the problems of limited exposure to stimuli from standard criteria for learning disabilities. Existing opinions are based primarily on anecdotal evidence, survey opinions, and limited empirical studies (Samar, Parasnis, & Berent, 1998). Attention deficit disorder (ADD) is also another problem category. Keeping in mind the sparse nature of the research, current evidence seems to suggest that deaf LD and ADD individuals have many of the same characteristics as hearing LD and ADD individuals. However, the primary etiologies of deafness—such as maternal rubella, Rh incompatibility, meningitis, anoxia, complications of prematurity, and cytomegalovirus infection—are also etiologies of LD (Mauk & Mauk, 1992). For this reason, the incidence of LD is probably higher in the deaf population than in the hearing population (Moores, 2001a). With ADD, an additional complicating factor may be the risk of misdiagnosis when deaf children exhibit restless behavior due to limited ability to understand their environment and get bored.

Because of the difficulties with diagnostic criteria, developing validated testing approaches for accurately diagnosing LD or ADD in deaf children continues to be a difficult task. Researchers have to contend with the lack of adequate norms on deaf children; inconsistent control over communication and language factors during evaluation, including how evaluators and deaf children communicate; and the potential reliance of deaf individuals on adaptive attentional and cognitive coping strategies in testing and learning situations that may mask true disabilities (Samar, Parasnis, & Berent, 1998; Samar, 1999). These are all aspects that impact on psychological evaluations, which we discuss later in this chapter.

CHILD ABUSE AND ITS CONSEQUENCES

Children with disabilities may be more at risk for various types of abuse, with incidences ranging from 4 to 10 times that of the general population (Ammerman & Baladerian, 1993 as cited in Burke, Gutman, & Dobosh, 1999). Precise figures are hard to come by because researchers use various criteria to determine whether behaviors can be defined as abusive and what constitutes a disability. Abusive behaviors can fall into physical, sexual, or emotional categories (Garbarino, Guttmann, & Wilson Seeley, 1986).

A review of the literature by Burke, Gutman, and Dobosh (1999) suggests that deaf children are at greater risk for abusive situations. Findings tend to be based on retrospective information asked of deaf individuals. Child abuse incidents in the deaf and hard-of-hearing youth population may actually be underreported due to various factors. These include fears of retaliation by the perpetrator and the system in which the abuse occurred (residential schools or/and home), fears of being stigmatized by those who view the reports of child abuse at residential schools as threatening the reputation of residential schools, and lack of understanding on the part of the victim (Schott, 2002).

Many deaf children may not know what abuse is. Thus, they may not understand that they are in abusive situations (LaBarre, 1998). They often have difficulty communicating about the abuse and do not know how to explain what has happened to them. They usually do not have the opportunity to learn what good and bad touching are, either from the family or school (LaBarre, 1998). Since they have less access to information, compared to hearing peers in general, particularly in terms of sexual abuse, they may more readily be victimized by pedophiles (Gannon, 1998).

In view of the limited research findings currently available, one may assume that deaf abused children suffer consequences similar to those of their hearing peers (Burke, Gutman, & Dobosh, 1999). When abuse, whatever the nature, is hidden, there can be grave physical, emotional, cognitive, and social consequences, particularly if the abuse is ongoing. For hearing children, these consequences can include delayed speech (Coster, Gersten, Beeghly, & Cicchetti, 1989), poor cognitive functioning and behavior problems (Eckenrode, Laird, & Doris, 1993), poor social skills and few friends, as well as negative and distorted self-concepts (Price, 1996). Most abused children do not become delinquent, criminal, or mentally ill, although this may be more likely (NRC, 1993). Low self-esteem and fearfulness often continue into adulthood. This group can be prone to depression, anxiety, anger, sexual difficulties, and alcohol and drug abuse (NRC, 1993). Although most abused children do not grow up to abuse children, the potential for perpetuating abuse is higher (USDHHS, 1999). And likewise, some abused deaf victims will become perpetrators themselves (Vernon & Rich, 1997). Many maltreated children are incredibly resilient, however—especially if they have been able to form an attachment to a supportive person, have help available, receive therapy, and experience good marital or love relationships (Kaufman & Zigler, 1987; Egeland, Jacobvitz, & Stroufe, 1988).

Abuse prevention and intervention programs will go a long way toward ameliorating any potential consequences. *No-Go-Tell* is an example of a well-known sexual abuse prevention curriculum for schools, designed by Elizabeth Krents and Dale Atkins at the Lexington Center for the Deaf in New York, in order to provide self-protection training to deaf and hard-of-hearing children (Sullivan, Brookhouser, & Scanlan, 2000). It teaches children what to watch for as well as teaches standard vocabulary to describe sexual abuse incidents that may have occurred. Achtzehn's (1987) *PACES: Preventing Abuse of Children through Education for Sexuality* has the same goal. Intervention programs have the intent of protecting the child, restraining the offender, and rehabilitating all involved parties, including the school or/and the family (Strand, 1991).

Unfortunately, there are no data on the effectiveness of prevention and intervention programs in preventing abuse or for effective post-abuse intervention. Sullivan and Knutson (1998) recommend careful screening and training of staff, providing staff support programs, and close monitoring and supervision of children to curtail sexual abuse in residential school settings, together with an external advocacy system for monitoring residential schools.

TREATMENT PROGRAMS

Deaf children in need of psychological treatment, particularly inpatient programs have few resources (see Chapter 2). Most treatment is provided by psychologists or school counselors within school settings, by mental health providers in private practice, or through structuring educational programs to meet the needs of the child as reflected in the IEP. Adequate communication with the deaf child becomes a critical factor in treatment success.

PSYCHOLOGICAL EVALUATION OF DEAF CHILDREN

Deaf children are tested frequently, starting with audiological assessments, intelligence and achievement testing, and psychosocial evaluations. Such testing is periodically repeated throughout the years, as required by IDEA legislation. This legislation specifies nondiscriminatory testing and requires that materials and procedures used for the evaluation and placement of special needs children be selected and administered in a manner that is neither culturally nor racially discriminating (Blennerhassett, 2000). The law further states that these materials and procedures must be administered in the language or mode of communication that the child uses. This means using oral communication and some form of sign communication/language, including ASL, or cued speech, depending on what the child is most comfortable with. Tests must be selected and administered in a manner that does not focus only on limitations or penalize deaf children for their linguistic difference (Lane, 1999; Lane, Hoffmeister, & Bahan, 1996). The child's strengths should be taken into account in the evaluation report.

Psychologists must obtain adequate training and knowledge of language issues, as these pertain to deaf children in order to objectively and accurately evaluate them. School psychologists who take a few sign language classes or attend inservice workshops are *not* qualified to evaluate deaf children (Blennerhassett, 2000). It takes far more training and experience to deal with the wide variation in which deaf children communicate and use language. If psychologists cannot match the linguistic and communication needs of the deaf child, they ethically should not proceed with the evaluation, since they could render an inaccurate picture of the deaf child's skills and abilities. This requires ongoing evaluation for each case, considering that each child is different.

However, communication and linguistic competence alone is not sufficient to assess deaf children. The National Association of State Directors of Special Education (NASDE) requires that psychologists be knowledgeable about the sociological and psychological aspects of deafness in addition to the linguistic and cultural factors related to deafness (Blennerhassett, 2000). Gallaudet University's clinical and school psychology programs (www.gallaudet.edu/psychology) and NTID/RIT's school psychology program (www.rit.edu/~schpsych) offer specialized training.

Language-appropriate testing for deaf children is an area ripe for research. More language-assessment tools for accurate evaluation of deaf children's language-specific processes are needed. There are no standard tests that examine fluency in ASL or its relation to academic and vocational achievement, as there are for fluency in spoken languages such as English.

This leads us to consider the challenge of discriminating language deficits from cognitive deficits when deaf children have varying levels of exposure to English. Many cognitive measures are heavily weighted in English. To assess cognitive skills in deaf children, psychologists who are sensitive to measurement issues should use multiple forms of assessment that include nonverbal measures. Braden (2001) divides those assessment approaches into four categories:

1. *Observations* are helpful for developing hypotheses regarding the deaf child's cognitive abilities. Psychologists must be cautious about the inferences they make from observations pending additional evidence.
2. *Interviews* provide a window for assessing the level of cognitive functioning within the parameters of dialogue between the psychologist and the child.
3. *Informal tests* are tests with no deaf norms, which can be utilized as a way of developing hypotheses about cognitive functioning for possible diagnosis and treatment. However, caution must be taken when using such tests due to reliability and validity concerns (see Chapter 9).
4. *Intelligence tests* are formal standardized tests that provide important information about an individual's functioning and ability levels. The use of nonverbal intelligence tests rather than verbal intelligence tests is recommended due to the limitations many deaf children have in accessing spoken language.

Information from these procedures should be combined into a total picture of the child's abilities that will lead to appropriate recommendations for educational placement and psychosocial development.

CONCLUSION

Generally, deaf and hearing children have the potential for similar developmental milestones, other things being equal. Early intervention programs can help parents learn optimal strategies for communicating with their deaf infants and promote positive psychosocial development. Social competence programs such as PATHS can benefit deaf children. Healthy identity development is facilitated when deaf children feel comfortable with being deaf and are exposed to deaf role models. More research into psychopathology in deaf children will facilitate appropriate treatment planning. In order to provide optimal assessment services, psychologists must be knowledgeable about psychological, linguistic, cultural, and social aspects of deafness and effectively communicate with deaf children.

SUGGESTED READINGS

Sheridan, M. (2001). *Inner Lives of Deaf Children: Interviews & Analysis.* Washington, DC: Gallaudet University Press.
   This book is about deaf children's social development and their formations of self-concepts. Deaf children between the ages 7 and 10 were interviewed. Each child comes from a unique background and uses different communication modes. Written by a social worker, this book provides rare insights into the minds of young deaf children, from their point of view.
Spencer, P., Erting, C., & Marschark, M. (2000). *The Deaf Child in the Family and at School.* Mahwah, NJ: Lawrence Erlbaum.
   This edited book contains contributions by noted authors that cover psycho-educational-social development of deaf children. It contains much useful information about family and school influences impacting on the deaf child that will facilitate optimal growth.

CHAPTER NINE

BEING A DEAF ADULT

Viewpoints from Psychology

*There are vastly more well-adjusted, psychologically
healthy, and effective deaf people than there are not.*
—Sussman and Brauer, 1999, p. 9

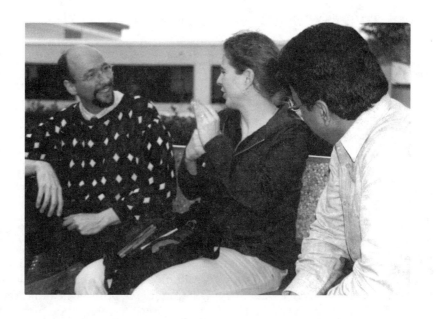

The stereotypical image of deaf people as a psychologically homogenous entity, limited in the ability to fully take advantage of the world around them, is changing. Recent psychology and deafness publications increasingly show the resilience, strengths, and capabilities exhibited by deaf adults in dealing with life. Their psychological functioning is influenced by innate factors, differences in familial and educational experiences, exposure to varied communication approaches, and other variables. Researchers, professionals working with deaf persons, and the general public are improving in their ability to recognize the variability in psychological functioning exhibited by deaf persons.

CHAPTER OBJECTIVES

This chapter explores the functioning of deaf adults using the lens provided by models of positive psychology, positive health, and wellness. The meaning of "normalcy" as applied to the deaf population will be analyzed. The roles of deaf identities and self-concept are highlighted as contributory factors to psychological well-being. The reader will be introduced to psychological assessment and mental health issues that are critical to appropriate service delivery.

POSITIVE PSYCHOLOGY AND POSITIVE HEALTH

The field of psychology is undergoing a transformation. Historically, psychology was preoccupied with negative, pathological, or problem-focused frames of reference such as mental illnesses or the inability of human beings to function as expected. For example, much work was done in the areas of psychopathology, negative emotions such as hostility and depression, and individual deficits (e.g., cognitive factors) that limited one's functional abilities. Starting in the 1940s and onward, luminaries such as Erich Fromm, Abraham Maslow, and Carl Rogers argued that the field of psychology was focusing too much on what the individual was doing wrong or on internal factors that hindered optimal adaptation to daily life, while ignoring the variables that enhance people's ability to actualize their potential in living "good" lives.

Recent publications indicate that positive psychology is now regaining momentum as psychologists start to examine biological, environmental, and cultural factors insofar as these separately and interactively influence positive development or optimal functioning (Sheldon & King, 2001; Seligman & Csikszentmihalyi, 2000). Seeman's (1989) model of positive health further specifies that optimal functioning is based on an organismic integration process that encompasses all of the person's behavioral subsystems: the biochemical, physiological, perceptual, cognitive, and interpersonal dimensions. Psychology's task, then, is to understand how these subsystems contribute to the positive psychological health of the individual and develop wellness models that focus on psychological growth.

THE DEAF ADULT:
PSYCHOLOGICAL PERSPECTIVES

Research findings have historically depicted deaf persons as being at risk for psychological problems (Marschark, 1993; Vernon & Andrews, 1990). The lack of hearing was blamed for problems in perception, cognition, and interpersonal functioning. In the early 1980s, psychologists such as Edna Levine, Allen Sussman, and Barbara Brauer suggested that it was time to move beyond these inimical and often invalid research findings and look at the survival strengths of deaf adults, many of whom were able to fashion satisfactory lives for themselves. Unfortunately, Sussman and Brauer (1999) observe that psychotherapists, and in turn, societies in general, still pathologize deafness and are hard put to describe healthy deaf personalities. Deaf adults too often encounter professionals who are inadequately informed regarding deafness, and therefore perpetuate the problems of inaccurate diagnoses. This occurs despite improvements in disseminating information to professionals on how to provide appropriate psychological evaluations of deaf adults (Brauer, Braden, Pollard, & Hardy-Braz, 1999; Leigh, Corbett, Gutman, & Morere, 1996; Pollard, 1998). Psychological evaluators must consider strengths and specific test factors (described in this chapter) in order to minimize negative and inaccurate interpretations for deaf clients. For psychotherapists to work effectively with deaf clients, using wellness models that focus on client assets and strengths in fashioning a positive adjustment to life is strongly recommended (Sussman & Brauer, 1999).

Normalcy: A Paradigm in Need of Clarification.   *Normal* is a highly pervasive word in U.S. society. Few realize that the idea of a "norm" entered the English language only as recently as the nineteenth century (Davis, 1995). Prior to that time, individuals were perceived as imperfect and different in some way as compared to an unattainable ideal of perfection. Today, *normal* is defined as synonymous with average intelligence or development. The implication is that the majority of the population is expected to fall within the standard bell-shaped curve that reflects probabilities. As such, being "average" or "normal" has become the yardstick as opposed to different, deviant, or abnormal characteristics.

Consequently, parents may have difficulty accepting their deaf child as someone who is "different" (Leigh, 1999a). Some will write about, for example, their deaf child becoming "a true hearing child" (Parents and Families of Natural Communication, Inc., 1998, p. 33), or being treated as such, as if being treated as a deaf child implies abnormality. If some of these deaf children end up not following typical hearing communication behaviors as adults, and rely instead on signed communication or use typical Deaf culture behavior such as tapping others to get their attention, they could at times be perceived as not quite normal (Davis, 1995; Lane; 1999; Pollard, 1998) or as objects of curiosity or pity.

Even though the typical hearing person may see deafness as not necessarily "normal," there are many deaf adults who see themselves as normal individuals who happen to be deaf. Davis (1995) argues that it is time to shift from the implicit hearing standard of normalcy to a standard of "differentness" as a part of the human condition. With this frame of reference, it is possible to view deaf people as part of the diversity spectrum that encompasses all human beings (Leigh, Corbett, Gutman, & Morere, 1996).

The Psychologically Healthy Deaf Adult.   A multitude of books (see the end of this chapter for a partial listing) and media publications, as well as improved television dissemination (including the CBS Sunday Morning presentation of *Sign City* on January 13 and 20, 2002, which showed the deaf people of Rochester, New York, going about their daily lives) have allowed the greater public to learn about the normal lives of deaf people. Many understand that deaf people are not necessarily objects of pity or curiosity, but rather people who are competent individuals, pretty much able to take care of themselves like most others. They are more or less capable of parenting deaf and hearing children like their hearing counterparts (Meadow-Orlans, 1997; Mohay, 2000; Preston, 1994; Swisher, 2000), and they hold down jobs. Barnartt and Christiansen (1996) present data that demonstrate the ongoing improvement of occupational status for deaf workers, even though deaf individuals continue to lag behind their hearing counterparts, particularly those who have not graduated from high school (see Chapters 2 and 10). Based on a national longitudinal survey of deaf and hard-of-hearing college graduates, most respondents were relatively successfully employed and satisfied with life (Schroedel & Geyer, 2000). In the intelligence domain, Braden (1994) reports on a meta-analysis of the literature that reinforces the similarity between deaf and hearing comparison groups in nonverbal intellectual functioning. Based on a lifetime of observations, Sussman and Brauer (1999) conclude that deaf adults have positive self-esteem, are comfortable with being deaf, can assert themselves, ask for help as needed, have effective interpersonal relationships and social skills, and demonstrate a positive zest for life. This happens despite the fact that many deaf adults often have had to deal with the stress of handling negative attitudes in facilitating communication access, as discussed in Chapter 11. Yes, there are deaf adults with problems in living, and we will discuss them when we cover mental health issues later in this chapter, but again, they are not ubiquitous.

Identity.   Very often, the word *deaf* appears when deaf adults are asked to describe themselves. *Deaf* (capital *D*) is a characteristic that a good number have internalized in formulating their self-representations or identities. People have different identities depending on their environment and what is most salient at any moment in time. These identities emerge through one's perceptions of similarities and differences in comparison with others, depending on attributes such as gender, ethnicity, occupation, educational level, cultural affiliation, and a host of other variables (Corker, 1996). The construction of these identities is created through the process of interaction within different social contexts—for example, the family, the school, the workplace, social settings, religious institutions, the sports arena, and so forth (Camilleri & Malewska-Peyre, 1997; Harter, 1997). Depending on the setting, people are parents or grandparents, teachers or students, congregants or religious leaders, and so on.

Identity constructs influence personal development (Waterman, 1992). Because of the recent increase in cultural diversity within the United States and other countries, interest in cultural or ethnic group membership and social identity has exploded (Sue & Sue, 1999). The goal of current research on the meaning of social identity and how it is measured is that of facilitating individual adjustment between and within cultural groups. What does this mean for deaf persons?

According to Corker (1996), deaf identity is not necessarily a core identity; rather, its development depends on the extent to which deafness is salient in one's daily life. If a deaf person is consistently exposed to Deaf culture—whether at school, within the family, or in social settings—the chances for identifying as a Deaf person increases. Those with less exposure may label themselves as *audiologically deaf, hearing impaired, hard of hearing,* or some other similar term (Leigh, 1999b). In the process of exploring how deaf identities develop and the implications for psychological health, researchers have noted that differences in the perceived quality of social experiences are related to one's social adjustment and identity as a person who is deaf (Leigh, 1999b; Stinson, Chase, & Kluwin, 1990). Generally, the stronger one's deaf identity, the more comfort there is in socializing with deaf peers.

Other researchers have taken advantage of different theoretical models to define deaf and hearing identities. Using a disability-based framework, Weinberg and Sterritt (1986) conceptualized hearing identity as able-bodied, deaf identity as disability-related, with dual identity reflecting identification with deaf and hearing peers. Dual identity was associated with more positive adjustment outcomes. Stinson and Kluwin (1996) used social orientation parameters in asking about socialization with deaf and with hearing peers, and with peers in general, in order to categorize one's social identity as deaf or hearing oriented. Using cluster analysis, Bat-Chava (2000) derived three identity categories—culturally hearing, culturally deaf, and bicultural, as based on four criterion variables related to communication and socialization: importance of signing, importance of speech, group identity, and attitudes toward deaf people.

Neil Glickman (1996a) explored cultural and racial identity stage development theories and developed a parallel model incorporating four different stages of deaf identity. In *Stage 1,* the culturally hearing stage, being deaf is seen as a medical condition or disability to be ameliorated, thereby minimizing the need for support services or sign language. Individuals adopt hearing ways of speaking, understanding, and behaving in ways that facilitate integration into hearing society. Those who typically fit this stage include late-onset deaf adults and oral deaf persons who grow up using spoken English, who interact primarily with hearing peers, and who may belong to organizations that advocate spoken language for deaf children. Since Glickman perceives this stage as reflecting some denial of deafness, he questions how psychologically healthy this stage is. *Stage 2,* which reflects cultural marginality, includes deaf persons who exist on the fringe of both Deaf and hearing cultures, unable to fully integrate into either. Close relationships with members of both groups are problematic. Deaf individuals in *Stage 3* immerse themselves within Deaf culture, identify as Deaf, and behave as they think authentic Deaf people are supposed to. Hearing values and deaf people with "hearing minds" who speak English are denigrated. In *Stage 4*, the bicultural stage, the deaf person can integrate the values of both hearing and Deaf cultures and positively relate with deaf and hearing people. In this stage, both ASL and English are respected.

Theoretically, the Stage 4 integrative stance reflects enhanced psychological health. Deaf individuals starting off in the culturally marginal stage may progress to the bicultural stage as the final one in the process of deaf identity development, whereas Deaf children of Deaf parents, who usually reflect pride in being Deaf and can demonstrate comfort in dealing with both Deaf and hearing worlds, typically assume a bicultural identity early on. Because not every deaf person starts at the first stage, progression through the various stages is not necessarily linear.

Glickman (1996a) developed the Deaf Identity Development Scale (DIDS), a 60-item measure that consists of four scales, each reflecting one of the stages just described. Follow-up studies indicate that the bicultural scale does not differentiate between deaf and hearing subjects (Fischer, 2000; Friedburg, 2000; Leigh, Marcus, Dobosh, & Allen, 1998). Social desirability may be a factor for both groups of subjects. As deaf people interact more often with hearing peers at work, through the Internet, or via other avenues, biculturalism is increasingly seen as socially desirable (Padden, 1998).

Taking another approach, Maxwell-McCaw (2001) developed deaf identity categories based on the acculturation model. This model posits that acculturation patterns for immigrants will vary according to the level of psychological (or internalized) identification with the culture of origin and the new host culture, as well as the degree of behavioral involvement and cultural competence in each culture. Paralleling this, Maxwell-McCaw theorizes that the acculturation patterns for deaf persons can vary in terms of the level of psychological identification with Deaf culture and with the culture of their hearing society and the extent to which they are behaviorally involved and culturally competent in each culture. To test this idea, she developed the Deaf Acculturation Scale (DAS) and demonstrated its reliability and validity with 3,070 deaf and hard-of-hearing adults. It is made up of two acculturation scales: a Deaf Acculturation Scale and a Hearing Acculturation Scale, each consisting of five subscales that are parallel to each other and measure acculturation across five domains covering psychological identification, cultural behaviors, cultural attitudes, cultural knowledge, and language competence related to deaf and hearing environments. Individuals can score as hearing acculturated (high scores in hearing acculturation and low scores in deaf acculturation), marginal (low scores in both hearing and deaf acculturation), deaf acculturated (high scores in deaf acculturation and low scores in hearing acculturation), and bicultural (high scores in both deaf and hearing acculturation). Maxwell-McCaw found that deaf acculturation and biculturalism were equally associated with higher self-esteem and satisfaction with life, more so than for those who were hearing acculturated. Marginalism was found to be the least adaptive of the four acculturation styles.

As this book emphasizes, the deaf community is increasingly multicultural. Identity formulations cannot ignore the ethnic dimension. In fact, Corker (1996) claims that ethnic identity takes precedence over deaf identity because of family influences in the early years. Those individuals to whom the deaf child is exposed depend very much on whom the family members interact with in daily life. Usually, these are members of the family's ethnic group. With increased exposure to deaf people in later years, one can expect an interactive effect between ethnic identity and deaf identity categorizations depending on the situation (Parasnis, 1996). The multicultural deaf person tends to integrate membership in at least four communities: the larger deaf community, the ethnic hearing community of origin, the ethnic deaf community, and the predominant majority community (Corbett, 1999; Wu & Grant, 1999). This requires altering behaviors to fit the specific community as explained by the alternation model, which focuses on code-switching or alternating behaviors appropriate to the cultural situation. Theoretically, the stress level would be lower than for the assimilation model, which requires giving up one culture (and identity) in order to assimilate into another (LaFromboise, Coleman, & Gerton, 1993). With the changing ethnic composition of the deaf community, the topic of cultural identities in deaf persons and their psychological adjustment is an area ripe for research, considering that 60 percent of the studies published in selected general psychology journals over a five-year period report ethnicity data (Case & Smith, 2000).

Self-Concept and Self-Esteem.   Researchers have long been interested in the self-concept or self-esteem of deaf people and how these might be influenced by relatively negative attitudes toward deafness. Both terms have often been used interchangeably in the literature, although their meanings differ (Harter, 1997). *Self-concept* is defined as a relatively stable cognitive structure that reflects subjective awareness of one's stable attributes such as beliefs, moods, intentions, and actions, or, in essence, self-perception or self-knowledge (Kagan, 1998). *Self-esteem* reflects positive or negative feelings about one's attributes and as such has a more emotional component (Kagan, 1998). These mental representations of the self regulate and influence psychological well-being (Harter, 1997).

Based on a review of studies covering self-concept and self-esteem continuing into the 1970s, Vernon and Andrews (1990) conclude that the self-concept of deaf people tends to be more negative than that of the general population. However, many studies from that period are generally not considered to be valid because of measurement issues (as mentioned in Chapter 1 and explained later in this chapter).

The theme emphasized in more recent studies is that self-perceptions (self-concept, self-esteem, self-image, etc.) of deaf adults vary depending on different factors. There have been numerous studies on the self-concept of deaf children and adolescents, but very few have focused on deaf adults. In a seminal meta-analysis of 42 empirical studies investigating self-esteem in deaf children, college students, and adults, mostly from the late 1970s through the early 1990s, Bat-Chava (1993) notes lower self-esteem in comparison to hearing people. Further scrutiny indicates that higher self-esteem in deaf adolescents and adults appears to be associated with several variables: having deaf parents, communicating with one's family using sign language, and using sign language in school (Bat-Chava, 1993, 1994, 2000; Desselle & Pearlmutter, 1997). Also, as mentioned earlier, higher self-esteem is associated with culturally deaf as well as bicultural identities in comparison to hearing or marginal identities (Bat-Chava, 2000; Maxwell-McCaw, 2001). These findings represent a significant change when one considers earlier studies such as Sussman's (1974), which noted lower self-esteem in those deaf adults who felt they did not speak well in contrast to deaf adults who described themselves as being able to communicate orally.

Bat-Chava (1993) interprets the current findings to mean that deaf people are not necessarily passive recipients of the majority's negative attitudes. Rather, they may adopt psychological mechanisms that facilitate positive self-esteem, such as comparing themselves with deaf peers and not with hearing peers, or valuing sign language and other deaf community attributes. Recent events—including the recognition of ASL, increased awareness that a Deaf culture exists, and the Gallaudet University Deaf President Now movement of 1988—had a profound influence in reshaping the self-perceptions of many deaf people in a more positive direction (Maxwell-McCaw, 2001).

Bat-Chava (1993) finds that the level of self-esteem in the studies she reviewed varied as a function of the measure, its format, and the way in which instructions were conveyed to research participants. Unmodified measures or written instructions (even if supplemented by sign language) resulted in lower self-esteem scores for deaf participants, whereas modified measures or instructions administered in sign language yielded similar scores for hearing and deaf participants. This leads directly to the consideration of psychological measurement issues and how these impact on the portrayal of deaf adults.

PSYCHOLOGICAL ASSESSMENT OF DEAF ADULTS

Psychological assessment is essentially a process in which individuals are evaluated for the purpose of describing behavior and obtaining a diagnosis that will lead to some type of intervention or recommendation for services (Braden, 2001). For deaf adults, these evaluations are usually requested or conducted by social or vocational service agencies to determine eligibility for social, vocational, or educational (remedial or postsecondary) services, to assess mental status and the capacity to take care of oneself, or to evaluate competency to stand trial (Braden, 2001). When deaf adults themselves request psychological assessments, this is usually because they are concerned about whether they have conditions such as learning disabilities or attention deficit disorders. There may also be medical concerns related to the aging process or some form of trauma that affects one's behavior (Braden, 2001).

As this book emphasizes, deaf adults differ from hearing counterparts to varying degrees in hearing acuity, communication method, linguistic use, cultural identity, and the presence of additional disabilities depending on etiology, among other things. These all influence how the psychological evaluation is conducted, which psychological tests are used, and how they are interpreted.

The Assessment Process.   Psychological evaluations typically involve observation of the client to determine behavioral characteristics; interviewing the client to obtain a history that covers information on medical, developmental, and past as well as current functioning; administering psychological instruments that will address the referral question; and interpreting the results. With the client's permission, information can also be requested from educational, medical, or social service institutions with which the client may have been involved.

Effectiveness of Psychological Tests.   Tests are selected depending on the purpose of the assessment (e.g., cognitive, socioemotional, vocational, or neuropsychological) and individual characteristics such as age, language and culture, and ability to understand questions and respond as required. No psychological evaluation can take place without checking whether tests consistently or *reliably* measure the constructs being assessed (e.g., depression, identity, or performance-based intelligence) and whether these tests are *valid* for different groups of people (i.e., they actually measure the constructs they are supposed to measure in those different groups).

Test Reliability.   Test reliability refers to the degree of stability, consistency, predictability, and accuracy of tests (Groth-Marnat, 1999). With good reliability, one can assume that a test score will not significantly change if the person is tested at different times, even though it is acknowledged that results will vary depending on mood, alertness, or problems in test administration. Usually, the variability is greater for personality measures than for ability measures such as academic achievement, aptitude, or intelligence.

Test Validity.   A test is valid when it accurately measures the construct or variable it is supposed to measure (Groth-Marnat, 1999). Establishing test validity is difficult, particularly when the constructs are abstract concepts, such as intelligence, anxiety, or creativity. For example, do items on an intelligence test actually reflect the test-taker's intelligence?
    Three main methods of establishing validity are as follows:

1. *Content validity* often involves comparing the new items with the content of similar tests, or checking that the items clearly reflect the skills or knowledge area being measured. For example, a test on handling money needs to match the person's actual skills in handling money.
2. *Criterion validity* is determined by comparing test scores with performance on a related measure, either at the same time for concurrent validity, or some time later, as in comparing test scores of job applicants with job status one year later, for predictive validity.

3. *Construct validity* reflects the extent to which a test actually measures a theoretical construct or trait. This requires analyzing the trait and how it should relate to other variables, and testing whether these relationships hold up. Good engineers should be able to obtain high scores on a test of spatial relationships, for example. This would indicate that the test actually reflects a construct necessary for good engineering.

Based on meta-analyses of test validity, a group of psychologists recently documented strong and compelling evidence of psychological test validity and its similarity to medical test validity (Meyer et al., 2001). They also demonstrated that distinct assessment methods provide unique sources of information in contributing to the picture of the client. Unfortunately, for individuals from different cultures and for deaf adults in general, reliability and validity continue to be thorny issues, as witnessed by the literature covering assessment of multicultural groups and people with special needs whose backgrounds differ from those groups on which tests were standardized (e.g., Groth-Marnat, 1999; Sandoval, Frisby, Geisinger, Scheuneman, & Grenier, 1998). When people with special needs are members of different cultural groups, interpretation of test results becomes that much more complicated.

The Use of Norms.   To evaluate and interpret the meaning of scores on a psychological test requires comparing these scores with test norms. Test norms are scores obtained by large numbers of individuals who represent the population being studied. One frequent difficulty is that different normative samples from the same large population group may result in different interpretations for any one score on specific tests because of lack of uniform representation within each sample (Mitrushina, Boone, & D'Elia, 1999), including differences in ethnic groups. Therefore tests such as the popularly used Wechsler Adult Intelligence Scales (WAIS) are increasingly incorporating norms that include members of different ethnic groups (Groth-Marnat, 1999).

Additionally, the WAIS III has mean scores for a sample of 30 deaf and hearing impaired adults, based on an ASL version of the WAIS III (Psychological Corporation, 1997). Tests often do not provide such data. Tests with deaf norms are believed to be more fair in that deaf individuals are compared to other deaf peers rather than hearing peers (Braden, 2001; Vernon & Andrews, 1990). This may be relevant for tests that tap into, for example, specific visual functioning abilities, which often result in deaf persons doing better than their hearing counterparts (Emmorey, 1998). Since deaf and hearing nonverbal intelligence norms do not differ significantly, Braden (2001) argues that deaf norms are unnecessary for nonverbal intelligence tests but are more appropriate for academic achievement tests. If a deaf woman reads better than most deaf people, and her reading level is comparable to the average hearing reader, we can infer that her English comprehension is exceptionally adequate considering the circumstances and make relevant recommendations.

Linguistic and Communication Factors.   Knowing the deaf adult's linguistic and communication preferences will facilitate test selection and administration with the goal of understanding the person's current functioning. Responses based on the deaf person's "best language" or primary mode of communication will also more accurately reflect individual strengths as opposed to deficiencies or weaknesses (Braden, 1994; Leigh, Corbett, Gutman, & Morere, 1996). The use of verbal (e.g., English) measures of intellectual functioning, memory, and personality are most often inappropriate unless reading and writing test scores provide evidence of adequate English proficiency (Freeman, 1989), even if the person prefers spoken language, signed English, or some combination of sign and speech. Reading scores generally tend to be slightly below the fourth-grade range for 17- and 18-year-old students (Johnson, 2001), though the range of verbal language competency may be broad (Johnson, 2001; Marschark, 1993).

On the other side of the coin, it can be important to assess the deaf adult's competency in English language usage (whether it is the first or second language), depending on the referral question. For any deaf adult, including ASL users, the clinician must weigh the need for careful evaluation of a deaf person's skills in verbal (i.e., English) information against the possibility of creating misleading impressions about the client's cognitive limitations because of verbal difficulties (Braden, 2001). Evidence of competency in other domains of intelligence and achievement should be emphasized. Generally, for cognitive assessment, language-reduced measures meeting one's language level are most appropriate.

Personality instruments often are at the sixth-grade or higher levels. They can have a number of items with linguistic properties that might be misinterpreted by deaf persons for whom ASL rather than English is the first or primary language (Bradley-Johnson & Evans, 1991; Freeman, 1989). For example, if an item asks about the potential for *carrying out some plan of action*, this might mistakenly be interpreted as *carrying* something instead of *doing* something because of unfamiliarity with the idiomatic use of "carrying out a plan."

Revising or Translating Tests.   Measures that are either linguistically revised or translated into ASL to meet the needs of deaf adults must be reassessed for reliability and validity to gauge if the constructs being measured are still being tapped, since linguistic changes can result in changes in the meaning of items (e.g., Brauer, 1993; Cohen & Jones, 1990; Leigh, Robins, & Welkowitz, 1988). For example, if the test item containing the phrase *carrying out a plan* is linguistically rephrased as *doing something planned,* the extent to which both phrases convey exactly the same meaning must be evaluated.

For those contemplating videotaped ASL translations of written measures, the goal is to ensure translation equivalence. This covers not only linguistic equivalence but also conceptual and functional equivalence (meaning that a construct can be applied meaningfully for both ASL and non-ASL users) (Brauer, 1993; Hui & Triandis, 1985).

To maximize equivalence, criteria have been developed for developing ASL translations of written measures to ensure that item meanings have not been altered and that equivalency of items is maintained (Brauer, 1993; Cohen & Jones, 1990; Crowe, 2002). These criteria include back-translation procedures that involve translating English into ASL and then back into English. This can be a challenging process. As cited in Cohen and Jones (1990, p. 46), *It's alright for my child to have an imaginary friend* could be translated using ASL signs for fantasy, pretend, or not real to represent the imaginary friend concept. However, after back-translation into English, the sentence became: *It's ok if my child doesn't have any real friends.* To correct for the lack of conceptual equivalence, signs for *imagine + envision + friend* can be incorporated.

There have been suggestions that deaf adults would be better served with the use of ASL-based psychological measures developed specifically for ASL users, based more on the deaf experience (McGhee, 1996). This would avoid the pitfalls of translations. None have been developed as of yet.

Using Sign Language Interpreters in Assessment.   The consequences of communication problems during the psychological evaluation can result in invalid conclusions about individual functioning. Therefore, it is best to check with the deaf client or referring agency to ascertain communication needs and make appropriate arrangements. If the psychological evaluator is not a fluent signer, or is not easily understood by the client, certified sign language or oral interpreters should be called in as needed. Direct signing or interpreted administration is preferable to poorly articulated (spoken), written, or gesturally based communication (Braden, 1994; 2001; Leigh, Corbett, Gutman, & Morere, 1996). Certified interpreters are trained to assess the client's communication needs, adjust communication to suit client preferences, provide ongoing English-ASL translations, and maintain confidentiality. Administering psychological measures with the use of a sign-language interpreter carries some risk because of the lack of standard ASL procedures that could compromise test integrity and test results. Even if certified, interpreters may vary in how they interpret test instructions without a standard protocol. In mental status evaluations of deaf individuals (discussed later), distinguishing ASL variations from psychotic distortions requires specialized mental health training, which certified interpreters do not necessarily have (Brauer, Braden, Pollard, & Hardy-Braz, 1998). The field lacks methodologically sound studies that indicate whether the use of interpreters is equivalent to direct signing with the client in assessment situations (Braden, 2001).

Socioemotional Assessment Issues.   The personalities of deaf adults have historically been portrayed as causing significant problems in daily functioning due to immaturity, egocentrism, impulsivity, concreteness, and similar negative appellations (e.g., Lane, 1999; Levine, 1981; Pollard, 1992–93; Vernon & Andrews, 1990). Professionals now know that the psychological functioning of deaf clients in mental health agencies is not the same as that of the psychologically healthy deaf adult (Lane, Hoffmeister, & Bahan, 1996; Pollard, 1992–93). Considering the fact that most socioemotional measures are English based, their use in differentiating deaf individuals with varying levels of psychological problems and psychopathology from the "normal" deaf adult requires understanding of the psychometric and linguistic issues that we have already described. Recent research in this area is sorely lacking compared to the relative wealth of studies up until the 1970s (as reported in Moores, 2001a). Nonetheless, there have been some relatively recent reliability and validity investigations of popular socioemotional measures using deaf adults whose English is adequate for these measures.

Reliability and content validity problems were identified in the Sixteen Personality Factor Questionnaire (16PF), which measures various personality traits and requires good English (Jacobs, 1987). The linguistic revision of the popular Beck Depression Inventory (BDI) resulted in lower internal consistencies (reliability) than those reported for normal hearing samples (Leigh, Robins, & Welkowitz, 1988; Watt & Davis, 1991). Interestingly, in a small sample of depressed deaf and hard-of-hearing adults, those with more severe depression diagnoses assigned by therapists had higher revised BDI scores than those with less severe diagnoses (Leigh & Anthony, 1999). Using a deaf college student sample, the reliability (internal consistency) of the new BDI-II, which did not require revision due to improvement in item clarity, was .88, which is good (Leigh & Anthony-Tolbert, 2001). Brauer (1993) found her ASL translation of the MMPI (Minnesota Multiphasic Personality Inventory) to be psychometrically feasible. The newer MMPI-2 has been translated into ASL but requires validation studies to evaluate its clinical usefulness (Brauer, Braden, Pollard, & Hardy-Braz, 1998).

Projective methods are an alternative procedure for assessing socioemotional functioning or personality in deaf adults. These are designed to elicit information on how one responds to ambiguous stimuli. The use of drawings—such as the Draw-a-Person test, the House-Tree-Person test, and the Kinetic Family Drawing test—are among the most popular of the projective techniques because they can be done quickly and are useful for global ratings of socioemotional functioning despite the fact that questions about validity persist (Groth-Marnat, 1999; Handler, 1996). A pilot study of the House-Tree-Person test using a small sample of deaf adults demonstrated encouraging reliability and validity results (Ouellette, 1988).

Other frequently used projective tools include the Thematic Apperception Test (TAT) and the Rorschach Inkblot Test. Both instruments require that the examiner write down responses to test items made by the examinee. For this reason, examiner bias becomes a problem when responses are translated from ASL to English or filtered through a sign-language interpreter before being written down, heightening the danger of inaccuracies. Schwartz, Mebane, and Malony (1990) compared signed and written administrations for a small group of deaf adults with college-level education who were administered the Rorschach. They concluded that signed administration was preferable to the subjects writing responses, since the latter could lead to underreporting of several Rorschach variables. They noted visual-perceptual differences between deaf and hearing persons and provided deaf sample mean scores for the variables investigated. Based on experience, Siedlecki (1999) considers the Rorschach useful for deaf psychiatric patients with limited ASL skills, and recommends additional research.

Computer-Assisted Assessments.   Psychological assessment has been strongly influenced by the increased use of computerized assessment, which enhances efficiency through rapid scoring, reduction in the length of face-to-face time needed between evaluator and client, and quick generation of explanations for results (Groth-Marnat, 1999). Although the general assumption is that these computerized tests are equally as valid as paper-and-pencil tests, not every test has been subjected to empirically based research for verifying validity (Groth-Marnat, 1999).

Psychological assessments of deaf adults often include standard computerized tests, yet research into their validity and reliability for a deaf population is lacking. Since the effectiveness of interactive video technology for surveying deaf ASL users has been demonstrated (Lipton & Goldstein 1997), a computerized interactive video version of a psychiatric diagnostic interview measure translated into ASL was developed (Eckhardt, Steinberg, Lipton, Montoya, & Goldstein, 1999). The assumption that this measure would elicit valid diagnoses was tested by comparing these diagnoses obtained from the self-administered ASL version with those obtained from a face-to-face clinician ASL-administered version of the same instrument. The investigators found that some diagnostic sections demonstrated greater reliablilty than others—specifically, the sections on depression and alcohol abuse (Eckhardt, Goldstein, Montoya, Steinberg, under review). More work on this type of measure is needed.

Advances in Neuropsychology.   Neuropsychology involves the study of brain-behavior relationships that are elicited through the use of neuropsychological test batteries (Groth-Marnat, 2000). Behavioral responses to test items help neuropsychologists extrapolate information about brain functioning and how it influences a person's ability to perform certain tasks. There is evidence that deaf persons demonstrate different cortical functions in comparison to hearing peers, basically because they rely more on vision than audition (e.g., Corina, 1998; Levanen, Jourmaki, & Hari, 1998; Neville et al., 1998; Nishimura et al., 1999).

The ability to create computer-based stimuli for research projects has made it possible to create new avenues for exploring how deaf people process information neuropsychologically. For example, Emmorey, Kosslyn, and Bellugi (1993) used computer-generated visual imagery tasks to demonstrate that using a visual-spatial language from an early age may affect the way the brain develops for particular visual imagery tasks. Additionally, technological innovations in brain scanning capabilities will advance the understanding of how the brain becomes activated in response to various stimuli. Recent studies in this area have been initiated. To cite a few, Bavelier and colleagues (2000) found more activation of the visual motion processing area of the middle temporal visual area in their deaf subjects compared to hearing subjects with the use of functional magnetic resonance imaging (fMRI). In a magnetoencephalograpy (MEG) study of sign-language processing, results indicated that within specific brain regions, neuromagnetic activity differed for deaf signers and hearing nonsigners (Levanen, Uutela, Salenius, & Hari, 2001). In another preliminary MEG investigation, Baldwin (2001) concluded that the auditory cortex showed activation for functions other than hearing in deaf-signing people. This did not happen with hearing nonsigning individuals. These findings and more will enhance the ability to sharpen neuropsychological assessment tools and in this way contribute to the understanding of the cognitive functioning of deaf adults.

Mental Status Examinations.   Mental status exams are observations and interviews conducted by qualified mental health service providers in order to assess one's current cognitive, emotional, and interactive functioning for psychiatric diagnosis purposes (Trzepacz & Baker, 1993). To avoid misdiagnosis, assessing the mental status of deaf adults requires special considerations, including communication skills and an awareness of the day-to-day realities of deaf persons (Pollard, 1998). Behavior such as flailing hands or hysterical outbursts have been cited as confirming evidence for psychiatric diagnoses when in fact such behavior may represent frantic attempts to communicate in situations where the deaf adult is feeling very misunderstood. Certified sign-language interpreters can facilitate accurate diagnosis if they are trained in mental health interpreting and can accurately convey, for example, psychotic productions within ASL discourse. However, the reality is that deaf people in need of mental health services are typically underserved because of communication difficulties and the small number of mental health service providers who are linguistically and culturally competent in diagnosing and dealing with deaf adults (Morton & Christensen, 2000; Steinberg, Loew, & Sullivan, 1999).

PSYCHOPATHOLOGY

Prevalence

Deaf adults are affected by mental health problems, just as the rest of humankind is (Pollard, 1998; Robinson, 1978). Using figures extrapolated from current gross estimates, Dew (1999) projects that approximately 687,951 Americans with hearing loss have psychiatric disabilities. If one adds those with less severe forms of mental illness who can benefit from mental health interventions, the numbers would climb. Even though the percentage of deaf clients per se who actually receive mental health services continues to be a very low percentage of those in need of such services (Pollard, 1998; Vernon, 1983), current levels of service have improved due to the increase in trained clinicians, as noted in Chapter 1.

   Based on previous reviews of epidemiological studies and clinical observations, the general perception is that the prevalence rates for deaf adults with different psychiatric diagnoses appear to be quite similar to those for hearing adults (Pollard, 1994, 1998; Robinson, 1978; Vernon & Andrews, 1990). The most recent epidemiological statistics on psychiatric diagnoses for deaf and hard-of-hearing persons are from Pollard's (1994, 1998) study of public mental health records in Rochester, New York, which boasts a large deaf population. His findings confirm the similarity of both deaf and hearing samples for psychiatric diagnosis rates related to adjustment, mood, organicity, psychosis, anxiety, and personality. There were some differences, however. Specifically, the proportion of substance abuse disorders was significantly lower for the deaf and hard-of-hearing sample. Also, the range of diagnoses was restricted. This means that the less common psychiatric disorders were less frequently diagnosed. Additionally, deferred or missing diagnoses were more frequent. Pollard does not consider this to represent real differences in the prevalence of psychiatric disorders. Instead, he attributes these differences to clinician error based on unfamiliarity with deaf clients as well as differences in the way these clients use mental health services. As mentioned in the mental status examination section, experienced mental health clinicians who confront communication barriers with deaf clients are not as able to do thorough diagnostic interviews, even with sign-language interpreters, unless they have some knowledge of how deaf people communicate and view the world. In the case of psychiatric disorders such as schizophrenia, a thorough understanding of deaf ways of communicating will facilitate the recognition of language atypicalities in the signing of deaf persons that can help clinicians do accurate diagnoses (Trumbetta, Bonvillian, Siedlecki, & Haskins, 2001).

Clinician error may also be a factor in the higher mental retardation rates found with this sample (Pollard, 1994, 1998; Vernon & Andrews, 1990). Misdiagnosis of mental retardation can be attributed in part to inappropriate use of verbal intelligence measures, a problem that continues to this day (Leigh, Corbett, Gutman, & Morere, 1996; Vernon & Andrews, 1990). However, there is an increased risk for mental retardation, as well as neurological impairment and developmental disorders associated with *some* etiologies for deafness (keeping in mind that this risk does not hold for many etiologies that may cause deafness).

Substance abuse diagnoses, including alcohol and chemical dependency, may be underreported (Guthman, Sandberg, & Dickinson, 1999; Pollard, 1998). The desire of the deaf community to present a positive image may mask the true level of substance abuse. This is also compounded by limited access to information, such as televised public service announcements that are not captioned, or prevention curricula in mainstream education programs, for example. Also, there are fears about "coming out" in the deaf community because of small community dynamics where "everyone knows everyone." Guthman, Lybarger, and Sandberg (1993) note that a significant proportion of deaf and hard-of-hearing clients exhibit dual diagnoses of substance abuse and psychiatric conditions in the Minnesota Chemical Dependency Program for Deaf and Hard of Hearing Individuals, the best-known such program in the United States. Such dual diagnoses make it easier to identify those in need of treatment, but access to treatment continues to be difficult due to scarce resources (Guthman, Sandberg, & Dickinson, 1999; Schonbeck, 2000).

Deaf survivors of sexual abuse "have been largely invisible" (Burke, Gutman, & Dobosh, 1999, p. 279). Based on evidence suggesting that children with disabilities may be at higher risk for such abuse (see Chapter 8), available information suggests that the incidence figures may be high for deaf persons in comparison to the general population. Sexual abuse is generally known to result in long-term emotional symptoms. One study reveals that sexually abused deaf adults report symptoms similarly to hearing counterparts (Dobosh, 1996, as cited in Burke, Gutman, & Dobosh, 1999).

Service Delivery

Specialized mental health services for deaf persons were nonexistent before 1955 (Altshuler, 1969). Since that time, the number of mental health service programs that have professionals trained to work with deaf individuals has grown (Pollard, 1992–93). Neil Glickman, cofounder of the Mental Health Unit for Deaf People at Westborough State Hospital in central Massachusetts, estimates that there are between 12 and 15 inpatient units for deaf patients in the United States today, including his unit (Schonbeck, 2000) and facilities such as Dorothea Dix Hospital in North Carolina, Rockland Psychiatric Center in New York, Springfield State Hospital Center in Maryland, St Elizabeth's Hospital in Washington, DC, and Western State Hospital in Virginia (Wax, Haskins, Ramirez, & Savoy-McAdory, 2001). Typically, these units have 18 beds and waiting lists.

Although there are many mental health outpatient clinics advertising services for deaf clients, as indicated in Morton and Christensen's (2000) resource directory of mental health services for deaf people, these are located mostly on the East and West coasts. Most areas continue to be underserved and accessibility to community mental health clinics serving local communities is limited. Additionally, Pollard (1994) considers the use of small community mental health centers specializing in deaf clients to be discriminatory, even though they do provide valuable services. In part, this is because these clients are not referred to larger centers with more comprehensive services that are available to the general public, such as staff psychiatrists on site, or different programs that match individual treatment needs by offering different therapy options, including medication, various types of individual psychotherapy approaches, family/group therapy, day treatment, and evening activities, to name a few. The low incidence of deaf persons makes it difficult for general mental health clinics to recognize the need for accommodations such as a TTY (teletypewriter) to communicate directly with deaf clients or using relay services, which exist in every state to facilitate communication between telephone users and TTY users. Cost factors complicate the use of sign-language or oral interpreters (see Chapters 10 and 11).

Disseminating information about accommodations can be facilitated by the use of meetings, such as the October 2000 conference for mental health agencies throughout New York state that was set up with the goal of improving equal access (Leigh, 2000). Additionally Myers (1995) developed a standards of care manual illustrating how mental health centers can be culturally and functionally accessible with the addition of visual emergency alert systems, signing staff, and TTY setups, to name a few.

Psychotherapy approaches include psychoanalysis, Eriksonian therapy, cognitive-behavioral therapy, humanistic-oriented therapy, and clinical hypnosis, among others. Sussman and Brauer (1999) emphasize that being deaf does not preclude the use of any of these approaches. It is crucial to recognize that therapeutic approaches, in order to be culturally affirmative and empowering for individuals and families, must be matched to individual needs, sociocultural factors, and individual communication requirements, whether the person is deaf or hearing (Glickman, 1996b; Pollard, 1998; Sussman & Brauer, 1999). Relying on medication alone, although tempting when there are communication problems, is not sufficient in most cases without psychotherapy to reinforce emotional self-regulation and more positive ways of functioning.

Deaf adult perceptions of mental health service delivery can provide insight into areas in need of improvement. Steinberg, Loew, and Sullivan (1999) interviewed deaf adults about their beliefs and attitudes regarding mental health. They report that communication issues were seen as central to mental health, with respondents recognizing that effective service delivery is facilitated when communication barriers are dealt with appropriately. Many do anticipate communication barriers, and prefer signing mental health personnel for direct communication. However, respondents are generally willing to work with sign-language interpreters but were concerned about the ways in which interpreters might convey information that would facilitate diagnosis and therapy. As Pollard (1998) indicates, how these interpreters may affect the psychotherapy process and outcome continues to be subject to debate. The presence of a third party (the interpreter) in situations privy to confidentiality and emotions will alter psychotherapy dynamics (Harvey, 1989; Pollard, 1998; Stansfield & Veltri, 1987; Turner, Klein, & Kitson, 2000). When psychotherapists get training in how to handle interpreter influences during the course of psychotherapy, they can use these influences to facilitate the process of therapy (Harvey, 1989). Additionally, specialist training in mental health interpreting will minimize the potential for misrepresenting the statements made by deaf adults.

Diversity

Because of the increasing multicultural nature of the deaf population in the United States, mental health service delivery to deaf persons must take the ethnic dimension into account. It is known that deaf persons who have received public mental health services are less likely than hearing persons to be from racial/ethnic minority groups (Pollard, 1994; Trybus, 1983). The lack of cultural sensitivity and the presence of racism, either conscious or unconscious, on the part of service providers as well as the negative implications of being labeled as one in need of "mental health services" detracts from the feeling of safety and support that mental health professionals would like to convey to clients (Corbett, 1999).

Professionals should examine their racial psychohistory in order to understand their attitudes toward their own and other race/ethnic groups (Corbett, 1999). This will help them to work productively with deaf persons of diverse cultural backgrounds. Such a process represents the first step toward cultural sensitivity and, in turn, cultural competence. Cultural competence includes awareness not only of Deaf culture, but also the deaf person's culture of origin, in order to provide culturally appropriate mental health treatment. Corbett (1999), Hernandez (1999),

Wu and Grant (1999), and Eldredge (1999) respectively have written about appropriate mental health interventions for deaf persons with African American, Latino, Asian American, and American Indian backgrounds.

CONCLUSION

Deaf adults run the gamut from those who are psychologically healthy, with positive self-perceptions and strong identities, to those who struggle with psychopathology. Positive psychology encourages one to look at the strengths of those individuals and their ability to manage in a complex world, while taking into account areas where they need support or help as well. As noted in Chapter 1, mental health, psychology, and research training programs specializing in deaf populations are now graduating professionals who are well prepared to advance the understanding of the psychological make-up of deaf adults and improve service delivery to this population. This understanding will be enhanced by the addition of researchers who are deaf and trained to critically examine the ways in which psychological constructs are applied to deaf populations.

SELECTED BOOKS ABOUT DEAF PEOPLE

Deaf in America: Voices from a Culture (Padden & Humphries, 1988). Cambridge, MA: Harvard University Press.

Deaf Persons in the Arts and Sciences (Lang & Meath-Lang, 1995). Westport, CT: Greenwood Press.

A Journey into the Deaf-World (Lane, Hoffmeister, & Bahan, 1996). San Diego, CA: Dawn Sign Press.

Lessons in Laughter: The Autobiography of a Deaf Actor (Bragg & Bergman, 1989). Washington, DC: Gallaudet University Press.

Orchid of the Bayou: A Deaf Woman Faces Blindness (Carroll & Fischer, 2001). Washington, DC: Gallaudet University Press.

A Phone of Our Own (Lang, 2000). Washington, DC: Gallaudet University Press.

Silent Alarm: On the Edge with a Deaf EMT (Schrader, 1995). Washington, DC: Gallaudet University Press.

Sounds Like Home: Growing Up Black and Deaf in the South (Wright, 1999). Washington, DC: Gallaudet University Press.

Train Go Sorry: Inside a Deaf World (Cohen, 1994). Boston: Houghton Mifflin.

Voices of the Oral Deaf (Reisler, 2002). Jefferson, NC: McFarland.

What's That Pig Outdoors: A Memoir of Deafness (Kisor, 1990). New York: Hill and Wang.

When the Phone Rings, My Bed Shakes (Zazove, 1993). Washington, DC: Gallaudet University Press.

CHAPTER TEN

BEING A DEAF ADULT

Viewpoints from Sociology

In a variety of ways, Deaf people have accumulated a set of knowledge about themselves in the face of the larger society's understanding—or misunderstanding—of them. They have found ways to define and express themselves through their rituals, tales, performances, and everyday social encounters.
—Padden and Humphries, 1988, p. 11

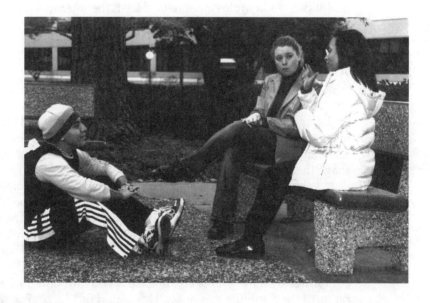

How do deaf people live their lives as part of a larger society? Their collective consciousness and broadly shared understandings have served as a basis for their coming together as a sociological entity, even taking into account the heterogeneity within this group. Communities of deaf people have been documented since at least the 1700s (Van Cleve & Crouch, 1989). When deaf persons come together, they do not feel weighted down by inadequacy. Rather, throughout time they have been able to internalize a dynamic sense of identity and comfort in themselves as a minority group with their own traditions and organizations. The 1988 Deaf President Now movement (see Chapter 1) highlighted the coming of age of the deaf community as a proud sociopolitical entity (Christiansen & Barnartt, 1995).

CHAPTER OBJECTIVES

This chapter briefly outlines sociological perspectives of the deaf community. It explores the role of the Deaf President Now movement in influencing the deaf community's sociopolitical evolution. The chapter then presents information on various deaf organizations, their roles in the lives of deaf people, and the political context for some of these organizations. It is important to recognize that the deaf community, as a microcosm of society at large, is not immune to sociocultural and technology changes. Those will be described as the text looks at deaf clubs and other avenues for socialization, deaf venues for athletic and religious activities, and health care and employment issues. Last, the interaction of deaf persons with the legal system is explored.

SOCIOLOGICAL PERSPECTIVES OF THE DEAF COMMUNITY

Sociology involves the study of how humans interact, and the evolving values and ideas that form the basis of these interactions. Both the medical/disability and sociolinguistic/cultural models (see Chapter 2) have sociological elements that shape the self-perceptions of groups of deaf people.

Within the medical model, the sociological implication is that the deaf person needs to accommodate to the larger hearing society in the interest of *better* social relationships with hearing peers. This requires changing the nature of the hearing loss by altering or minimizing it through the use of speech lessons, auditory training, and technology assistance such as listening devices. This model reinforces the concept that deaf individuals (or individuals with disabilities) rely on professional authorities with the goal of creating a pathway to some sort of recovery or amelioration of the disabling condition. This is part of a larger framework in which these authorities sometimes impose a benevolent paternalism (tendency to protect) on those who differ, who appear unable to fend for themselves, or who are "a disturbance to society" (Malzkuhn, 1994, p. 781). According to Lane (1996, 1997), when professionals with vested interests take on the mantle of paternalism, it becomes very difficult for deaf persons to throw off this paternalistic shield and take charge of their own lives. Sociologically, this creates the notion that the deaf person who "overcomes" deafness is more acceptable in society. However, to give the medical model its due, there are many deaf individuals who use professional help well and function very independently in hearing society with effective compensatory tools, even when they or those around them perceive deafness as a significant disability (e.g., Oberkotter, 1990).

In exploring the sociopolitical implications of disability definitions, activists are challenging the notion that disability is an individual problem (Lane, 1997; Mackelprang & Salsgiver, 1999; Olkin, 1999; Shapiro, 1993). From their perspective, society's typically negative attitude toward people with disabilities and its failure to accommodate them by enhancing environmental access has created the problem of disability. Sociologically, instead of welcoming individuals with disabilities as individuals with different notions of environmental access, society generally sees them as problems. In explaining this phenomenon further, Olkin (1999) points out that people without disabilities cite physical limitations as major problems for people with disabilities, whereas people with disabilities themselves tend to focus on social barriers and negative attitudes. In the case of culturally Deaf people, being Deaf has very little to do with one's ears. For these individuals, being Deaf means enhancing visual access. If society cooperates in enhancing visual access, social barriers will then be eliminated. Since deaf persons know what they need in order to manage daily lives, it is they, not the professionals who "serve" them, who are the ultimate authorities on their needs. (See Chapter 11 for additional discussion.)

For these reasons, many deaf people see themselves as a minority group, struggling to gain equal opportunity with nondisabled citizens. Increasingly, this group is defined more as a sociolinguistic group of people who are culturally Deaf and less as individuals with disabilities. Through their language, cultural traditions, and organizations, they have coalesced into a community of people, many of whom see deafness as part of the spectrum of diversity. Together with other deaf and hard-of-hearing people who do not identify with Deaf culture, they have created social and political momentum in critical arenas. For example, they work together to fight for parity in civil rights, access to optimal educational environments for deaf children, upward mobility in employment, and communication access (including interpreter services, functional equivalence in access to telecommunication, etc.). The implications of the 1988 Deaf President Now (DPN) movement go beyond the recognition that a deaf person could successfully take the helm of Gallaudet University.

DEAF PRESIDENT NOW: IMPLICATIONS FOR THE DEAF COMMUNITY

During the 1988 DPN movement at Gallaudet University, the only liberal arts university for deaf students, the Board of Trustees' choice of a hearing rather than a deaf candidate to head Gallaudet sparked a campuswide uprising against what

Schein (1989, p. 4) termed "a prejudice dramatized by the university's own board of directors." Those who participated in the uprising wanted to validate the inherent capabilities of qualified deaf candidates as a means of counteracting the traditionally low expectations held of them by hearing decision makers (Christiansen & Barnartt, 1995; Gannon, 1989; Schein, 1989; Shapiro, 1993). Their collective action took the needs of deaf people out of the disability framework and reframed these as a civil rights issue (Barnartt & Scotch, 2001).

The ability of deaf persons, both within Gallaudet University and throughout the nation, to get information, communicate with each other, and collaborate as a community during this movement was enhanced by demographic, social, and technological influences (Bateman, 1994; Christiansen & Barnartt, 1995). The 1964–65 rubella epidemic swelled the ranks of deaf people. Sign-language interpreting changed from the stop-gap measure of using family members or friends to a professional service. This allowed deaf people the opportunity to understand and participate when interacting with hearing persons in schools, on the job, and with medical and other service providers. Technology, too, played a prominent role. In the 1970s and 1980s, television captioning drastically increased the amount of information deaf people could access (Bateman, 1994). Deaf people were more directly exposed to media portrayals of groups fighting for self-determination. This heightened their sense of unfair treatment and oppression when being continually passed over for increased employment and policy-making responsibilities. Additionally, instantaneous communication was now possible due to the proliferation of text telephones (TTYs) (Lang, 2000), which provided deaf people with access to telephone communication. Previously, the major means of communication had been via face-to-face and mail contact.

Through widespread media publicity, DPN awoke the nation and the world to the existence of a vibrant deaf community and increased the awareness of U.S. society regarding the needs of deaf people. As Jankowski (1997, p. 131) states, "Indeed, for Deaf people, a victory meant the creation of a new image. A new vision for Deaf people and the world watching them was that indeed, Deaf people 'can.'" This translated into more positive self-images and increased feelings of empowerment.

The political involvement of deaf people began in the late 1800s, when the National Association of the Deaf (NAD) was organized (Gannon, 1981; Jankowski, 1997; Schein, 1989). There were intermittent periods of effective political activity, but after DPN, the political acumen and strengths built up by the NAD and other deaf organizations came of age as more deaf people learned to capitalize on the political process to campaign for a variety of goals and objectives. More frequently, they engaged in political action (Bateman, 1994). Various protests were held to emphasize the need for additional deaf administrators, teachers, and staff at residential schools throughout the country, to defend ASL usage, to lobby for the use of deaf instead of hearing actors for deaf roles in films, and to fight for emergency information captioning on TV stations (Christiansen & Barnartt, 1995; Jankowski, 1997). Deaf groups gained more influence in shaping social policy to incorporate barrier-free environments, most notably with reference to the Americans with Disabilities Act of 1990 and the Telecommunications Act of 1996, among others.

Sociopolitically, in the eyes of deaf people, the most important thing about these laws (which legislated different types of accommodations) is that society acknowledges their right to the various types of access enjoyed by the majority society. Now, legislators and others are more willing to work politically both with deaf organizations and with organizations of people with disabilities. For example, in order to win support from both the deaf community and groups of people with disabilities, sponsors of the Telecommunications Act of 1996 agreed that provisions mandating the accessibility of telecommunications for all people with disabilities would be included in the act (A. Sonnenstrahl, personal communication, September 18, 2001).

However, the struggle continues. Mandating accommodations does not necessarily guarantee their implementation. Architectural accommodations for individuals with mobility disabilities involve a one-time cost, but communication accessibility requires ongoing economic support. This becomes a disincentive that can easily engender "hidden discrimination." Proving that it exists is no easy task. The amount of money devoted to attempts to "eliminate" deafness remains greater than the amount spent to ensure equal access for deaf persons. For example, more funds are directed toward a cure for deafness than toward enhancing accessibility of 9-1-1 emergency centers for deaf persons. This requires the installation of TTYs and the ongoing training of new personnel to respond appropriately to emergency TTY calls. Limited 9-1-1 center TTY accessibility is due in part to the small number of deaf people in various locations, but the implication is that their lives are that much less valued.

To cite another example, because of cost factors, medical settings have often limited the hiring of sign-language interpreters for deaf patients seeking medical consultation, ADA provisions notwithstanding (Harmer, 1999; Raifman & Vernon, 1996a). Deaf patients have instigated complaints and lawsuits in order to remedy the lack of equal access, most of which have been decided in their favor (Harmer, 1999).

Political barriers are not only external to the deaf community. Some are internal, too. In a survey of deaf leaders in Rochester, New York, Bateman (1994) concludes that deaf community political activism is diluted by:

- Limited understanding of the political process
- Apathy and a sense of disenfranchisement
- A sense of powerlessness to enact changes

There is a fear that being too politically active may translate into setbacks when hearing people may balk at accommodating deaf people's requests. For example, eliminating communication barriers may be seen as a moral obligation in U.S. society. But if demands for costly accommodations continue, some may claim that deaf persons have an obligation to accept responsibility for some of these costs if they choose not to minimize or eliminate deafness if and when that becomes an actuality (through medical advances) (Tucker, 1998a, 1998b).

The deaf community that instigated the 1988 DPN movement had a largely white face. There were no African American deaf leaders, even though Washington, DC (where Gallaudet University is located), has a large African American community. Many minority deaf people and their leaders did not perceive themselves to be a significant part of this historic movement. However, the infusion of multiculturalism into the deaf community in recent years, fueled by the increase of multicultural students in settings where deaf children and youth are educated (Holden-Pitt & Diaz, 1998), has reinforced the need to acknowledge diversity in the deaf community. The publication of books such as *Black and Deaf in America: Are We That Different?* (Hairston & Smith, 1983), *The Hispanic Deaf* (Delgado, 1984), *Sounds Like Home: Growing Up Black and Deaf in the South* (Wright, 1999), *Psychotherapy with Deaf Clients from Diverse Groups* (Leigh, 1999c), and *Deaf Plus: A Multicultural Perspective* (Christensen, 2000), as well as various chapters on multiculturalism in deafness-related texts show that the deaf community is changing, as American society is changing. The empowerment message emerging from the DPN protest now involves multicultural deaf groups. Dr. Glenn Anderson, a prominent African American deaf leader became Chair of the Gallaudet University Board of Trustees after the resignation of Phil Bravin, a well-known deaf community member who was the first post-DPN Chair. The Gallaudet University Board of Trustees now has a larger number of multicultural deaf persons.

DEAF ORGANIZATIONS

The commonality of deafness does not override the pluralism of U.S. society, which is also reflected within the deaf community (Bateman, 1994; Jankowski, 1997; Leigh & Lewis, 1999). Existing groups of deaf people have different interests and different goals, various communication beliefs and cultural backgrounds, and multiple understandings of how to be deaf. We now provide brief descriptions of some of the major deaf organizations that have shaped the nature of the deaf community. These organizations have united for common causes but have gone their separate ways when consensus fails. Many of them are connected with local chapters or groups.

■ In 1880, the National Association of the Deaf (NAD), the oldest organization founded and run by people with disabilities, came into being (Schein, 1989; Van Cleve & Crouch, 1989). The goal of the NAD was to bring deaf people throughout the United States together to deliberate on their needs, and eventually to advocate for basic rights. Today, it is a federation of state associations of the deaf, which is governed by a national board. Politically, its ability to advocate successfully throughout the years has varied. Currently, the NAD works on the federal level to ensure that the accessibility and civil rights of deaf and hard-of-hearing persons are safeguarded. It advocates for the educational, vocational, legal, and social concerns of its deaf constituents. Recent NAD monthly publications (now called *NADmag*) have reported on a wide range of issues such as educational policy, telecommunications access, cochlear implants, sign-language interpreter certification, and the changing nature of vocational rehabilitation services. The law center provides legal advocacy, assistance, and education related to the rights of deaf people. To achieve its political goals, the NAD works closely with other national deafness and disability organizations and coalitions. Its membership base was historically white male. It is now shifting to a more diverse base that reflects U.S. demographics (Bloch, 2001). This can be seen both at the board level and in outreach work. There is also a youth division, the Jr. NAD, which uses leadership training activities to encourage the development of new deaf leaders among young deaf students from both residential and mainstream programs.

■ On the international front, the NAD is affiliated with the World Federation of the Deaf (WFD), which is made up of associations of deaf people from all over the world that contribute to the enhancement of cultural, social, and economic status of deaf persons. The WFD was established in 1951 with the goal of increasing global cooperation.

■ State associations of the deaf carry on political activities to ensure that legislation and services are favorable for deaf persons. For example, a number of these associations have worked to establish permanent state offices or commissions to serve deaf and hard-of-hearing citizens who require better access to state programs and services, improve television captioning, and institute local emergency warning systems, as noted in regular *NADstates* publications (National Association of the Deaf, 2001). These associations keep deaf people within each state linked as a community. Opportunities for political action are often combined with social events at biennial conferences.

■ The National Fraternal Society for the Deaf (NFSD) celebrated its 100th anniversary in 2001 (Suggs, 2001a). Next to the NAD, it is the oldest organization of deaf members, having come into being when a group of deaf men decided to get around the arbitrary denial of insurance coverage and overcharges common at that time by providing life insurance to deaf people at low cost (Gannon, 1981; Schein, 1989). Since the membership base is aging, the NFSD has begun an aggressive marketing campaign to attract new members.

■ The Deaf and Hard of Hearing Section (DHHS) is one of three sections within the Alexander Graham Bell Association for the Deaf and Hard of Hearing (2001a). The other two sections are for parents of deaf children and for professionals working with deaf children and adults. The primary objectives of this association include those of advocacating to pass legislation that supports the rights of children and adults utilizing the auditory approach, disseminating information of auditory approaches to language learning and advances in hearing technology that will benefit people with hearing loss, and providing assistance to ensure the availability of appropriate education that meets the communication and academic needs of children with hearing loss. Although this organization is historically seen as opposed to the use of sign language for educational purposes, it has collaborated with other organizations (e.g., the NAD) in the interest of achieving common political goals, such as universal newborn hearing screening and telecommunications access. The association includes young people and adults who have the opportunity to interact at biennial conventions.

Specialized Organizations

More recently, a number of organizations have emerged in response to specific needs expressed by diverse groups of deaf people, reflecting different constituencies and different goals, paralleling what happens in the hearing community. This attests to the commonality of social interaction processes and the push toward banding together for similar purposes within deaf and hearing communities. Following is a description of some of those specialized organizations.

■ The American Association of the Deaf-Blind (AADB) grew from a correspondence club into a national consumer advocacy organization for individuals who are deaf and have visual impairments (American Association of the Deaf-Blind, 2001). Its goals are to encourage independent living for those who are deaf-blind. Toward that end, it provides technical assistance, advocacy, and networking opportunities for deaf-blind individuals, since many of them are isolated (American Association for the Deaf-Blind, Summary, undated; Miner, 1999). Conventions are held to encourage interaction, with deaf-blind interpreters available to facilitate communication during sessions. Family members are welcome.

■ People deafened after childhood banded together in 1987 to form the Association of Late-Deafened Adults (ALDA). It enables members who are seeking a community that understands what it means to be deafened later in life to band together. In addition to encouraging a sense of community, ALDA's mission is to support the empowerment of late-deafened people (Association of Late-Deafened Adults, 2001).

■ The Cochlear Implant Association, Inc. (CIAI), formerly known as Cochlear Implant Club International, was originally formed in 1981 as a self-help group to facilitate ways to meet challenges in living with hearing loss and cochlear implants (Cochlear Implant Association, 2001). Together with a network of local chapters and support groups, CIAI provides information, referral, education, support, and advocacy efforts to its members, professionals, special-interest groups, and the general public. Due to the increasing numbers of deaf individuals with cochlear implants, it is anticipated that CIAI as a consumer organization will assume a leadership role in the field of cochlear implants. It is important to note that cochlear implant usage is increasing among those deaf persons who rely on signed communication or ASL (Christiansen & Leigh, 2002). These individuals are now being welcomed within the deaf community instead of being rejected outright. Although CIAI currently is the premier organization for cochlear implant users, other organizations, including the NAD (National Association of the Deaf, 2000b) and AG Bell (Alexander Graham Bell Association of the Deaf, 2001b), have developed position papers and informational activities related to the topic of cochlear implants.

■ Deaf Seniors of America (DSA), which was organized in 1994 (Deaf Seniors of America, 2001), reflects the presence of a large group of deaf seniors, paralleling the increasing number of Americans who are elderly. Many seniors look forward to socializing at the biennial conventions, where DSA performs its mission of informing members about advocacy efforts and resources to improve their participation in deaf and mainstream society.

■ Deaf Women United (DWU), founded in 1985, is devoted to ensuring that deaf women have access to a community of support and increased recognition of their contributions to society (Deaf Women United, 2000). Considering that deaf women are unique to the extent that they encounter both gender and deafness discrimination and oppression (Wax, 1999), DWU endeavors to affirm these women's experiences in a positive light. It is involved in advocacy, education, and outreach to ensure that gender and access issues do not deprive deaf women of the opportunities available to others. Biennial conferences provide a platform for deaf women to network and provide support.

■ The establishment of the Rainbow Alliance of the Deaf (RAD) in 1977 created a national organization that focuses on the educational, economical, and social welfare of deaf gays and lesbians (Rainbow Alliance of the Deaf, 2000). Deaf gay men and lesbians need to navigate the worlds of hearing people, heterosexuality, work, differing ethnic communities, and gay and lesbian people. Each setting represents differing contexts for discrimination or acceptance (Gutman, 1999). Support such as that provided by RAD facilitates the acquisition of skills needed to manage the situations and issues that may emerge in these different settings. The organization fosters fellowship opportunities through biennial conferences, which enable members to discuss solutions to problems related to social and legal issues. Major metropolitan areas also have deaf gay and lesbian communities that facilitate networking and social support (Gutman, 1999).

■ Self Help for Hard of Hearing People, Inc., was established in 1979 as a nonprofit educational membership organization with the goal of enhancing the quality of life for hard-of-hearing people (Self-Help for Hard of Hearing People, 2001). Its mission is to open the world of communication through education, information, support, and advocacy. Its members tend to be primarily individuals who do not see themselves as part of the deaf community. Advocacy efforts involve collaboration with deaf organizations when common goals are identified.

■ TDI, formerly known as Telecommunications for the Deaf, Inc., appeared on the scene in 1968 when members of AG Bell and NAD joined forces to contribute and service teletypewriters for deaf people (Lang, 2000). Members of the deaf community volunteered to condition and distribute the first machines. Since then, TDI has become a premier organization for promoting visual access to entertainment, information, and telecommunications through education, networking, collaboration, advocacy, and national policy development. It publicizes information about new technology and new policies to ensure equal access to communication.

Ethnic Deaf Groups

Ethnic groups emerged as the deaf community became more diverse and as deaf people of different ethnic origins sought each other out. For example, deaf African Americans established their own social clubs and sports teams even though similar clubs for deaf people were nearby (Hairston & Smith, 1983; Jankowski, 1997). In part, this was engendered by a history of segregated schooling and segregated white deaf organizations (Aramburo, 1994; Lane et al., 1996; Rittenhouse et al., 1991). Additionally, the experiences of black deaf persons and deaf persons of other ethnic origins clearly differed from the experiences of white deaf persons despite the common bonds of deafness. This was due to the racist attitudes, both overt and subtle, that have continued to prevail in white American society (Cohen, 1991; Corbett, 1999; Lopez, 2001). For these reasons, and because people with common ethnic origins tend to bond together and affirm their unique cultural heritages, local and statewide groups were formed. The next logical step was to establish national organizations.

The first to appear on the scene was the National Black Deaf Advocates (NBDA), founded in 1982 (Schein, 1989). Its goal was to create role models and a vision of success for black deaf youth as part of the process of empowering this group. Glenn Anderson (1994), mentioned earlier in this chapter, writes about the importance of networking and self-help as part of the African American tradition of survival in the face of discrimination and oppression. He views these functions as a critical part of the mission of NBDA. This organization holds biennial conferences during which attendees interact and develop agendas for empowerment.

The Intertribal Deaf Council, founded in 1994, has adopted as its goal the carrying out of traditions and cultures of Native American deaf people and improving the appreciation of these cultures on the part of members and the public at large (Intertribal Deaf Council, 1999). In 1997, the National Asian Deaf Congress came into being in order to recognize and preserve Asian Deaf culture, heritage, identity, and history for Asian American deaf people (National Asian Deaf Congress, 2001; Wu & Grant, 1999). Both organizations hold regularly scheduled conferences to reaffirm their missions and follow up on agendas that will help their members. The National Hispanic Council of the Deaf and Hard-of-Hearing is currently inactive (Deaf Latino Organizations, 2001), but there is an online resource for the deaf Latino/a community called Deaf AZT-LAN (Across the Nation Newsbriefs, 2001; Deaf Latino Organizations, 2001). Interested readers may refer to the end of the chapter for Internet addresses.

Religious Groups

Religious interest in deaf people goes back to the time of the Old and New Testaments and the Talmud (Van Cleve & Crouch, 1989; Zwiebel, 1994). Religious institutions have worked to enable members of the North American deaf community to participate in the practice of religion since the 1800s (Schein, 1989). Nowadays, "no religion is without deaf members" (Schein, 1986, p. 85). Deaf religious leaders—

including Catholic priests, Jewish rabbis, and Protestant ministers—have been trained to take their place along with hearing religious leaders in leading deaf congregations (Gannon, 1981; Schein, 1989). Deaf ministries are scattered throughout the United States (Deaf Churches, 2001). National religious organizations such as the Lutheran Church-Missouri Synod: Deaf Missions, United Methodist Congress of the Deaf, International Catholic Deaf Association–US, and the Jewish Deaf Congress collaborate with local religious settings and organizations. With the influx of immigrants, the deaf community is beginning to take notice of deaf members who follow Buddhism, Hinduism, Islam, and other religions that are now taking root in the United States.

Deaf Clubs

Deaf people have maintained contact through national, regional, and state organizations, but it was the Deaf clubs that historically formed the mainstay of local Deaf communities (Lane, Hoffmeister, & Bahan, 1996). These clubs provided opportunities for Deaf friends to continue socializing after they had left the environs of residential schools. Not only did the clubs provide opportunities for activities that encourage interaction—such as dances, celebrations, sports events, workshops, and so on—they also provided a means for the transmission of Deaf culture, customs, history, and worldviews. At these clubs, Deaf members served as mentors and educators as they welcomed young members. These clubs also created supportive environments, or what Hall (1994) describes as a safe haven without the communication barriers that typically existed beyond the club settings.

With the advent of television captioning and the Internet, as well as accessible telecommunication devices such as TTYs and pagers, deaf persons no longer strongly feel the need to convene in Deaf clubs to maintain the sense of community. Anecdotal evidence indicates that many such clubs may be on the wane (Lane et al., 1996). Occasional events such as Deaf Awareness events or Deaf Festivals are now serving as new venues for Deaf community interactions. The boundaries that separated Deaf events from the hearing community are no longer as firm, as Deaf events take place in hotels, convention centers, and sports arenas where hearing people mingle as well (Padden & Rayman, 2002). With deaf persons having more opportunities to interact with hearing peers because of improved telecommunications and sign-language interpreters at work, in school, and at recreational activities, the boundaries of Deaf groups have become more permeable, even while these groups maintain strong Deaf culture orientations.

Sports

The role of sports looms large in the lives of deaf people (Gannon, 1981; Schein, 1989; Stewart, 1991). Deaf community publications and media devote sections to sports events organized by deaf organizations and deaf sports competition results. There are numerous international, national, state, regional, and local organizations that sponsor deaf sports activities. Jerald Jordan, former president of the Comité International des Sports des Sourds (CISS) (International Committee for Deaf Sports), which serves functions similar to those of the International Olympic Committee, writes that the sense of deaf people taking charge of their own lives is strongest in deaf sports (Jordan, 1991, p. vii). Through managing the sociocultural contexts of sports, deaf athletes and volunteers are able to ensure social gratification and self-actualization, as well as a sense of belonging and ease of communication, when everyone understands everyone else. Deaf athletes can be mentors and role models within a wide variety of sports, including baseball, basketball, skiing, soccer, and wrestling. Consequently, they serve as athletic inspirations for deaf youth.

The premier national sports organization in the United States is the USA Deaf Sports Federation, formerly known as the American Athletic Association of the Deaf (USA Deaf Sports Federation, 2001). Founded in 1945, this organization is linked with regional and local sports groups as well as with the CISS. It sends U.S. teams to the Deaflympics (formerly World Games for the Deaf) every four years. There is also a European Deaf Sports Organization, formed in 1983 (EDSO History, 2001).

HEALTH CARE ISSUES

Deaf and hard-of-hearing patients are less likely to have updated information about health issues such as AIDS, and are less likely to receive preventive information in general from physicians (Langholtz & Ruth, 1999; Woodroffe, Gorenflo, Meador, & Zazove, 1998). Communication barriers on the part of physicians may be a contributory factor (Harmer, 1999; Witte & Kuzel, 2000). Ralston, Zazove, and Gorenflo (1995) suggest that physician reactions are a result of lifelong conditioning to negative stereotypes about deaf people, which are based on limited knowledge. Decisions to limit communication accessibility are often based on cost, ADA requirements notwithstanding (Gianelli, 1999). All these contributory factors led Harmer (1999) to conclude that deaf and hard-of-hearing individuals often receive inadequate, inappropriate, and unethical health care. Research on the health care needs of minority deaf persons is sorely needed. Harmer recommends randomized surveys of current health status and health care utilization, assessment of barriers to service, and comparison of the fiscal costs of providing accessible health care with the long-term costs of failing to provide full health care information.

If health care providers were sensitive to the communication needs of their deaf and hard-of-hearing patients, and aware of how to modify written communication and when to utilize sign language interpreters, they would do a far better job of addressing their obligations to serve those in need of good health care services. Information on resources for health care, including mental health care and community resources, can be found by accessing http://www.deafhoh-health.org/.

Like their hearing counterparts, aging deaf persons require increased contact with health care professionals. In the United States, where old age tends to be devalued, these deaf individuals are at an even greater disadvantage because of communication barriers to health information and emotional support (Andrews &

Wilson, 1991; Munro-Ludders, 1992). Additionally, when they require assisted care or health care facilities, including nursing homes, there are few residential facilities designed specifically for elderly deaf persons where deaf community connections are maintained. Many of those needing residential placements will end up isolated in mainstream facilities because of staff misconceptions about their ability to comprehend information (Andrews & Wilson, 1991). In other words, staff will assume they are being understood, when in fact this may not necessarily be the case.

When facing challenges related to the dying phase of life, Munro-Ludders (1992) describes the confusion and uncertainty that elderly deaf people experience when they do not get full information about their physical condition or services in hearing health care facilities due to inadequate communication. He comments on their resiliency and patience during this phase because of their lifelong experiences in coping with communication barriers. Nonetheless, loneliness is still a factor to be reckoned with, as it is for many hearing elderly Americans.

THE WORLD OF WORK

One only has to pick up the books *Deaf Persons in the Arts and Sciences* (Lang & Meath-Lang, 1995), *Hollywood Speaks* (Schuchman, 1988), *Deaf Women: A Parade through the Decades* (Holcomb & Wood, 1989), and *Deaf Heritage* (Gannon, 1981), to see that occupational possibilities for deaf persons now border on the infinite. Stockbrokers, physicians, cooks, architects, engineers, printers, lawyers, woodcarvers, baseball players, poets, actors, museum curators, chemists, janitors, computer technicians—deaf women and men have entered these fields and more. Deaf individuals have climbed into the upper echelons of government, a premier example being Dr. Robert Davila, former Assistant Secretary of Special Education and Rehabilitative Services in the Department of Education during the first Bush administration (Lang & Meath-Lang, 1995). Deaf workers are found in settings ranging from those specialized in providing services to deaf children and adults, where they may have numerous deaf co-workers, to those settings where they may be the only deaf employee (Schein, 1989). Success stories of break-throughs in fields originally perceived as closed to deaf persons are legion.

But not all is rosy. Robert Buchanan's book, *Illusions of Equality* (1999), outlines the struggles deaf people have had in trying to achieve stature or even employment in the workforce, benefiting primarily from times of economic expansion such as those following both world wars. All too often, when deaf people access entry-level jobs, they are not provided the same opportunities for advancement available to hearing peers (Buchanan, 1994; Christiansen, 1994; Schein, 1989). Additionally, Lang and Meath-Lang (1995) express distress at the relative lack of deaf minority career successes.

Historically, deaf people have more frequently been found in jobs ranging from unskilled to skilled labor (Christiansen, 1994). One popular and prestigious occupation was printing, in part because residential schools for the deaf had strong vocational training programs in printing (Christiansen, 1994; Gannon, 1981; Van

Cleve & Crouch, 1989). Today, skilled printing positions have drastically decreased due to changes within the industry, with advanced technology taking over various printing functions that formerly required experienced workers.

Another popular work area was the postal service (Lane et al., 1996). This field became feasible for deaf workers when training was provided to prepare deaf applicants for Civil Service examinations (*Deaf American*, 1969, 1970). Going back to 1906, access to these examinations had been limited for deaf people due to guidelines excluding deaf people, among others. It took years of strong political action on the part of deaf leaders to overturn these guidelines for various federal positions and to remove examination barriers (Buchanan, 1999; Gannon, 1981; Van Cleve & Crouch, 1989). For example, Al Sonnenstrahl (personal communication, September 18, 2001) recalls that the Civil Service examinations for post office positions included questions about music and vocabulary that essentially were unrelated to job performance abilities.

Today, there is no specific vocational area that deaf people are flocking to, illustrating that occupational choices and opportunities are now well diversified. Education has become increasingly important, with job requirements demanding higher skill levels for those desiring advancement. So how do deaf and hard-of-hearing people fare in this type of work environment?

Barnartt and Christiansen (1996) examined data collected on 478 prevocationally deaf adults who were part of National Health Interview Surveys in 1990 and 1991. They found that despite improvements in educational and occupational attainments, deaf adults were still somewhat disadvantaged compared to hearing adults, with the differences being larger for men than for women. Although deaf men increased their representation in white-collar jobs and decreased their representation in blue-collar jobs, they were still more likely to hold blue-collar jobs in comparison to hearing men. Deaf and hearing women were more similar in that most held white-collar jobs.

Results of a 15-year follow-up survey done by Schroedel and Geyer (2000) (briefly reported in Chapter 2) indicated that most of the 240 deaf and hard-of-hearing college graduates who participated in this survey were successfully employed and satisfied with life. Females earned one-third less than their male counterparts, who had more consistent earning gains throughout their employment. Nonetheless, deaf and hard-of-hearing college graduates earned less than their hearing counterparts. Even though more deaf women than men obtained higher degrees, women continued to be clustered in clerical occupations. Approximately 15 percent of the graduates surveyed were underemployed in 1999, with vocational degree recipients being at greater risk of underemployment. These results may be an underestimation, considering that 27 percent of hearing college graduates were underemployed nationally. The researchers recommend that occupational choices should be based on career rather than "job" considerations, with career productivity requiring learning new skills as jobs within a career area changes. Deaf women need to be challenged to maximize their potential. Because of traditional gender stereotypes, it has taken them time to follow deaf men in the effort to break down barriers to employment (Holcomb & Wood, 1989).

Most worrisome, however, is the 44 percent rate of high school drop-outs among deaf students (Blanchfield, Feldman, Dunbar, & Gardner, 2001, as reported in Chapter 2), when compared with a general population rate of 19 percent. State vocational rehabilitation agencies (VR) have facilitated the occupational training of deaf persons, most notably in the years after World War II. However, the number of those successfully employed through VR services declined during the period between 1989 and 1998, even though there were more deaf and hard-of-hearing persons than in previous years (Reichman, 2000). One possibility is that in the strong economy of the 1990s, employment opportunities were easier to find without VR assistance, employers were more willing to hire "nontraditional" workers, and the workplace became more accessible with the presence of sign-language interpreters, text-related technology such as emails and computer assisted real time captioning, and access to telephone relay services. On the other hand, VR counselors may be experiencing more difficulty in placing deaf clients with limited skills in English and mathematics. In addition to employer resistance, the automation of many work functions has hurt the deaf unskilled worker (Buchanan, 1999).

Information on ethnically diverse deaf workers is sorely lacking. In Schroedel and Geyer's (2000) survey, there were insufficient college graduates from ethnic minority backgrounds for analysis. A study of professionals in 349 deaf education programs revealed that 10.4 percent were from nonwhite or minority ethnic cultural backgrounds, primarily African American and Hispanic/Latino (Andrews & Jordan, 1993). Of that group, 11.7 percent were deaf, and 8 individuals were administrators. John Lopez, J. D. (2001), a prominent member of the Hispanic/Latino deaf community, expresses concern about this community's exclusion from community development programs, thus hindering upward mobility for qualified Hispanic Deaf individuals. He claims that the number of Hispanic Deaf professionals in decision-making positions can be counted on one hand. In sum, more needs to be done to encourage upward mobility for minority deaf persons.

The Americans with Disabilities Act of 1990 limits the ability of employers in settings with 15 or more employees to exclude job applicants on the basis of disability. Although the explicit message is that of encouraging employers to learn that persons with disabilities do make good workers with reasonable accommodations, enforcement continues to be a problem. Intent to discriminate can be difficult to prove. Willingness to hire deaf people exists, as does resistance, the ADA notwithstanding. Even though deaf workers as a group have long since proved themselves to be good workers, the struggle for equality in accessing the workplace continues.

Those deaf persons who remain unemployed have recourse to Social Security Disability Insurance (SSDI) and Supplemental Security Income (SSI). In 1993, almost 100,000 persons with *hearing losses considered severe enough to affect work* received either SSI or SSDI (Lane, Hoffmeister, & Bahan, 1996). It is not clear what "hearing losses considered severe enough to affect work" means, considering the fact many deaf people can hold jobs. Based on the results of a collaborative study between the Social Security Administration and the National Technical Institute for the Deaf (NTID) of young adults who were deaf and hard of hearing, Clarcq and

Walter (1997–98) concluded that the more education deaf individuals have, the less likely they will draw SSI. In addition to the findings from this study, a good number of SSDI or SSI recipients do have additional disabilities or are unable to internalize work requirements. Also, the rules for SSDI or SSI are a disincentive to work when entry-level or manual-type jobs may not pay more than what SSDI or SSI provides (Buck, 2000; Vernon, 1991). Some will resort to peddling as a potentially more lucrative venture.

Throughout the years, the deaf community has had an uneasy coexistence with deaf peddlers. The NAD used to have a slogan: "The deaf do not beg" (Gannon, 1981, p. 255). It was deleted after World War II when deaf peddler rackets became widespread. Campaigns against peddling were instituted by deaf organizations in order to dispel the notion that deaf people collectively needed charity (Buck, 2000; Gannon, 1981). Current perceptions are that peddling is less frequent due to greater awareness of training and employment options for deaf people in need. Self-respect and pride in the deaf community are also mitigating factors. The widely publicized 1997 discovery of an illegal network of deaf Mexican peddlers in the New York City borough of Queens who were subject to threats and violence in order to produce cash for the ringleaders testifies to the ongoing lucrative nature of peddling (Barry, 1997). The deaf perpetrators of this network were arrested and sentenced to prison terms (Fried, 1997).

As indicated in Chapter 6, to address the employment disparities that have been reported here requires that educational programs serving deaf and hard-of-hearing students incorporate transition efforts in their master plan. Critical juncture points include those from secondary schools to postsecondary education or employment, and from postsecondary education to employment. State vocational rehabilitation programs, employers, and community representatives, as well as the students and their families, need to be involved in chartering career and vocational pathways, creating learning opportunities in the community to facilitate the transition process, and ensuring employment opportunities (LeNard, 2001). Fostering job-related skills and a work ethic are integral parts of this process.

LEGAL ISSUES

Although persuasion and collaboration are the preferred techniques, the law has often been the court of last resource for deaf people in the United States who feel they have been deprived of their rights. The book, *Legal Rights: The Guide for Deaf and Hard of Hearing People,* fifth edition, was prepared by the National Association of the Deaf (2000a) in order to disseminate legal information to the deaf community and professionals advocating for deaf citizens. The goal is to counteract discrimination, unequal communication access, and stereotypical notions about the inabilities of deaf people. Legal action that has improved the lives of deaf people range from making laws to initiating lawsuits, ensuring the following:

- Appropriate education
- Access to telecommunications
- Removal of architectural barriers (e.g., lack of visual alerting systems)
- Equal access to health care and mental health services
- Equal employment opportunities
- Equal access to services within the criminal justice system

Deaf inmates have sued for reasonable accommodations (e.g., communication access within correctional systems). The NAD law center has sued city and county police departments to ensure communication access by law enforcement personnel. There is a NAD position statement on communication access by law enforcement personnel (National Association of the Deaf, 2000c) because of situations in which innocent deaf people were killed by police officers who did not know that these individuals were deaf and required special communication approaches. A number of court cases have concerned decisions about educational placement for deaf children because of differences of opinion about the type of educational services that public schools need to provide (e.g., Siegel, 2000). The list goes on and on.

Raifman and Vernon (1996b) recommend that mental health administrators develop contingency plans to serve deaf patients who request services. In this way they can avoid costly equal access legal challenges. In another article, Raifman and Vernon (1996a) describe court actions mandating that mental health service providers demonstrate ASL fluency in order to provide services to deaf clients.

Deaf persons who find themselves in the criminal justice system face a number of pitfalls, including communication difficulties emerging during basic legal processes, such as police interrogation, interactions with lawyers, determination of competence to stand trial, and other basic legal processes (Vernon, Raifman, Greenberg, & Monteiro, 2001). The problems start at the time of arrest or during investigations, since police agencies rarely implement procedures governing the use of interpreters and other support services with deaf persons (Miller, 2001). The fact that deaf suspects may be easily led to sign confessions or other legal documents beyond their understanding compounds these problems. Due to linguistic idiosyncrasies on the part of deaf people, making sure they understand the implications of due process and giving testimony can be difficult to achieve. Assessing linguistic diversity in order to communicate effectively with deaf criminal suspects, or providing sign-language interpreters who can match the person's linguistic needs, is essential in order to achieve due process for these individuals. Vernon, Raifman, and Greenberg (1996) list recommendations that help assure successful communication of the Miranda Warnings to deaf defendants.

CONCLUSION

The sociology of the deaf community is highly reflective of the larger society in terms of its complexity and its susceptibility to the dynamics of social policy that influence the ways in which society members interact. The more one understands about sociological factors as these apply to deaf people, the more one is able to develop strategies that will enable deaf people to optimally manage their lives. Considering the struggles of deaf people to achieve parity with hearing peers through the decades, their efforts to test the limitations imposed by hearing society, and their inherent resilience, deaf people have come a long way. More work remains to be done in order to lower barriers to opportunities that deaf people desire.

SUGGESTED READINGS

Buchanan, R. M. (1999). *Illusions of Equality: Deaf Americans in School and Factory: 1850-1950.* Washington, DC: Gallaudet University Press.
    This book describes strategies used by deaf community leaders to win and keep jobs during periods of high and low national employment. The focus on individual responsibility for job security hampered the possibility of advocating collective employment rights for deaf people.

Carbin, C. (1996). *Deaf Heritage in Canada.* Toronto: McGraw-Hill Ryerson, Ltd.
    The author provides a history of Deaf people in Canada. He describes Deaf people's contributions and the people and events that shaped their lives, their education, and their knowledge of culture, arts, and history.

Jankowski, K. (1997). *Deaf Empowerment: Emergence, Struggle, & Rhetoric,* Washington, DC: Gallaudet University Press.
    The Deaf social movement in the United States was strengthened by the use of tactics from the civil rights movement and other social protests, and also through a shift of focus from individuals with impaired hearing to a language minority within a dominant hearing culture. The author discusses how these strategies can enhance equal chances for diverse groups in a multicultural society.

■ ■ ■ ■ ■

ORGANIZATIONS' WWW ADDRESSES

Alexander Graham Bell Association for the Deaf and Hard of Hearing	http://www.agbell.org
American Association of the Deaf-Blind aadb.htm	http://www.tr.wou.edu/dblink/
American Deafness and Rehabilitation Association	http://adara.org
American Sign Language Teachers Association	http://aslta.org/national/index
Association of Late-Deafened Adults	http://www.alda.org
Children of Deaf Adults	http://www.coda-international.org
Cochlear Implant Association, Inc.	http://www.cici.org
Communication Services for the Deaf	http://www.c-s-d.org
Deaf Aztlan: Deaf Latino/a Network	http://www.deafvision.net/aztlan/ welcome.html
Deaf History International	http://depts.gallaudet.edu/DHI
Deaf Women United	http://www.dwu.org
Intertribal Deaf Council	http://www.bigriver.net/~rasmith/ idc/idc.html
National Asian Deaf Congress	http://www.nadc-usa.org/about.html
National Association of the Deaf	http://www.nad.org
National Symposium of Childhood Deafness	http://www.c-s-d.org
Rainbow Alliance of the Deaf	http://www.rad.org
Self Help for Hard of Hearing People	http://www.shhh.org
TDI, Inc.	http://www.tdi-online.org
USA Deaf Sports Federation	http://www.usadsf.org

DEAF-HEARING
RELATIONSHIPS IN CONTEXT

*Deaf futures hinge not only upon the recognition that stereotyped beliefs,
values and attitudes are the scourge of minority communities, but upon an
understanding that a restriction of diversity prevents growth and adaptability.*
—Corker, 1996, p. 202

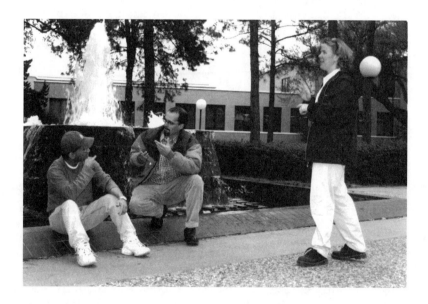

When Brenda Jo Brueggemann, who is hard of hearing, arrived at the Gallaudet University campus in 1991, every day she was asked, "Are you Deaf or Hearing?" (Brueggemann, 1999, p. 237). Daily she struggled with the answer.

The salience of this identity question is a powerful one, implying as it does that if you are one, you are not the other. For deaf persons firm in their Deaf identity, the answer is clear. For persons on the margin of the deaf community who are struggling to define their identity, this question may force them to navigate the unchartered territory of Deaf-Hearing community dynamics. For naïve hearing persons, the "Deaf or Hearing" question is outside the realm of their experience, since "hearing" tends to be an unconscious status taken for granted. Hearing people don't know that they are hearing until they encounter deaf people, and they do not know what "hearing" represents for deaf persons (Lane, 1996). Complicating matters, those who are hard of hearing may struggle with where they belong, and decide that they are neither and/or even both, depending on the situation, as Brueggemann (1999) finally decided. To say that one is "both" is to take a "bicultural" stance, which acknowledges a comfortable attitude toward both worlds. For hearing children of Deaf parents, the "Hearing or Deaf" question can reflect a minefield of confused answers. On the one hand, they are true inheritors of Deaf culture, having been born into the culture; on the other hand, they hear as hearing people do.

Whatever the choice, the decision carries with it not only the issue of deaf-hearing identity but also the assumption, either explicit or implicit, of how the relationship with the "other" culture is to be played out and how one is to behave with the "other." In short, we now confront the issue of hearing-deaf relationships and attitudes.

CHAPTER OBJECTIVES

This chapter explores the power of stereotyped reactions to deaf persons, based on typical perceptions, values, and attitudes of hearing society, exceptions notwithstanding. It also explores how deaf persons react to hearing persons. These typical responses can have an impact on hearing and deaf community, school, and work relationships. Professionals bear a heavy responsibility as shapers of how these relationships are constructed. The chapter also discusses the nature and influence of professionals' attitudes. Healthy deaf-hearing relationships are described. One must not forget that these relationships are also heavily influenced by sign-language interpreters. Their influence as conduits between deaf persons and the larger hearing society will be examined. The chapter takes a look at attitudes within the deaf community before concluding with the belief that through greater positive exposure to each other, attitudinal barriers between deaf and hearing people will continue to diminish.

"INTERESTING" ATTITUDES

■ During a job interview for an administrative position, one of the coauthors of this book, Irene W. Leigh, who is deaf and happens to be well versed in both spoken and written English in addition to ASL, was asked about her proficiency in written English because, as the interviewer put it, deaf people had serious problems with writing, and there was concern about how the written English requirements of this position would be handled. Additional questions covered how she would communicate with hearing contacts via telephone. This was in spite of the fact that Leigh already had her doctorate and her resume included listings of professional publications.

■ In an article on psychology internship accessibility issues, the majority of questions addressed to deaf applicants involved "inappropriate questions, comments, or challenges to their competency based on interviewers' negative perceptions of deafness or Deaf people" (Hauser, Maxwell-McCaw, Leigh, & Gutman, 2000, p. 570).

■ People have not stopped asking the Deaf superintendent of the Maryland School for the Deaf if he is married, has children, or possesses a driver's license, and want to know from him what Deaf children do when they become adults (Tucker, 2000).

■ In stories of mainstream experiences, even those students who are successful academically or very "hearing" oriented acknowledge experiencing different levels of rejection (Kersting, 1997; Leigh, 1994). Although deaf students with good speech and lip-reading skills can easily interact with hearing peers, relationships are often not perceived to be as close as they would have liked (Stinson & Whitmire, 1992).

■ As a hearing son of deaf parents, Lennard Davis (1995) wanted to escape "deafness" but eventually discovered that he really sought to flee the deafness constructed by hearing society. This was built on experiences of discrimination to which his deaf parents typically reacted by stating that they were as good as anyone else. In other words, they "knew" they had to prove they were equal to their hearing peers.

Yes, deaf people have come a long way. They have achieved far more than hearing persons ever thought possible, as witnessed by the number of deaf people in different prestigious occupations (Chapter 10). The public is much more familiar with deaf people than they were in the years before the Deaf President Now movement, thanks to mass media reports of the event (Christiansen & Barnartt, 1995). Deaf financial advisors are now counting both deaf and hearing people among their clientele, thanks to technology such as electronic mail and other Internet venues that reduce communication barriers. Patients who hear are comfortable about requesting advice from deaf physicians such as Carolyn Stern, M.D., who appeared in the January 13, 2002, CBS Sunday Morning production of *Sign City* that featured the deaf community of Rochester, New York. Deaf as well as hearing congregation leaders minister to both deaf and hearing members. The rehabilitation field led the move toward hearing staff working together with deaf supervisors and deaf administrators. The fields of education and mental health have increasingly followed suit and now there are more opportunities for deaf administrators.

THE INFLUENCE OF PERCEPTIONS

Unfortunately, experiences like those just described have not disappeared from the scene. They emanate from typical perceptions by hearing persons that, because deaf persons cannot hear, that suffices to classify them as having a disability, since communication using spoken language is blocked or limited. Despite the fact that deaf people through the centuries have found different ways to communicate, these different ways do not fit the parameters of spoken language to which hearing society is accustomed. Even if deaf people use speech, they are not always easily understood. Because they frequently cannot follow hearing discourse, they are often seen as living in a world of silence. As Baynton (1997, p. 143) states,

> The most persistent images of deafness among hearing people have been ones of isolation and exclusion, and these are images that are consistently rejected by deaf people who see themselves as part of a deaf community and culture. Feelings of isolation may even be less common for members of this tightly knit community than among the general population. The metaphors of deafness—of isolation and foreignness, of animality, of darkness and silence—are projections reflecting the needs and standards of the dominant culture, not the experiences of most deaf people.

Little wonder that hearing people extol the miracle of any device that supposedly restores hearing and brings the world of sound to deaf persons (Christiansen & Leigh, 2002), without recognizing that deaf people connect with the world in multiple ways.

The arts have been guilty of reinforcing negative stereotypical perceptions of deaf people. For example, Davis (1995) examined written literature and drama from the nineteenth century onward that included descriptions of deaf people. He found that these descriptions typically depicted deaf characters as ones who are ostracized from mainstream society, often ending up as the "butt of many 'eh-what??' jokes" (p. 114) or as melancholy characters in a world of silence. The entertainment industry's portrayals of deaf people have historically been ones that often do not resemble real-life deaf people, thereby perpetuating society's misunderstanding of deaf people and reinforcing discriminatory attitudes (Schuchman, 1988). For example, films reinforced the stereotypes of deaf people as "dummy characters," as perfect lip-readers and speakers, or as solitary, unhappy figures. Thankfully, that is changing today with films such as *Children of a Lesser God* and others (see Chapter 2) that portray intelligent deaf people confronting life issues like anyone else.

MEANINGS OF DISABILITY AND DEAFNESS

Deaf people have been typically seen as individuals on the margin of society by virtue of their inability to hear, even though for Deaf people this inability is not a major focus due to their common language and community background. Because of this inability to hear and their difficulties in learning spoken language, they become part of the construct of disability. When people talk about diversity, disability is practically never mentioned as part of the diversity spectrum (e.g., Corker, 1998; Davis, 1997; Linton, 1998; Shapiro, 1993). To literally translate *disability* is to say that one is *not* able. This logically leads to a response set that encourages thoughts about disability as a state of being that is not normal, that reflects loss, weaknesses, helplessness, or heroism in the face of adversity. This frame of reference is bound to encourage ambivalence toward disability, involving both compassion and callousness.

This ambivalence extends to deaf persons. Just like people with disabilities, they often become objects of pity, or they are treated as individuals who don't quite make the grade because they don't fit what society expects of hearing individuals. If they speak well and achieve in the world of work, they are regarded with admiration as having overcome a disability. This is tellingly captured in the title of the book, *Damned for Their Difference: The Cultural Construction of Deaf People as Disabled* (Branson & Miller, 2002). Branson and Miller illustrate the irony of a society that declares all people are created equal, and yet creates structured inequalities based on social class, gender, age, race, ethnicity, and ability/disability. Even though many culturally Deaf persons do not make much of having a disability and maintain some distance from the disability rights movement (the Deaf President Now movement was not a disability rights movement; rather, it was a civil rights movement [Barnartt & Scotch, 2001]), the vignettes at the beginning of this chapter show that hearing society does not readily distinguish between disability and Deaf. Nor is hearing society sensitive to the fact that hearing people with physical disabilities are not the same as people with hearing disabilities who are dealing specifically with communication access.

What hearing society tends to overlook is that a disability is not static. When a community makes a commitment to remove barriers, the disability is redefined. If a wheelchair user enters an accessible movie theater, and is watching the movie in the same seated position as theater patrons are, who is then disabled in the audience? If there are open captions on the screen, so that deaf theater attendees have visual access to the spoken dialogue, who is then disabled in the audience? If voice dialogue is deleted and the hearing audience coming to watch a play sees actors communicating in ASL, who is then disabled in the audience?

Despite the fact that disability is to some extent defined by the environment, leveling the playing field is often hampered by, for example, cost factors that become the prime argument against the widening of every door for wheelchairs or producing captions for every feature film. This point has been repeated in previous chapters. It essentially reflects a facet of discrimination that society does not own up to. To put it bluntly, society continues to reinforce the disability rather than create an equal playing field. In a society that runs on economic rules, the equal access of persons with disabilities is often seen as too costly. It took legislation in the guise of the Americans with Disabilities Act of 1990 (ADA) to require accommodations that can benefit all, deaf persons included. Considering that lawsuits to enforce the ADA are still entering the legal system (e.g., Raifman & Vernon, 1996a), it is clear that all too often society does not accommodate disabilities gladly and prejudiced attitudes toward deaf people continue to influence their daily lives.

With the ADA in place, and in the face of increasing tolerance accompanied by the recognition that society is responsible for those with disabilities as it is for all its able-bodied citizens, subtle discrimination against persons with disabilities has gradually begun to replace overt discrimination (Blotzer & Ruth, 1995). This is a more insidious form of discrimination, one that is difficult to prove and fight. When deaf persons in the workplace are not told information that may be critical for job performance, when deaf children are rarely called on to be team members by their hearing peers in mainstream or inclusion educational settings, or when 9-1-1 emergency calls via TTYs (defined in Chapter 10) are not followed up because operators have not been trained to respond to TTY calls, such incidents are frequently dismissed as oversights, even when the argument that these are examples of subtle discrimination could be made.

THE OTHER SIDE

So, in turn, how do Deaf people perceive hearing people? Their question, "Are you Deaf or Hearing?" is a powerful one. It asks, "Are you with us or with the other?" It highlights the issue of belongingness and the issue of cultural values. If the answer is, "Hearing," what does this signify? According to Padden and Humphries (1988), "Hearing" is not the central point of reference; rather, it represents the greatest deviation from "Deaf" and as such can be less than complimentary, or as representing the external world outside of the Deaf-World. This makes sense, considering the historically poor treatment of deaf individuals by hearing people in positions of power and control. This is poignantly illustrated by the section on Deaf/Hearing Interaction in *The Deaf Way* (Erting, Johnson, Smith, & Snider, 1994, pp. 660–718) that illustrates the resentment deaf people feel when they are defined by their inabilities instead of their strengths.

It comes as no surprise that Deaf persons who have to interact with unknown outsiders are more comfortable with foreign Deaf people than with hearing Americans (Woodward, 1989). Additionally, in an analogue study of preferences for hearing and deaf therapists, deaf respondents chose therapists who were identified as deaf over hearing therapists who were equally proficient sign-language users after viewing filmed initial interviews (Brauer, 1980).

As the "voices" of Deaf people grew stronger in recent decades, emboldened by the support of a Deaf culture frame of reference (Humphries, 1996), Deaf people began to articulate their needs for self-definition and equality with hearing peers. To accomplish this, they began telling hearing people to "back off," to let Deaf people assume more of a say in their destinies. Interestingly, Cumming and Rodda (1989) view this as an articulation of prejudice against hearing people. At some level, it really reflects efforts to gain some transfer of power, considering that hearing people have long been in the role of policy and implementation decision maker. Neil Glickman (1996a, 1996b) captured this sentiment when he described the immersion stage in Deaf identity development (see Chapter 9) as one in which Deaf culture values reign strong and the hearing world is disparaged. Deaf persons in this stage will accuse hearing people of treating them unjustly or unfairly.

When Deaf people assert themselves, they often confront bewildered hearing participants, who may say, "What is it with you deaf people? . . . What is it about deaf culture that makes you have a chip on your shoulder when the hearing world is trying to help you?" (Drolsbaugh, 2000, p. 12). These stereotyped responses reinforce the feelings of being misunderstood or maligned that many Deaf people have. At the same time, it reveals the difficulty hearing people have in seeing their own paternalistic attitudes and in recognizing that deaf people are trying to help themselves and be independent.

When deaf people identify more closely with an integrated or bicultural stance, the focus shifts toward that of supporting Deaf people rather than attacking hearing people (Glickman, 1996a). People in this stage are able to recognize that the "Hearing" category does not necessarily have to be one of denigration. Rather than simplistically reflecting a paternalistic force, Deaf people can also see "Hearing" to mean a person with a different set of experiences based on hearing, or who may be judged as a trustworthy ally (Hoffmeister & Harvey, 1996).

The boundaries between deaf and hearing individuals have become increasingly porous in recent years due in great part to increased communication using visual technology such as electronic mail and TTY relay services, greater use of mainstream settings for education, and the lowering of barriers to employment opportunities. Therefore, deaf people who "behave as hearing people do" are less often criticized as not being Deaf enough. In concrete terms, biculturalism has become increasingly acceptable (Grosjean, 1998). This is reflected by the greater number of hearing and deaf teams working together more or less as equal partners in various venues, including education, mental health, politics, policy making, and so on. That deaf people can be the "boss" in large organizations with hearing employees reached its epitome in 1989, when Robert Davila was appointed by President Bush as assistant secretary in charge of the Office of Special Education and Rehabilitative Services.

PROFESSIONAL ATTITUDES

However, considering the lingering and oftentimes blatant reluctance of hearing society to accommodate to the needs of deaf people, or even in some situations, the tendency to ignore deaf people, the task of defining how hearing-deaf biculturalism can be implemented in a sociologically healthy manner continues unabated. In the wake of the Fall 2001 anthrax threat within the postal system, postal employees, including deaf workers, were directed to meetings to obtain medical information during this emergency situation. Despite pleas for explanations, sign-language interpreters by and large were not made available to convey information to the deaf workers in what could potentially have been a life or death situation (Suggs, 2001b). In this case, such neglect is certainly not the answer. Professionals with responsibility for those they are leading, working, with, or educating must endeavor to maintain a mindset or attitude that incorporates awareness of and respect for the needs of these deaf individuals.

Despite documented changes for the better, the majority of individuals in charge of organizations and businesses serving deaf individuals continue to be hearing, to network within themselves and not with deaf professionals, and to feel that they have the best interest of deaf people at heart. This is what Lane (1999) means when he uses the term *mask of benevolence* (the title of his book) as a guise for oppressing deaf people and exploiting them for financial gain. He claims the presence of "a hearing way of dominating, restructuring, and exercising authority over the deaf community" (p. 43) that does not take Deaf perspectives or input into account. To describe this phenomenon, he uses the word *audism*, which was coined by Tom Humphries. Corker (1994) further clarifies this word to reflect social relationships constructed by the hearing-speaking majority on the basis of assumed superiority over deaf people. This in turn engenders oppressive stances toward this minority group. Although Lane does provide a disclaimer in his preface that some of the hearing professionals are unjustly accused of audism since they are in the business of empowering deaf persons, the book proper is a powerful indictment of these hearing professionals who are audist.

A point of clarification is in order. The deaf community typically takes its own counsel and expresses its opinion, most often through deaf organizations. For example, film studios will often claim that the best solution is to hire a hearing actor who will need to learn some signs for the role, even when deaf actors are available who could attempt the role and who would not need to learn sign language! When the hearing establishment claims that deaf actors cannot fulfill role expectations, they are taking on an audist stance. For this reason, deaf organizations have banded together to rally for the hiring of deaf actors as opposed to hearing actors for deaf roles in films.

Interestingly, Lane himself has been accused by Moores (1993a, 1993b) of audist tendencies in a devastating critique of *The Mask of Benevolence*. As a prime example, Moores uses Lane's narrative to illustrate how Lane himself made decisions regarding deaf education in Burundi without consulting deaf professionals, either white or African, or deaf organizations with expertise in African educational systems for deaf children. Clearly, however well-intentioned professionals may be, sensitivity to one's own potential audist tendencies requires being open to criticism and addressing blind spots.

Lane emphasizes the financial incentives for hearing professionals. This does not always play out on the individual level, since motives for entering the field of deafness are not always based on money but rather on complex factors and good intentions (Baynton, 1992; Moores, 1993a, 1993b; Vernon & Andrews, 1990). In moving from denunciations of hearing professionals to more individual scrutiny, Hoffmeister and Harvey (1996) recognize that people choose to work with deaf persons for a variety of reasons. Some have deaf family members or have encountered deaf people, some are intrigued by sign languages, some see the field as a challenge, and some will show a "missionary zeal" in that they feel deaf persons need their guidance. They could be altruistic, identify with the oppressed, or religiously inspired. What is important in the long term is how they relate with deaf persons in the course of their work. Do they immerse themselves in the Deaf community and then become disillusioned because they can never be Deaf? Do they intervene to help those deaf who are "less fortunate than hearing people," or become so jaded that they see deaf "victims" as ungrateful? Do they experience frustration because, contrary to their opinions, the deaf people they want to help have different notions of how to get things done? As members of the dominant hearing society, do they in some manner continue to oppress the deaf people they work with by imposing their perspectives or value systems on deaf persons who might "see otherwise"? Hoffmeister and Harvey warn that these hearing relational postures, or perceptions of deaf people, if not worked through, will interfere with potentially healthy hearing-deaf collaboration.

Deaf people have often commented on the negative and paternalistic attitudes of professionals they encounter. According to Vernon and Andrews (1990), it is the authoritarian personality that reinforces these attitudes and subsequently the existence of oppression. Authoritarians tend to be antagonistic to groups other than their own, equating deafness with being different and weak. Weaknesses provoke anxiety, and authoritarian persons project these feelings outward to others with whom they are not comfortable. In this way, they attempt to reinforce their own superiority over these individuals by determining how to deal with these differences. They tend not to intermingle with deaf people outside of working hours, and they set up barriers for the entry of deaf people into decision-making roles. This translates into "acts of benevolence" in working with deaf people and "acts of condescension" in working alongside them (Pollard, 1996, p. 393).

In education, it is common knowledge that the deaf community has long been excluded from decisions about the education of deaf children (Nover & Ruiz, 1994), although in some areas that is now changing. Nover and Ruiz accuse the "Politics of Disability" (the medical model) of forcing "hearization " (the use of spoken language) on deaf persons. For culturally Deaf persons, this smacks of oppression. Their resistance is manifested in their claims that Deaf people have a right to be part of Deaf culture and schools for deaf children should use ASL. Hearing people strongly invested in their spoken language values have had difficulty recognizing these claims (Jankowski, 1997). The conflicts between the hearing and deaf communities over educational methodologies and language approaches have created what Nover and Ruiz call the "Politics of Fear." They hope that eventually the "Politics of Possibility" will transcend such conflicts so that deaf children will not be defined by their limitations and that deaf people will be recognized as full participants in the educational process and in the community at large. This requires that professionals be more open to collaboration. We discuss this later in this chapter when we describe healthy ways of relating.

OPPRESSION

The word *oppression* has become a popular catchword to define the behavior of many hearing professionals. People who enter the helping professions tend to perceive themselves as enablers who want to empower those they help. For many of them, being told they are *oppressors* is mind-boggling. Why does the term *oppressors* keep appearing in the literature even with growing evidence of positive hearing-deaf interaction and the greater willingness of Deaf people to take on the mantle of biculturalism and display comfort with hearing people?

The process of oppression takes place in the guise of social, political, and economic relationships with marginalized groups, including people with disabilities and people who are deaf (Corker, 1998). Oppression happens when hearing persons control decision-making processes involving deaf people instead of working with them to enact accommodations that benefit all.

In industrialized societies, for example, jobs are power. When economic opportunities are limited because one is "deaf" despite the fact that there are ways to reconstruct jobs in order to focus on abilities instead of "disabilities," this reinforces the expectations of "inability" (Corker, 1998). When deaf people are repeatedly stymied in their efforts to make advances—whether in school, in training opportunities, on the job, or in the political arena—they may see society as unwilling to work with them and therefore oppressing them. When they attempt to criticize the advice of hearing persons, their points may not be seen as valid and they can be perceived as being ungrateful.

Deaf people can respond in different and complex ways to situations they perceive as oppressive. They may uncritically accommodate to hearing society, withdraw into Deaf culture where their attributes are seen as positive, or work with hearing society to change oppressive tendencies (Corker, 1998). Their responses may vary depending on the situation in which oppression takes place and their individual attributes and past experiences. In looking at the larger picture, Corker emphasizes the need to look at not only the oppressors and the oppressed but also the process of oppression—specifically, the dynamics of the power relationship between these two groups. The Deaf President Now movement required consciousness-raising to illustrate the dynamics of this power relationship and to upend the balance of power so that it did not remain fully in the hands of hearing decision makers (Jankowski, 1997).

Although perceptions of oppression do predominate, a counteracting perspective claims that deaf people are not necessarily oppressed by hearing people. Larry Stewart, a deceased deaf professional, ASL user, and prolific as well as outspoken author, ridiculed the paradigm of deaf people being oppressed or framed as victims of hearing society (Stewart, 1992). He claimed that although some hearing people do treat deaf people badly at times, they also treat other hearing people badly. He has explained that compared to other parts of the world, deaf people have been supported to a far greater degree in the United States, and do have many opportunities to achieve. He even went so far as to suggest that getting a taste of life in, for example, Iraq or Cuba, would teach people a new definition of the word *oppression*.

Stewart acknowledged that, compared to hearing counterparts, deaf people have had to struggle that much harder to overcome "ignorance, prejudice, and at times cruelty" (p. 141) and to achieve comparable linguistic, educational, and occupational achievement and equal community participation. He has reminded us that many groups of hearing people—of varied ethnic origins, size and shape, disabilities, religions, or whatever—have had to struggle against oppression by other hearing groups as well, and that deaf people are no different. According to Stewart, many deaf people are satisfied with the quality of their lives, so defining them as oppressed does not make inherent sense. And finally, he made a case for avoiding the needless splintering between deaf and hearing people, for which he laid blame on Deaf culture because of its "rejection" of those who differ in their perspectives.

The fact that deaf people in the United States do have it good in comparison to other places in the world, particularly when it comes to educational and job opportunities, does not obviate the need to examine the tensions between groups whenever that happens. All in all, for diverse groups, whatever their group affiliation, there is a critical need to work together in coalitions that respect the value of difference in order to advance opportunities for *all* people. Society needs techniques to minimize the continual discrimination and splintering among groups. At the same time, it is important to learn about the unique traits and the diversity within each group. Many hearing and deaf professionals are working toward that end.

HEALTHY WAYS OF RELATING

In order to establish trustworthiness in the eyes of deaf people, it is recommended that professionals undergo the admittedly difficult process of honest self-analysis in trying to understand why mistrust may exist and how they can ensure healthy relationships with "the other" (Corker, 1994; Hoffmeister & Harvey, 1996). In describing this process, Harvey (1993), a hearing psychologist, asks himself:

> I don't oppress.
> But how can this be? How can I NOT oppress? (p. 46)

He and other hearing professionals recognize that being hearing tends to afford them higher status and greater privileges than might have otherwise happened. Trying to become fully integrated into Deaf culture is not necessarily the answer. What works better is to examine one's own attitudes intensively, be sensitive to hearing-deaf relations in any arena, work toward a status of mutual respect, and understand that hearing professionals do not always have all the answers. Deaf professionals do not, either.

This process requires mutual teaching. Hearing and deaf people must be open to understanding and working with each other's perspectives as part of an ongoing educational dialogue. In cases of perceived discrimination, misunderstandings need to be discussed in safe places where neither the hearing or the deaf person feels threatened. Efforts to create mutual accommodation and compromise go much farther in terms of helping hearing and deaf people understand each other and working together in mutually beneficial ways. Lawsuits should be seen only as a last recourse, since these set up either-or situations and engender bitter feelings in the process, even though the end result may mean permanent changes for the better.

Many examples of positive hearing-deaf working relationships can be found in research groups and schools for the deaf throughout the country. For example, since 1997, the ASL/English Bilingual program, a U.S. Department of Education sponsored project, has formed collaborative deaf-hearing teacher/mentor groups that meet weekly to discuss ASL/English bilingual methodology (www.star-schools.org/nmsd). This has been an insightful process for both hearing and deaf professionals (Nover & Andrews, 2000). About 14 schools for the deaf, including more than 150 teachers, are involved in this project. From these positive deaf-hearing working relationships, deaf children will be the beneficiaries, as they can see and incorporate healthy ways of relating to hearing peers based on what they see of these relationships.

There are also many examples of deaf and hearing collaborative projects where both hearing and deaf authors and researchers share their perspectives, as witnessed by the collaborative efforts of this book's authors, each of whom have diverse opinions and beliefs. Such hearing-deaf collaborative research and teaching relationships are crucial in forging attitudinal changes and leveling the playing field for everyone.

Another way to promote healthy deaf-hearing relationships is to forge alliances between hearing and deaf groups, whether in the professional, political, or social arenas (Lane, Hoffmeister, & Bahan, 1996). This increases "cross-pollination" and encourages potential changes in attitudes when mutual respect is maintained. This is not always an easy process, considering that the issue of sharing and control will always be present. Such alliances were what enabled passage of the ADA and the universal newborn hearing screening act by Congress, which saw an united front composed of diverse constituents.

If both hearing and deaf professionals go about their work in a collegial and collaborative manner, giving careful consideration to each other's perspectives, this encourages healthy deaf-hearing relationships. It is up to these professionals to set examples and train future generations to recognize this as status quo. This is exemplified by programs such as the training program for deaf and hearing pre-doctoral and postdoctoral students in psychology, social work, and medicine set up at the University of Rochester Medical Center Department of Psychiatry. In this program, deaf trainees are not cordoned off into work with deaf patients only, but are exposed to training experiences throughout the department alongside hearing faculty and hearing patients as well, thereby changing the culture of the institution in positive ways (Pollard, 1996).

In recent years, agency, organization, and educational boards with responsibility to deaf constituents, for example, have drastically increased deaf membership in the interest of parity, setting a precedent for others to follow. Examples include the Gallaudet University Board of Trustees, the Lexington School/Center for the Deaf Board in New York City, and the board of the Alexander Graham Bell Association for the Deaf, which had its first deaf president back in 1976. However, boards of other prominent organizations have yet to follow suit. For example, few deaf adults have been selected to serve on selected otolarngology, audiology, or speech and language boards to offer advice to professionals, hearing aid manufacturers, and researchers on various issues that involve policy, product, and service provision for deaf people.

There are more deaf teachers today, even though barriers in the guise of examinations make it difficult to obtain certification in some locations (Andrews, 1998/1999). Some examination sections might cover material unrelated to classroom practices or that make it difficult for deaf teachers to pass. Professionals today are scrutinizing this practice in the interest of ensuring that potential deaf teachers are not discouraged from entering the field and can join hearing peers in providing collaborative models for their students.

The fact that day programs for the deaf rarely feature deaf adults as administrators makes it that much harder to enhance hearing-deaf relationships in such settings. Individuals such as Kathleen Treni of New Jersey have broken through this barrier and held on to their administrative positions by virtue of good hearing-deaf collaborative approaches. In the field of audiology, Gallaudet University has enrolled deaf students in its audiology doctoral program. They will be able to work with hearing audiologists and help the field incorporate different perspectives about "hearing" in the course of evaluating audiological needs and providing amplification information.

INTERPRETER ISSUES

The development of healthy hearing-deaf relationships is very often contingent on how sign-language interpreter issues are resolved. Most hearing professionals and hearing peers do not develop sign-language proficiency and not all deaf persons develop proficiency in spoken English. During face-to-face interactions, it is the sign-language interpreter who serves as a bridge for the facilitation of hearing-deaf communication.

Sign-language interpreting, traditionally seen as a service for deaf adults, developed out of the need for deaf people to communicate in depth with hearing people. Early interpreters were family members who could sign, particularly hearing children of deaf parents, friends, and other local resources (Schein, 1989).

Although their social intentions were often above reproach, hearing people could intrude themselves into the dialogue, provide opinions, and, without being aware, inadvertently influence not only the outcome of such interactions but also reinforce how hearing people might perceive deaf people as inferior. And deaf people themselves found it difficult to complain because of their dependency on these volunteer interpreters.

Sign-language interpreting evolved into a professional field because of an increasing demand for interpreters by deaf adults and the inability of informal volunteers to meet this demand. The establishment of the Registry of Interpreters for the Deaf (RID) was a natural outcome of the professionalization of the field (www.rid.org). Because of ethical issues related to confidentiality and interpreter exploitation of information obtained through interpreted situations among other things, the RID developed a stringent code of ethics that covers the use of sign-language interpreters. This ensures confidentiality and accurate reflection of ongoing dialogue, whether it is voice to sign or sign to voice. The RID is also working with the National Association of the Deaf on interpreter certification issues (E. Pollard, 2002). This provides another positive example of hearing-deaf collaboration. Clearly, it is best to use certified interpreters who are fully qualified to handle many interpreter situations both linguistically and ethically. Throughout the United States, there are interpreter agencies, which are a valuable resource for providing sign-language interpreters as well as oral interpreters.

Many deaf people are acutely aware that their ability to develop positive relationships with hearing peers, whatever the context—the workplace, the social setting, the classroom, the conference—depends to a significant degree on the quality of the interpreters being used and their skills in formulating accurate translations. Deaf people see interpreting as a valued and cherished service. For many, this has provided entry into job opportunities that might have otherwise been unavailable, or into social, educational, and recreational situations that maximize the potential for participating in hearing society activities. However, there are ongoing issues that need to be acknowledged and dealt with in order to enhance hearing-deaf relationships.

Interpreters regularly deal with a variety of demands, including linguistic, environmental (e.g., court, classroom, business conference), interpersonal, and intrapersonal (role expectations, knowledge of specialized language relevant to the setting, such as medical or statistical terminology) demands. In addition, they are at risk for chronic physical disability such as carpal tunnel syndrome (Dean & Pollard, 2001). Interpreters must constantly judge appropriate responses, oftentimes in difficult situations. Recurrent frustrations include, for example, situations when deaf persons are unfamiliar with interpreter roles or when hearing people start talking to interpreters instead of focusing on the process of communicating with deaf persons through these interpreters. Unfortunately, some deaf persons are not particularly sensitive to interpreter stress, considering their dependency on interpreters and their expectations of how interpreters perform their duties. For both hearing and deaf parties, training will facilitate the comfort of interpreting situations and sensitivity to the role of the interpreter.

Admittedly, sign-to-voice interpreting is more difficult than voice-to-sign interpretation. Adequate translation requires a true understanding of linguistic nuances in whatever way the deaf person chooses to express himself or herself, especially in individual facial nuances, gestures, and signs. When the interpreter's first language is spoken English and not ASL, there can be considerable stress in working through the translation process, particularly when interpreters know that they are responsible for how the deaf person is represented to the hearing public.

In turn, what is extremely frustrating for deaf persons themselves are situations when they recognize that they are not being accurately interpreted. Interpreters are *not* neutral conduits. Instead, they significantly affect interchanges through their ability to understand, their knowledge of terminology, and their translation selections (Dean & Pollard, 2001; Metzger, 1999; Roy, 2000). These issues are manifestations of how interpreters potentially control situations and affect hearing perceptions of deaf people.

For example, excellent speeches by deaf presenters may sound less than excellent when poorly interpreted. Hearing listeners will then develop poor opinions of the presenters. When professional terminology is translated incorrectly, this can negatively affect perceptions about the sophistication level of deaf professionals. During a professional meeting, a deaf sociolinguist used the term *language acquisition* in the course of his lecture (S. Nover, personal communication, January 15, 2002). The interpreter interpreted this term as *language pick-up.* By selecting this phrase, the interpreter unwittingly created false impressions that put the deaf sociolinguist at a disadvantage in the minds of hearing scholars at this academic conference.

Multiplied many times over, such situations leave sign-language users at the mercy of interpreters and without any means of evaluating whether they have been accurately interpreted. All too often, deaf people are not aware that they have not been accurately interpreted. As more deaf adults earn advanced degrees, the need for more highly educated and sophisticated interpreters to minimize such mistakes will increase.

To rectify mistakes, deaf people need to become extra-sensitive to hearing respondent dialogue, correct misunderstandings as these emerge, and obtain feedback from trusted hearing colleagues. When real-time captioning is available, deaf people can verify interpreter translations by checking text as they go along. These tactics demand a level of sophisticated awareness that the typical deaf person may always not possess, and training efforts in this direction will help.

In addition to questions of interpretation, some deaf professionals may be wary of the hidden ambitions of some sign-language interpreters. Based on on-the-job informal networking and exposure to job duties, hearing coworkers and supervisors may feel that interpreters understand both the subject matter and the roles of the deaf persons for whom they are interpreting. People, deaf or hearing, are more comfortable in situations that involve direct communication. Thus, having to work through an interpreter requires some adjustment. There have been stories of job openings being filled by the interpreter instead of qualified deaf applicants. Deaf professionals who rely on sign language see this as a thorny issue, reflecting ongoing oppression. Training of hearing personnel about interpreter roles and boundaries may help rectify this situation. Other than that, there is no clear resolution apart from recourse to the ADA. People who might think of suing have to deal with concerns about their professional reputations as potential troublemakers with negative implications for future job possibilities.

It is important to remember that many sign-language interpreters embrace interpreting as a lifelong career and establish excellent reputations. Some use their interpreter training and interpreting work to obtain in-depth understanding of deafness and related issues. Others pursue higher education to improve their qualifications for working in different capacities with and for deaf people. Their abilities to form positive relationships with deaf colleagues is a key factor in their being accepted by deaf people.

Are sign-language interpreters adequately sensitized to the perceptions of deaf consumers in the course of whatever training they receive? Considering the lack of consistency in criteria for interpreter training programs and the fact that the term *qualified* has yet to be specified throughout the country (Dean & Pollard, 2001), training and subsequent experiences should involve ongoing feedback regarding performance, particularly from deaf consumers themselves.

One overriding issue regarding interpreters is cost. Many administrators may be willing to accommodate deaf people, but they are concerned about this ancillary expense. This is a valid concern that needs to be addressed (see, for example, Gianelli, 1999; Hauser et al., 2000). For example, many medical providers and hospitals continue to deny communication access or interpreters for patients and claim that writing is sufficient, based solely on economic or profit considerations, thereby inviting lawsuits (Harmer, 1999). This is a blatant example of oppression in which hearing perspectives about the communication needs of deaf people are superimposed over the perspectives of the deaf consumers. What is overlooked is that cost effectiveness as part of the greater picture can be argued when deaf people in most typical situations fully understand their medical issues, take care of themselves, and reduce their need for medical attention and in turn for medical insurance payment. It is heartening to hear reports of medical offices inquiring about communication preferences when deaf patients call to schedule appointments so that interpreters can be on site if needed.

To look at the cost issue from a different perspective, a hearing organization may automatically include sound systems that enhance communication for hearing people as part of operating costs, but will question whether to enhance communication access for deaf persons as an integral part of operating costs. Admittedly, this is an expensive proposition. Some effort to consider creative financial solutions will go a long way in conveying the message that accessibility is important for *both* deaf and hearing people. Not making this effort does deaf people an enormous disservice and perpetuates discrimination. The Americans with Disabilities Act of 1990 has provisions that apply to both privately and publicly funded settings as well as an undue hardship provision that covers settings having 15 employees or more. If settings claim undue hardship, both the program or subdivision resources and the resources of the entire institution or agency are examined in order to ascertain whether operating costs for interpreting services do justify denying accessibility because of undue hardship.

ATTITUDES WITHIN THE DEAF COMMUNITY

Although this chapter focuses on hearing-deaf relationships, we cannot leave the topic of attitudes without very briefly touching on attitudes within the deaf community. Yes, the deaf community is diverse, and one can find a multitude of deaf members of various ethnic and racial groups, members who are gay, lesbian, bisexual, deaf-blind, affiliated with various religious groups, and so on, mingling amicably at large deaf community events (Lane, Hoffmeister, & Bahan, 1996). The commonality of being deaf does facilitate cohesiveness in these diverse groups of deaf people, even to a greater extent than may be found in hearing gatherings.

However, the deaf community is also a microcosm of the larger hearing community. It has factions that do not always coexist in full harmony or that exhibit bigotry (Erting et al., 1994; Lane, Hoffmeister, & Bahan, 1996; Leigh & Lewis, 1999). And, sadly, some deaf people absorb the discriminatory values of the societies in which they develop, and perpetuate the ongoing oppression of deaf peers on the basis of religion, race or ethnicity, sexual orientation, language preference, and disability.

Take the case of deaf-blind persons, among the most isolated of all people. Many deaf people understandably harbor some fear of vision loss, and seeing deaf-blind persons will ignite that fear (Miner, 1999). Even more, there is the stigma of additional disability. To deal with this, sighted deaf persons will often minimize social contact with deaf-blind people, thus perpetuating their isolation. Openly gay deaf people still confront varying types of rejection, ranging from snide remarks to overt rejection by heterosexual deaf people (Gutman, 1999; Langholtz & Ruth, 1999). American Indians who are deaf have been beaten up by their peers in schools for the deaf (Eldredge, 1999). The black and white deaf communities have historically gone their separate ways because of institutionalized racism (Aramburo, 1994; Corbett, 1999; Jankowski, 1997). Deaf people who object to oral values have ostracized deaf people who prefer spoken English, even if they can sign (Leigh, 1999b). The history of deaf women approaching parity with deaf men in running deaf organizations is relatively recent (Lane, Hoffmeister, & Bahan, 1996; Holcomb & Wood, 1989).

In coming to terms with the fact that we are a diverse society, we can turn to models of deaf people who reject such behavior, and who strive for common causes that bring deaf people together. These causes include civil rights and empowerment, employment equity, and access to communication, whether face to face or via technology. Just as society struggles with discrimination as an ongoing process, the deaf community is engaged in a parallel struggle to learn about respect for diversity in the face of an increasingly multicultural deaf component. It is the schools, ranging from preschool through postsecondary settings, that bear most of the burden for increasing sensitivity to diversity. Many have responded to this call by instituting multicultural programs that teach about respect for diversity.

Even though deaf people have worked hard to ensure their places in society, it has taken them a long time to learn that if they are not seen as a united front, they will fail to achieve desired political agendas. The number of organizations in the deaf community is large in proportion to the small size of the community (Van Cleve & Crouch, 1989). All of these organizations have their own mission and objectives, and historically they were seldom united on issues related to the lives of deaf people (Christiansen & Barnartt, 1995). This often sabotaged political possibilities.

The Deaf President Now movement showed that the deaf community was capable of media manipulation, a united front, and political saavy. Since then, national organizations of deaf people, including some of those listed in Chapter 10, have banded together to form the Consumer Action Network (CAN) (Christiansen & Barnartt, 1995). Organizations composed of hearing people who work to serve the interests of deaf people can be associate members but do not have voting rights. The network engages regularly in the political process and produces position statements related to different legislative initiatives that affect the educational, rehabilitation, mental health, occupational, social, and political lives of deaf people. In doing so, CAN not only informs hearing society of the perspectives and goals of deaf people but it also draws deaf organizations together and limits the potential for infighting.

CONCLUSION

When deaf and hearing administrators of schools and programs for deaf and hearing children are seen as equally desirable, when no eyebrows are raised at the announcement of deaf professionals heading major institutions and corporations, when the expectation is that deaf people from diverse backgrounds can contribute as much to society as hearing people, and when subtle discriminatory biases that reinforce the perception that deaf people are limited in some way because of their deafness are eliminated, then one may say that the potential for healthy relationships between deaf and hearing colleagues has been fully achieved. The possibility of that happening today is far greater than it was decades ago, but, as indicated throughout this book, there still is room for improvement.

We believe that through recurrent positive exposure to each other, deaf and hearing people will continue to work together in dismantling attitudinal barriers that hamper healthy coexistence. This requires ongoing education and sensitivity in view of the fact that society at large is still engaged in the process of breaking free of lingering stereotypical perceptions of deaf people.

SUGGESTED READINGS

Branson, J., & Miller, D. (2002). *Dammed for their Difference: The Cultural Construction of Deaf People as Disabled*. Washington, DC: Gallaudet University Press.

This book explains the different constructions of the word *disabled* and attempts to address why deaf people have been repeatedly discriminated against. The authors analyze cultural, social, and historical contexts to provide an explanation for this phenomenon.

Jepson, L. (1992). *No Walls of Stone: An Anthology of Literature by Deaf and Hard of Hearing Writers*. Washington, DC: Gallaudet University Press.

This is an anthology of poetry written by deaf persons, primarily those who lost their hearing in later childhood, youth, or adulthood. The emotional intensity of the poems and prose pieces can startle and shock but they can also amuse and please.

Wrigley, O. (1996). *The Politics of Deafness*. Washington, DC: Gallaudet University Press.

This book, in the author's words, "is about the political meanings of deafness, about the politics of Deaf identity, and about what it costs to be 'unusual.'" It couches the conflicts between deaf and hearing people in a historical context and therefore provides insight to the present and future needs for productive deaf-hearing collaborative relationships.

CHAPTER TWELVE

TO THE FUTURE

The basic reason for becoming involved with deaf adults: we are
your children grown. We can, in many instances, tell you the
things your child would like to tell you, if he had the vocabulary
and the experiences to put his feelings and needs into words.

—Schreiber, 1969, cited in Schein, 1981

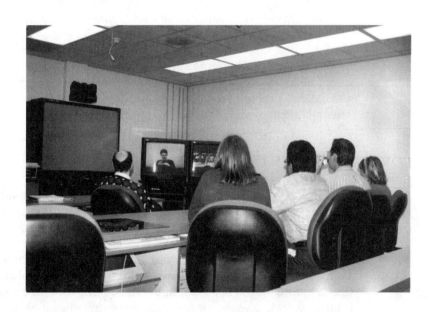

In the Preface, we introduced questions about deaf people. Throughout the book, we have attempted to answer these questions, starting in the first chapter with an exploration of the field of psychology and deafness. The issues discussed in that chapter—including intellectual testing, mental health services, changes in standards of care, professional training, and the effects of Deaf culture—illustrate how the field has evolved. Chapters 2 though 11 provide additional information to help us answer the questions posed in the Preface. This chapter briefly reviews critical points and uses this as a stepping-stone to envision what the future may bring in terms of research and development.

Nationwide, almost 28 million people have hearing loss ranging from mild to profound. This can affect speech and language comprehension to varying degrees. Some causes of hearing loss can be treated medically, but the majority of profoundly deaf persons have a sensorineural hearing loss that is permanent (Chapter 3). Each year in the United States, approximately 5,000 infants are born with moderate to profound, bilateral, permanent hearing loss. Approximately 400 types of genetic deafness have been identified (Gorlin, Toriello, & Cohen, 1995). About one out of every 1,000 children is born deaf. Another one person in 1,000 becomes deaf through infections such as meningitis. Roughly one in every 10,000 to 15,000 persons will experience sudden sensorineural hearing loss, primarily in the 50- to 60-year-old range (Muller, 2001). Acoustical trauma and damage from loud noises, especially at industrial and military settings, also cause hearing loss. Presbycusis, a specific type of hearing loss that emerges in the later stages of adulthood, affects almost 25 percent of the population by age 65 and 50 percent by age 80. Hearing loss for the elderly population can be socially isolating. Older Americans can also suffer from Meniere's disease, which affects the vestibular system and results in hearing and balance problems. In this book, we have focused on deaf persons with sensorineural deafness starting in the early years.

ADVANCES IN MENTAL HEALTH SERVICES

Historically, deaf people were perceived as less than mentally competent. In the past 50 years, society has learned that deaf people have similar ranges of intellectual abilities as hearing persons do. This discovery was accomplished by professionals who recognized that intelligence can be defined in a variety of ways. It was not necessary to rely solely on verbal testing to measure intellectual functioning. Using performance tests to assess cognitive and intellectual abilities facilitated professional recognition of the strengths and abilities of deaf people. This was a significant advance in that the professional community began to perceive deaf people not as deficient human beings, but as persons with different types of capabilities. Professionals now know that with optimal innate factors and environmental stimulation, deaf people can maximize their potential. This meant that services were necessary to facilitate that process. This also meant that professionals had to internalize the expectation that deaf people could benefit from mental health services (Chapters 1, 8, and 9).

In their work with deaf individuals, counselors and therapists can take advantage of the wide range of therapy approaches that have been developed. In the general population, outcome results for some of these approaches have been investigated relative to various mental health problems. It is time to start investigating the effectiveness of specific treatment processes that are used with culturally and linguistically diverse deaf people. One example of such research is that of Guthman (1996), who evaluated the effectiveness of different interventions for chemically dependent deaf adults enrolled in the Minnesota Chemical Dependency Program for Deaf and Hard of Hearing Individuals. She found that participation in 12-step programs, a communicatively accessible support system, and employment significantly increased the chances of maintaining sobriety.

The evolution of telehealth services should improve mental health service delivery to deaf clients in far-flung areas. South Carolina now uses videoconferencing to enable a signing psychiatrist to communicate with deaf clients throughout the state (Afrin & Critchfield, 1999). The University of Rochester Medical Center recently started offering cost-effective sign-language interpreting for medical settings using remote sign-language interpreting services available through videoconferencing (www.urmc.rochester.edu/strongconnections/). How this will impact counseling and psychotherapy services provided by nonsigning clinicians remains to be seen.

Psychologists have used a variety of psychological tests with deaf children and adults. Only a few measures have deaf sample population norms. The field could benefit from the rigorous evaluation of numerous existing measures to determine their validity and reliability for deaf test-takers. Much work is needed to develop ASL-based measures that can appropriately assess psychiatric symptoms. Additionally, research is needed to evaluate the use of sign-language interpreters in test administration. Researchers need to learn if test results based on interpreted information can accurately reflect how a deaf person functions in the different domains being tested. Finally, it is time to take a closer look at computerized testing and assess its reliability and validity for deaf test-takers.

The move away from dealing with deaf people as a homogenous entity has resulted in the need to understand the unique influences of various factors that differentiate deaf people from each other. Today, people know that understanding the impact of these influences and using this knowledge to treat deaf people requires professional training. Without such training, mental health services, or any other type of human services, such as rehabilitation counseling, will not be effective. Psychologists, psychiatrists, social workers, and counselors need to be able to communicate with deaf clients. They also must understand communication issues and how these interact with differing cultural backgrounds. In the early years, those professionals with adequate training were minuscule in number. This has changed. Today, there are a number of graduate programs in psychology, social work, and counseling with specialization in deafness. These programs have trained many hearing and deaf professionals who have worked to improve the quality of mental health and allied services. A critical training priority is that of recruiting and training mental health service providers from different ethnic backgrounds.

Another important training issue involves the appropriate use of psychological assessment by psychologists. This is a particularly important issue, since assessment results depend greatly on the competence of the psychological evaluator. Familiarity with deafness and communication issues will improve the chances that psychological test results accurately portray the strengths and weaknesses of deaf children and adults who are evaluated (Chapters 1, 8, and 9).

AMERICAN SIGN LANGUAGE

Another advance has been the recognition and acceptance of American Sign Language (ASL), not only as the language that Deaf people use but also as a language worthy of formal research. The use of ASL is being explored through research into its role in psychological functioning, best practices in education, bilingualism and second language learning, psycholinguistics, neurolinguistics, and literacy learning (Chapters 1, 4, 5, 7, 9, and 10). The study of cognitive processing and learning styles in deaf children has gone in new directions with the addition of ASL as an investigative tool (Chapter 4). In mental health, analyzing the ASL expressions of Deaf people who are psychotic will facilitate accurate diagnosis of deaf persons confronting mental illnesses.

The use of ASL has enabled neuroscientists to explore the frontiers of the brain in order to understand where sign language is processed and to develop more accurate hypotheses about how the brain is organized for language. Previously, linguists relied on studying deaf stroke victims with brain damage to learn more about language lateralization. Using measurements of proficiency for understanding and producing signs, scientists have found that stroke victims using speech and those using signs had similar localized brain damage. A significant finding was that the brain's left hemisphere is dominant for sign language, just as it is for speech (Poinzer, Klima, & Bellugi, 1987).

Today's noninvasive brain imaging techniques, including magnetic resonance imaging (MRI) and positron-emission tomography (PET), have allowed neuroscientists to explore the brains of Deaf individuals who communicate in ASL with the goal of probing for the neural roots of signed languages. In their attempt to clarify the role of the right hemisphere for sign-language processing, scientists have reported surprising findings. Even though sign language has visual-spatial organizational features, the neural organization of sign language has more in common with that of spoken language than it does with the neural organization of visual-spatial processing. Based on this new information, researchers at the Salk Institute are now investigating the activity of sign language processing in both left and right hemispheres (Hickok, Bellugi, & Klima, 2001) (Chapter 4).

Language teaching approaches for deaf children have been developed based on the use of signs in general and ASL in particular. Total communication, which uses ASL signs superimposed on English word order and speech, was developed to take advantage of visual ways to use English. It was introduced into the homes of deaf children, infant programs, and classrooms. Additionally, several sign systems using English word order were invented and used with deaf children. Although these approaches led to better face-to-face communication skills compared with spoken communication alone for many deaf children and their families, researchers did not see major gains in language and literacy achievement test scores (Chapter 7).

In the early 1970s and again in the 1990s, researchers turned to an examination of the links between the acquisition and use of ASL and English reading and writing abilities (Butler & Prinz, 1998; Chamberlain, Morford, & Mayberry, 2000). Teachers and researchers are now studying the bilingual and second language literature with the purpose of using these theoretical and practical frameworks to better understand the language learning needs of deaf students. Interactive literacy lessons are a recent development that can assist deaf readers in moving from ASL, a language that uses space and movement, to English, a phonetically based sequential language (Bailes, 2001; Gallimore, 1999). The use of finger-spelling and signs as a bridge to understanding literacy is also being explored (Padden & Ramsey, 2000). Just as Shirley Brice Heath, in her book, *Way with Words* (1983), provided profound insights into how culture affects children's literacy learning, Deaf culture elements—such as ASL narratives and storytelling, ABC stories, and visual and spatial strategies—are increasingly being used in deaf children's literacy lessons (Lane, Hoffmeister, & Bahan, 1996).

The gains reported in speech production for deaf children with cochlear implants lead us to wonder whether this will translate into ease in mastering phonological approaches to reading. Considering that some deaf children with cochlear implants are now entering schools for the deaf that use the bilingual-bicultural approach, we are curious to learn whether relying on auditory information to facilitate phonological awareness is in fact compatible with the use of ASL strategies to enhance reading. Specifically, would the use of both ASL and auditory strategies provide the deaf reader with additional tools to decode words, or would using both of these strategies lead to confusion?

As we pointed out in Chapter 4, deaf children and adults can provide insights regarding the nature of the so-called critical period, because many deaf persons are delayed in their exposure to language. Scientists have yet to fully understand the mechanisms responsible for the "critical period" in first and second language acquisition, with some arguing in favor of this period and some against it (Emmorey, 2000). However, ongoing study of how deaf children acquire their first and second languages can provide further data on this controversial theory.

Research on speaking-signing bilingual children acquiring two languages—sign language and spoken English—can shed light on childhood bilingualism in general. Research studies done by Petitto and colleagues on dual language bilinguals and signing-speaking bilinguals show that very early simultaneous bilingual language exposure does not cause young children to be delayed in achieving the classic milestones nor does it cause children to confuse their semantic and conceptual learning of language. In other words, hearing children can easily learn two languages early, whether it be two spoken languages or a signed and a spoken language (Petitto & Holowka, 2002). How this research translates to deaf children learning ASL and English remains to be explored. But these new research findings of childhood bilingualism may provide insights to develop more effective early intervention programs for deaf bilingual children learning ASL and English.

CHANGES IN THE DEAF COMMUNITY

To many, the culture of Deaf people has historically signaled repression, isolation and dependence. Hearing people not intimately acquainted with deaf people have traditionally seen the deaf community as a ghetto apart from the "real world," hence the urge to "bring deaf children into the hearing world." But deaf people are full participants in their community, just like hearing people are participants in their own communities. The world is full of communities to which people gravitate, depending on their origins and their life experiences.

In addition to the traditional model of deafness as a disability, recent literature has increasingly incorporated sociocultural models of deafness that reflect different feelings and perspectives about deafness as a way of life. Recent efforts by Allen Sussman to develop a wellness model that portrays psychologically healthy deaf adults provides a fresh perspective of who deaf people are, how society views them, and how deaf people identify themselves (Chapters 2, 9, and 11). This challenges the age-old stereotypical version of deaf people as people with problems in living. Many deaf individuals manage to live productive lives and some don't—just like their hearing counterparts. Additionally, the faces of deaf people have changed from the traditional picture of white deaf males to pictures of deaf women, men, and children who are members of the diverse ethnic and racial groups that now make up the population of the United States. The demographic shifts currently taking place in the United States are mirrored in the deaf community as well (Chapters 2 and 9).

Deaf culture serves to draw all these diverse deaf people together with a set of shared experiences and worldwide social and educational networks (Chapters 2, 9, and 10). It is a vibrant culture vividly expressed at the many Deaf cultural festivals occurring in cities, and through Deaf art, ASL storytelling, and Deaf theater and literature. For Deaf people, such artistic expressions provide an opportunity to share the "Deaf perspective." In particular, these cultural expressions serve as a forum to vividly illustrate their experiences at the hands of hearing society, in particular their feelings of oppression. This is a form of empowerment. One end result of these expressions has been to provide hearing viewers with new perspectives that counteract their natural and traditional urges toward ethnocentric and egocentric behaviors when it comes to Deaf people. In essence, these cultural expressions serve to reinforce the fact that Deaf people want to be understood. In turn, we also want to emphasize that not only culturally Deaf people, but also deaf people who have different types of affiliations with the deaf community, and outside the deaf community want their views and opinions considered as well in the larger hearing society (Chapter 11).

Historically, in their choice of occupations many deaf persons were limited to blue-collar jobs such as printing, shoe repair, factory work, peddling, and barbering.

With today's proliferation of interpreter services, wireless and digital technologies, relay services, positive media representations, free and appropriate education, and legal protections from discrimination, deaf people intermingle in the broader society as never before. They increasingly benefit from the larger society's offerings in education, employment, and recreation. Gallaudet University has a deaf president (I. K. Jordan) and NTID has a deaf vice president (Robert Davila) who holds that rank under the umbrella of RIT and its president. The numbers of deaf teachers working in schools for young deaf students has increased exponentially. Hundreds of deaf adults are now studying for graduate degrees and teacher certification at various universities in the country (Chapter 6). With postsecondary and graduate education accessibility enhanced by the use of interpreters, voice-to-text software, video relay, real-time captioning, and distance learning and tutoring, many deaf adults are succeeding in higher education and in various professions and trades. Today, even more occupations are accessible to deaf people (Chapters 2 and 10). Many are employed as computer programmers and software developers, educational researchers, scientists, inventors, physicians, religious leaders, lawyers, teachers, administrators, CEOs of companies, stockbrokers, chefs, auto mechanics, ad infinitum. Although automation continues to hinder the deaf unskilled worker, job opportunities in an increasing number of fields are open to them (Chapter 10).

There is a dark side, too. The deaf community is plagued by illiteracy, underemployment, and underachievement (Chapter 10). Many deaf persons get caught in the criminal justice system and need special services (Miller, 2001). Some refuse to work, and abuse the social security system. Some cannot get work. Learning to read and write continues to be difficult for many (Traxler, 2000). The wide gap between many deaf persons' intelligence levels as indicated on intelligence tests and their low academic performance remains. All of this is very discouraging. But looking at the big picture, it is not difficult to see how many hearing Americans are struggling with same issues. Like many Deaf Americans, African American, Hispanic, Asian American, Native American, and immigrant communities struggle daily to survive economically, get a good education, enjoy all the freedoms and benefits the United States offers, and assimilate into U.S. society without sacrificing their cultural identities.

The media continually reflect ongoing debate about the best ways to resolve these complex issues. But solutions can be effective only when the strengths of the people involved are utilized. With deaf people, their problems can more readily be addressed when instructional programs are built on their sensory, cognitive, and survival strengths rather than on their limitations. Framed in this way, there is hope that future research can alleviate the problems that continue to plague deaf people. Cross-cultural studies of ethnic communities and deaf communities that focus on the skills they use to succeed may be one way to address these issues. With the inclusion of more deaf professionals on research teams, different perspectives and creative solutions have the opportunity to emerge.

Historically, the community of deaf people expanded as graduates of residential schools for the deaf entered its ranks. That is changing. Today, increasing numbers of deaf children are being educated in the public schools, more often with hearing peers. Many will not form social networks with deaf people until a much later age, if at all (Chapter 2). This clearly influences psychosocial development in general, and the development of deaf identities in particular (Chapters 8 and 9). Furthermore, this new development will change the face of the deaf community to one that is more diverse in terms of experience.

Additional factors include the fact that the ways in which deaf people socialize has moved beyond the traditional structure of Deaf clubs. These clubs appear to be on the decline due to home TV captioning, email, and other technologies. There is a rising middle class of deaf professionals who have enjoyed the benefits of increased postsecondary and graduate school opportunities (Padden, 1998). They tend to engage in different types of socializing that is not necessarily Deaf club based. As noted in Chapters 2 and 10, there has been a proliferation of organizations of deaf persons representing different constituencies in recent years. These include, for example, organizations of deaf people having diverse ethnic origins; deaf persons with cochlear implants; gays, lesbians, and bisexual persons who are deaf; deaf senior citizens; deaf religious groups; and many others, each of which encourages group bonding.

When people enter the deaf community, they will find that this involvement fosters strong interdependence among its members. This continues from early childhood into old age. Elderly deaf persons from residential schools typically maintain lifelong friendships developed in childhood. Those who enter the deaf community during adolescence and adulthood also develop close bonds within the community. Their social networks sustain them, even after they have retired. The number of deaf retirees has greatly increased, and they have banded to form a national organization, Deaf Seniors of America (Chapter 10). Many of the deaf retirees are now clustering in areas such as Las Vegas, Nevada, and Boynton Beach, Florida. There are some rest homes and retirement villages throughout the United States that have been set up for deaf senior citizens.

The issue of tolerance in the face of increasing diversity within the deaf community is one that demands attention. Although the community has traditionally been known to welcome this diversity, tolerating different types of people still continues to be an issue on the local level. Research into effective ways of fostering tolerance, particularly in the schools, will ameliorate the insidious effects of discrimination. Leadership training will encourage the development of effective leaders that will model tolerance for a widely diverse deaf population.

There is also a need to reinforce the perception, both professionally and on the lay level, that there are psychologically healthy deaf adults who choose the hearing world or the deaf world, or, most commonly, who gravitate between both worlds. We repeat this observation yet again because too many tend to forget that these adults, who are able to confront life and to fashion satisfactory adjustments for themselves, are more the norm than the rarity (Chapter 9). Studying these psychologically healthy deaf adults will help develop parameters of normalcy within the deaf population as contrasted with those who struggle with mental illnesses and other significant difficulties. This can also contribute to improvements in differential diagnosis in the psychiatric realm.

ADVANCES IN MOLECULAR GENETICS AND
COCHLEAR IMPLANTATION

The deaf community is now facing critical developments that have the potential for radically influencing the lives of its members and future generations of deaf people. These developments are related to advances in molecular genetics and cochlear implantation. The work in both areas raises profound and complex biological, ethical, and social issues.

The issues pertinent to genetics and deafness are not new. There is a history that is filled with controversy and tragedy (Chapter 3). The recognition of familial-based hearing loss goes way back to the late 1800s, when schools for the deaf noted the existence of large numbers of families with deaf siblings and relatives. In his book, *On a Deaf Variety of the Human Race*, Alexander Graham Bell (1883) recommended that, in order to eliminate deafness, deaf people should not marry each other or bear children. This and other work contributed to the early policies of the Nazi Germany regime that ordered the sterilization and eventual extermination of deaf children and adults. These crimes are well documented. In particular, Biesold (1999) poignantly describes the long-term effects of these sterilization policies on deaf survivors in his book, *Crying Hands*.

Scientists are making major strides in identifying and locating the genes involved in hereditary deafness. Currently, the field now has access to the biochemical and molecular characteristics of the genes involved in the composition of more than 30 forms of genetic hearing loss (Grundfast, Siparsky, & Chuong, 2000). Genes have been located and identified for specific syndromes that include hearing loss. The recent identification of connexin 26 represents a significant development in the investigation of genes for nonsyndromic deafness (Arnos, 2002) (Chapter 3). Testing for connexin 26 is relatively easy in comparison to other more complex genes for deafness. Overall, genetic research has resulted in practical applications of this new knowledge, improved testing, and better access to genetic counseling for deaf individuals and their families (Arnos, 1999).

Today, experts know that genetic deafness occurs more often in hearing families than in deaf families. Chapter 3 describes the various ways in which genetic deafness is transmitted. With the Human Genome Project, vast amounts of data are made available to scientists who are identifying and mapping genes. Currently, there are hundreds of publications and websites that focus on the dissemination of information on genetics and hearing loss (Gerber, 2001). Certainly, genetic information, when properly used, can offer many benefits to hearing people, deaf people, and their families.

But what does "proper use of genetic information" really mean? Extensive publicity about the unknown and potentially fatal consequences of gene therapy leads one to seriously consider the ethical issues of this procedure. Should the goal be to prevent deafness altogether by using genetic engineering to modify the structure of the gene that causes hearing loss through adding, replacing, or repairing the gene? Could and should deafness be prevented with the use of fetal testing in the early months of pregnancy? If findings are positive for deafness, parents will be confronted with decisions related to keeping or aborting the fetus. Such prevention techniques are highly controversial (Gerber, 2001).

More acceptable and viable prevention measures are already in place in the guise of early intervention programs. These encourage appropriate environmental stimulation to ensure that deafness does not result in language disability. However, a difference of opinion exist on what form early intervention should take for infants diagnosed through newborn hearing screening (Chapter 8) (Thompson et al., 2001). One side argues for the use of early auditory input as early as possible to facilitate language development. The opposing view suggests that during infancy, attachment behaviors such as nonverbal communication, joint attention, shared experiences, and mutual understanding are more important than having the infant hear and produce sounds, at least in the first six months of life. The field needs to determine the best practices in early intervention for newborns and for those diagnosed later, as well as how to minimize false positives and negatives.

Another difference in viewpoints relates to genetic pathology versus genetic diversity. The medical desire to enhance the human condition by eliminating genetically based pathology often clashes with the view that genetic diversity is an expected and acceptable part of the human condition. Gerber (2001) expresses concern about the potential implications for genetic manipulation in eliminating groups of people with inherited conditions, including genetically transmitted hearing loss. From an ethical perspective, this conflict raises issues related to self-determination and autonomy on the part of those most directly affected. As indicated in Chapter 3, Arnos (2002) recommends that deaf people empower themselves through learning more about the genetics of deafness and analyzing how new developments in the field will potentially impact the lives of deaf people. Deaf organizations are beginning to explore this issue. Ongoing debate on the ethics of genetic treatment for hereditary forms of deafness will be fueled by the development of gene therapy that can manipulate genes to prevent hearing loss. Whether it means the eradication of Deaf culture in the future is subject to conjecture at this time. Who will decide whether gene therapy should be available—the medical community, the potential parents of the deaf children, or the deaf people themselves?

Still another subject for debate is that of cochlear implants. Cochlear implants have been on the scene for several decades. Researchers are now studying the effects of pediatric cochlear implantation, particularly in the areas of speech and language development. Some researchers are beginning to consider the possibility that the exact genetic condition and pathology in the cochlea may influence the recommendation to proceed with cochlear implantation. This knowledge could ensure that only those children who can optimally use the cochlear implant get it.

It is important to acknowledge, however, that there are many other factors extraneous to the genetic basis of deafness, including individual variability and environmental input, which play significant roles in predicting whether individuals will benefit from using the cochlear implant (Chapter 7). At this time, research data indicate considerable variation in how well children learn to decipher and understand the information they receive through the cochlear implant. Some will have optimal access to information that can help them understand spoken language and speak intelligibly. Their numbers are growing. Others will only react to environmental sounds.

Parents of children with cochlear implants who participated in surveys eliciting their perspectives on the procedure indicated that for the most part they were happy with their decision to implant their child (Christiansen & Leigh, 2002). They found it made their daily lives easier in ways that ranged from being able to call their children from the next room to ease in spoken communication. Many of those parents who were already signing to their children pre-implant have not stopped using signs with their implanted children. They see their children as deaf and support contact with deaf friends in addition to hearing peers. The Clerc Center at Gallaudet University is experimenting with bilingual classrooms for implanted children that provide speech and auditory training in conjunction with the use of ASL for academically based information.

With the increase in the number of individuals getting cochlear implants, some people express concern that this process could lead to the demise of the Deaf world if deaf children with cochlear implants in fact functioned much like hearing children did. Interestingly, in a survey of Gallaudet University faculty, staff, students, and alumni related to cochlear implants, Christiansen and Leigh (2002) found that the majority of deaf, hearing, and hard-of-hearing respondents felt that the Deaf world would not disappear. Based on a breakdown of the respondents, half of the deaf sample concurred, as did over 70 percent of the hearing and hard-of-hearing sample.

Considering the variable results with cochlear implant use, we agree that Deaf culture is not in imminent danger of extinction, particularly in view of financial roadblocks for many, including minority members and those in third world countries. Corollary with this perspective, the National Association of the Deaf (2000a) revised its position paper. It now accepts the implant but provides cautious guidelines for parents, the medical community, and manufacturers. It is possible that the deaf community will change in response to the infusion of individuals with cochlear implants, as it has changed in response to other technological innovations such as the hearing aid, the TTY, email, and so forth.

EDUCATION ISSUES

Today, 46 percent of deaf children are from nonwhite homes (GRI, 2002). Almost 22 percent of deaf children are from Hispanic homes. In many of these homes, Spanish is spoken. There is also an influx of deaf immigrants from Mexico, South and Central America, and Southeast Asia. Many of these individuals arrive in late childhood or during the teenage years without having had much formal education in their home country. These deaf immigrants pose a unique educational challenge to U.S. schools. Sign-language immersion and job training programs are needed for them. Training educational researchers, teachers, and administrators who are deaf and persons of color will facilitate the ability of educational institutions to meet this critical challenge.

Since the enactment of Public Law 94-142 and subsequently the Individuals with Disabilities Education Act (IDEA), parents legally have had access to a continuum of school placements for their deaf children. These placements cover public schools that provide inclusion experiences, mainstream settings, self-contained classrooms, day schools for deaf children, and state residential schools for the deaf. Each type of placement has its advantages and disadvantages (Chapter 6). The bottom line is that each deaf child deserves a quality and communication-driven program.

Deaf children need a setting where they can develop age-level language skills in their first language, whether it is spoken English, the non-English spoken language of the home, or ASL, together with corresponding skills in English literacy. In addition, deaf children need a critical mass of communication, age, and cognitive peers in order to develop healthy self-perceptions (Stinson & Leigh, 1995). Teachers and staff should be able to communicate directly with deaf students. Interpreters, note takers, captioning, speech and audiology services, school counseling, and school psychology services with expertise in deafness, tutoring, and opportunities for inclusion in extracurricular activities are services that can improve the performance of deaf students in public schools. Administrators need to be sensitive to the unique needs of deaf children. Those children need exposure to adult deaf and hard-of-hearing role models employed at the school. Parents should use the availability of these services as criteria when selecting a school program for their deaf child (Chapter 6). Legally, they have the right to demand support services.

With IDEA, the trend toward educating all disabled children in schools with their nondisabled peers accelerated. Educating deaf children in these settings was often seen as inclusive, and therefore preferred to segregated education. Placing deaf children in public school settings is legally inclusive, but it may in fact be an exclusion setting for far too many deaf children (Siegel, 2000). Although well intentioned, this law has created a situation where many deaf children are now in hearing classrooms without access or with limited access to the support services that are essential for effective communication, language development, and academic learning. Consequently, many are deprived of an appropriate visual and linguistic classroom that is culturally friendly for deaf children. These children are at risk for experiencing academic failure and feelings of isolation, rejection, and negative self-worth (Stinson & Leigh, 1995). Unquestionably, with appropriate services in place, whatever the setting, the chances for academic success and optimal psychosocial development are far greater.

Self-contained classrooms can be a boon in that these bring deaf children together within mainstream settings. However, especially in rural areas where the number of deaf students is low, teaching becomes more complicated. For example, a teacher may have several children in the classroom, each one of different ages and having different language backgrounds and communication needs. Even though children benefit from interacting with each other during group teaching situations (Vygotsky, 1978), such instructional practices in this case may be less than ideal. For instance, what does the teacher do when the class contains children who have cochlear implants and require speech and auditory training, a hard-of-hearing child who uses a total communication or simultaneous (speech and sign) approach, and a profoundly deaf child who benefits from an ASL/English bilingual approach? These are just some of the myriad of issues teachers of the deaf in the mainstream face.

Currently, there are no standards for providing educational and support services that apply to teachers and administrators in public schools, day programs, and residential settings for deaf children and youth. These standards might minimize some of the difficulties teachers currently face. Such standards need to be developed and evaluated for effectiveness by sophisticated educational researchers. Additionally, there is a need for more research that examines the effectiveness of using state or county curriculum in residential schools for the deaf to improve academic quality. With the emergence of new language approaches for teaching deaf children, it is extremely important to accurately reflect the level of success for each approach in facilitating language development. Now that high-stakes testing is rapidly becoming the criterion for successful completion of elementary and high school education, appropriate measures to evaluate the academic progress of deaf students becomes even more critical.

TECHNOLOGY

Currently, the use of new technology for medical, research, and educational purposes is in high gear. As already mentioned, brain imaging technologies are now used to locate how and where spoken and signed languages are processed in the brain (Chapter 4). With more than 30 states mandating universal newborn hearing screening, hospitals and clinics are testing infants using technology that can measure electrical activity in the auditory nerve through auditory brainstem responses (ABRs). In addition, otoacoustic emissions (OAE) now allow for the study of cochlear functions in humans.

Today, many deaf people take advantage of auditory technology, including digital hearing aids, assistive listening devices, and cochear implants (see Chapter 7 and the appendix at the end of Chapter 3). Visual technologies include real-time captioning, captioning software, note-taking software, and systems such as CAN (computer assisted note-taking), CART (Communication Access Real-time Translation), and C-Print can also be used in classrooms, in courtrooms, and at professional meetings to provide verbatim or summary transcriptions of all spoken communications that take place. Communication technologies such as TTYs, TTY relay systems, email, wireless pagers, listserves on the Internet, and videoconferencing—all provide access. SmartBoards, LCD projectors, captioned movies, multimedia software with text, graphics, animation and ASL movies, CD-ROMs and DVDs with ASL movies, signing avatars, virtual reality adventure games, electronic books, digital cameras and camcorders, web-based courses, wireless laptop labs, document projects, and computer software all can be used to present both languages—ASL and English-- to deaf students. With improved bandwidth, the Internet will be used more easily to transmit ASL. Such technology, and new technology yet to be developed, will continue to shape and reshape deaf people's communication experiences (Chapters 5 and 7).

Understanding hearing loss has definitely been enhanced by the use of increasingly sophisticated technologies. However, one must be cautious in expecting that technology will totally eliminate the communication challenges deaf people confront when interacting with hearing people, and also with other deaf people. Technology is ever-changing, but human needs change as well and pose new challenges for technology. For example, we anticipate a significant increase in the use of voice recognition software in computers. Consequently, new technology will have to be installed to eliminate the access problems deaf people will encounter with voice recognition software.

CONCLUSION

In this book, our goal was to present many of the issues that deaf persons face in society at large. We focused on interactions with hearing families, at school, at work, and during recreation. We emphasized the critical need for professionals to take advantage of deaf people themselves as a valuable resource. This will enhance professional insight into the needs of the deaf children, youth, and adults with whom they work. Using Deaf culture represents an additional resource for professionals. We reflect on the observation of Frederick Schreiber, former executive director of the National Association of the Deaf, that deaf adults are our deaf children grown up. Deaf adults know what worked for them during different periods in their lives. Professionals who listen to deaf adults have the potential to be more successful in creating optimal interventions, whatever their area of specialization.

We began this book with questions. And we end this book with additional questions. How can society continue to improve mental health, social, education, and support services for families, deaf children, and deaf adults? In what ways will molecular genetics affect the deaf community? Where are the empirical data showing the results of monolingual, language-mixing, and ASL/English bilingual language approaches? Are researchers careful to eliminate bias when investigating the various approaches? What are the model literacy teaching methods that work? How will the deaf community change in the future? Will deaf persons with implants eventually dissociate from the deaf community? How can more deaf-hearing partnerships be forged in education and research? With new technology, is it possible for deaf children to develop intelligible speech and effective auditory skills after having acquired a strong ASL foundation? These questions and more will encourage ongoing debate and highlight areas that warrant further study. We invite you, the reader, to join us in this ongoing endeavor to expand our understanding in these areas.

WEBSITES

American Sign Language (ASL)

American Sign Language Links: www.swarthmore.edu/SocSci/Linguistics/
asl/links.html
ASL Access: www.aslaccess.org/basic ASL.htm
Basic Dictionary of ASL Terms: www.hoh.org/~masterstech/ASLDict.spml
Interactive ASL Guide: www.disserv.stu.umn.edu

Art

Deaf Art: www.deafexpo.org/artist_forum.html

Charter, Residential, and Day Schools

Jean Massieu Academy: http://jeanmassieu.com
The Lexington School for the Deaf: http://lexnyc.org
The Magnet School of the Deaf: www.colorado.edu/CDSS/MSD/
National Deaf Academy: http://nationaldeafacademy.com
The Ohio Valley Oral School: www.oraldeafed.org
Note: A listing of U.S. schools for the deaf: http://clerccenter.gallaudet.edu//
InfoToGo/schools-usa.html

Cochlear Implants

Cochlear Implant Association, Inc.: http://www.cici.org/historyciai.html
Cochlear Implant Education Center at Gallaudet: http://clerccenter.
gallaudet.edu/CIEC/
Cochlear Implants: www.nidcd.nih.gov.

Deaf Organizations

Alexander Graham Bell Association for the Deaf and Hard of Hearing:
www.agbell.org
American Association of the Deaf-Blind: www.tr.wou.edu/dblink/aadb.htm

Association of Late-Deafened Adults: www.alda.org
Deaf Latino Organizations: http://www.deafvision.net/aztlan/resources/
   index.html.
Deaf Women United: http://dwu.org.
Intertribal Deaf Council: www.bigriver.net/~rasmith/idc/idc.html
National Association of the Deaf: www.nad.org
National Asian Deaf Congress: http://www.nadc-usa.org/about.html.
Rainbow Alliance of the Deaf: www.rad.org
Self Help for Hard of Hearing People: www.shhh.org

Education

Council on Education of the Deaf, Office of Program Evaluation:
   www.deafed.net
Deaf Education information: www.educ.kent.edu/edu, www.deafed.net
Oral Deaf Programs: www.oraldeafed.org

Educational/Research Organizations

National Task Force on Equity in Testing Deaf Individuals: www.gri.
   gallaudet.edu/TestEquity

General Information on Deafness

Deaf World Web: www.dww.org
Gallaudet's National Information Center on Deafness: www.gallaudet.edu

Hearing

American Speech-Language and Hearing Association: http://www.asha.org/
   professional.asha.org/news/nihs.cfm.
Hearing Health Magazine: www.hearinghealthmag.com
Infant Hearing: www.infanthearing.org
Late Deafened Persons: www.gohear.org
Self Help for Hard of Hearing People: www.shhh.org.

Literacy

Assistive Technology: www.asel.udel.edu/at-online/assistive.html
Deaf Children: http://deafworldweb.org/dww.kids/internet.html
Literacy: www.learner.org/the guide/deaf.html
National Clearinghouse for ESL Literacy Education: www.cal.org/ncle
NTID High Technology Center: http://htc.rit.edu
Sign Writing: www.signwriting.org
Star Schools Project: 4 Reports: www.starschools.org/nmsd

Programs to Prepare Psychologists Working with Deaf People

Gallaudet University School Psychology and Clinical Psychology Programs: www.gallaudet.edu
National Institute for the Deaf School Psychology Program: http://www.rit.edu/~schpsych

Psychology Topics

American Psychological Association: http://www.apa.org
Clerc Center, Gallaudet University: http://clerccenter.gallaudet.edu/infotogo/491.htm
Mental Health Net: http://www.cmhc.com
National Institute of Mental Health: http://www.nimh.nih.gov/home.htm
National Library of Medicine: http://www.nlm.nih.gov/
National Library of Medicine-free MedLine: http://www.nlm.nih.gov
Psychology Central: http://www.mentalhealth.com
Psychology and Law: http://www.psyclaw.org
Stanford University Online Full Text Science Journals: www.highwire.stanford.edu/lists/largest.dtl

Religion and Organizations

Deaf Churches: http://members.aol.com/deaflist/deafch.htm.
United Methodist Congress of the Deaf: www.UMCD.org

Service Organizations

American Deafness and Rehabilitation Association   http://www.adara.org
National Alliance of Black Interpreters: www.naob.org
Registry of Interpreters for the Deaf, Inc.:   www.rid.org/edu.html
TDI, Inc.:   www.tdi-online.org

Special Education

ADA & Disabilities Information: www.public.iastate.edu/~sbilling/ada.html
Council for Exceptional Children Homepage: www.cec.sped.org
National Information Center for Children & Youth with Disabilities: Gopher://aed.aed.org:70/11/disablity.nichcy
Postsecondary Education Consortium: www.pepnet.org
SERI: Special Education Resources on the Internet: www.hood.edu/seri/serihome.htm

Sports

European Deaf Sport Organization: http://www.edso.net/histo.htm
USA Deaf Sports Federation: http://www.usadsf.org/About_Us/
   What_is_USADSF/what_is_usadsf.html

Syndromes and Medical Websites

Medline Database on Cochlear Implants: http://www.nlm.nih.gov/databases/
   freemedl.html, http://igm.nlm.nih.gov/
Salk Institute: www.salk.org
Usher Syndrome: www.deafblind.co.uk/index.html, www.tr.wou.edu/dblink/
   links.htm

REFERENCES

■ ■ ■ ■ ■ ▬▬▬▬▬▬▬▬▬▬▬▬▬▬▬▬▬▬▬▬▬▬▬▬

Achtzehn, J. (1987). *PACES: Preventing abuse of children through education for sexuality.* Workshop presented at a conference on Preventing Incidence of Sexual Abuse among Hearing Impaired Children and Youth, Department of Education, Gallaudet University, Washington, DC.

Acredolo, L., & Goodwyn, S. (1994). Sign language among hearing infants: The spontaneous development of symbolic gestures. In V. Volterra & C. Erting (Eds.), *From Gesture to Language in Hearing Children.* Washington, DC: Gallaudet University Press.

Across the Nation Newsbriefs. (2001, April). Deaf AZT-LAN. *Silent News,* 3.

Afrin, J., & Critchfield, B. (1999). Telepsychiatry for the deaf in South Carolina: Maximizing limited resources. In B. Brauer, A. Marcus, & D. Morton (Eds.), *Proceedings of the first world conference on mental health and deafness* (p. 27). Vienna, VA: Potiron Press.

Ahmad, W., Darr, A., Jones, L., & Nisa, G. (1998). *Deafness and ethnicity: Services, policies and politics.* University of Bristol: The Policy Press.

Ainsworth, M. D. S., Blehar, M. C., Waters, E., & Wall, S. (1978). *Patterns of attachment: A psychological study of the Strange Situation.* Hillsdale, NJ: Erlbaum.

Al Muhaimeed, H., & Zakzouk, S. (1997). Hearing loss and herpes simplex. *Journal of Tropical Pediatrics, 43,* 20–24.

Alexander Graham Bell Association for the Deaf and Hard of Hearing. (2001a). Retrieved September 27, 2001, from http://www.agbell.org.

Alexander Graham Bell Association for the Deaf and Hard of Hearing. (2001b). *AG Bell position statement on cochlear implants.* Unpublished paper.

Altshuler, K. (1969). New York State program of mental health services. In K. Altshuler & J. D. Rainer (Eds.), *Mental health and the deaf: Approaches and prospects* (pp. 15–23). Washington, DC: U.S. Department of Health, Education, and Welfare.

American Academy of Audiology. (1997). Audiology: Scope of practice. *Audiology Today, 9,* 12–13.

American Association of the Deaf-Blind (undated). *AADB summary.* Unpublished paper.

American Association of the Deaf-Blind. (2001). Retrieved September 27, 2001, from http://www.tr.wou.edu/dblink/aadb.htm.

Americans with Disabilities Act of 1990, 42 U.S.C.A. #12101 et seq. (West 1993).

Ammerman, R. T., & Baladerian, N. J. (1993). *Maltreatment of children with disabilities* (Working paper No. 860). Chicago: National Committee to Prevent Child Abuse.

Anderson, G. (1994). Tools for a wiser, healthier, black deaf community. In M. Garretson (Ed.), *Deafness: Life and culture, A Deaf American monograph.* Silver Spring, MD: National Association of the Deaf.

Anderson, G. (2001). *Diversity revolution in deaf education.* Paper presented at the National Symposium on Childhood Deafness, Sept. 29–Oct. 2, 2001, Sioux Falls, SD.

Anderson, J., & Werry, J. S. (1994). Emotional and behavioral problems. In I. B. Pless (Ed.), *The epidemiology of childhood disorders* (pp. 304–338). New York: Oxford University Press.

Andersson, Y. (1994). Deaf people as a linguistic minority. In I. Ahlgren & K. Hyltenstam (Eds.), *Bilingualism in deaf education.* Hamburg: Signum.

Andrews, J. (1986). Childhood deafness and the acquisition of print concepts. In D. Yaden & S. Templeton (Eds.), *Metalinguistic awareness and beginning literacy: Conceptualizing what it means to read and write* (pp. 277–289). Portsmouth, NH: Heinemann.

Andrews, J. (1998/1999). Deaf professionals in deaf education. In A. Farb (Ed.), *Unrealized visions: What's next for the deaf and hard of hearing community? NAD Deaf American Monograph, 48,* pp. 9–12. Silver Spring, MD: National Association of the Deaf.

Andrews, J., & Franklin, T. (1996/1997). Why hire deaf teachers? *Texas Journal of Audiology and Speech Pathology, 22(1),* 120–131.

Andrews, J., & Gonzales, K. (1992). Free writing of deaf children in kindergarten. *Sign Language Studies, 74,* 63–78.

Andrews, J., & Jordan, D. (1993). Minority and minority-deaf professionals: How many and where are they? *American Annals of the Deaf, 138*, 388–396.

Andrews, J., & Mason, J. (1991). Strategy use among deaf and hearing readers. *Exceptional Children, 57(6)*, 536–545.

Andrews, J., & Wilson, H. (1991). The deaf adult in the nursing home. *Geriatric Nursing, 12*, 279–283.

Andrews, J., & Zmijewski, G. (1996). How parents support home literacy with deaf children. *Early Child Development and Care, 127–128*, 131–139.

Anthony, D. (1971). *Seeing Essential English, Vol. 1 & 2*. Anaheim, CA: Educational Services Division, Anaheim School District.

Antia, S. D. (1999). The roles of special educators and classroom teachers in an inclusive school. *Journal of Deaf Studies and Deaf Education, 4(3)*, 203–214.

Aramburo, A. (1994). Sociolinguistic aspects of the black deaf community. In C. Erting, R. C. Johnson, D. Smith, & B. Snider (Eds.), *The Deaf way: Perspectives from the international conference on Deaf culture*. Washington, DC: Gallaudet University Press.

Armstrong, D., Stokoe, W., & Wilcox, S. (1995). *Gesture and the nature of language*. New York: Cambridge University Press.

Arnos, K. S. (1999). Genetic counseling for hearing loss. *The Volta Review, 95 (5, monograph)*, 85–96.

Arnos, K. S. (2002). Genetics and deafness: Impacts on the deaf community. *Sign Language Studies, 2*, 150–168.

Arnos, K. S., Israel, J., Devlin, L., & Wilson, M. P. (1996). Genetic aspects of hearing loss in childhood. In F. N. Martin & J. G. Clark (Eds.), *Hearing care for children* (pp. 20–44). Boston: Allyn and Bacon.

ASHA. (1999). *Universal screening gains mometum in states*. Retrieved October 12, 2001, from http://www.asha.org/professional.asha.org/news/nihs.cfm.

Association of Late-Deafened Adults. (2001, September). *Lost your hearing? Know someone?* Retrieved September 27, 2001, from http://www.alda.org.

Atkins, D. (1987). Siblings of the hearing impaired: Perspectives for parents. *The Volta Review, 89*, 32–45.

Bailes, C. (2001). Integrative ASL-English language arts: Bridging paths to literacy. *Sign Language Studies, 1(2)*, 147–174.

Baker, C. (2001). *Foundations of bilingual education and bilingualism* (3rd ed.). Clevedon, England: Multilingual Matters Ltd.

Baldwin, D. (1993). *Pictures in the air: The story of the National Theater of the Deaf*. Washington, DC: Gallaudet University Press.

Baldwin, R. (2001). *Functional reallocation of the auditory cortex in individuals who are deaf*. Unpublished doctoral dissertation, Gallaudet University, Washington, DC.

Bangs, D. (1987). Fairmont Theater of the deaf. In J. Van Cleve (Ed.), *Gallaudet encyclopedia of deaf people and deafness, Vol. 1* (pp. 421–422). New York: McGraw-Hill.

Barbour County Bd. of Educ. v. Parent (1999). 29 IDELR 848. *Individuals with Disabilities Education Act law report, 29(7)*, 848–852.

Barnartt, S., & Christiansen, J. (1996). The educational and occupational attainment of prevocationally deaf adults: 1972–1991. In P. C. Higgins & J. E. Nash (Eds.), *Understanding deafness socially* (2nd ed., pp. 60–70). Springfield, IL: Charles C. Thomas.

Barnartt, S., & Scotch, R. (2001). *Disability protests: Contentious politics 1970–1999*. Washington, DC: Gallaudet University Press.

Barrenas, M., Nylen, O., & Hanson, C. (1999). The influence of karyotype on the auricle, otitis media, and hearing in Turner Syndrome. *Hearing Research, 138*, 163–170.

Barry, D. (1997, July 22). Captive in Queens: The profits: Dollar bills laundered in casinos, U.S. says. *The New York Times*, p. B4.

Basilier, T. (1964). Surdophrenia: The psychic consequences of congenital or early acquired deafness. Some theoretical and clinical considerations. *Acta Psychiatrics Scandinavia: Supplementum, 180(40)*, 362–374.

Bat-Chava, Y. (1993). Antecedents of self-esteem in deaf people: A meta-analytic review. *Rehabilitation Psychology, 38*, 221–234.

Bat-Chava, Y. (1994). Group identification and self-esteem in deaf adults. *Personality and Social Psychology Bulletin, 20*, 494–502.

Bat-Chava, Y. (2000). Diversity of deaf identities. *American Annals of the Deaf, 145*, 420–428.

Bat-Chava, Y., & Deignan, E. (2001). Peer relationships of children with cochlear implants. *Journal of Deaf Studies and Deaf Education, 6*, 186–199.

Bateman, G. (1994). Political activism in the deaf community: An exploratory study of deaf leaders in Rochester, N.Y. In C. J. Erting, R. C. Johnson, D. L. Smith, & B. D. Snider (Eds.), *The Deaf way* (pp. 854–859). Washington, DC: Gallaudet University Press.

Bavelier, D., Tomann, A., Hutton, C., Mitchell, T., Corina, D., Liu, G., & Neville, H. (2000). Visual attention to the periphery is enhanced in congenitally deaf individuals. *The Journal of Neuroscience, 20* (RC93), 1–6.

Baynton, D. (1992, Fall). Book review: The mask of benevolence: Disabling the deaf community. *Gallaudet Today*, pp. 31–32.

Baynton, D. (1993). "Savages and deaf-mutes": Evolutionary theory and the campaign against sign language in the nineteenth century. In J. Van Cleve (Ed.), *Deaf history unveiled: Interpretations from the new scholarship* (pp. 92–112). Washington, DC: Gallaudet University Press.

Baynton, D. (1997). A silent exile on this earth: The metaphorical constructions of deafness in the nineteenth century. In L. Davis (Ed.), *The disability studies reader* (pp. 128–150). New York: Routledge.

Bebko, J. (1998). Learning, language, memory, and reading: The role of language automatization and its impact on complex cognitive activities. *Journal of Deaf Studies and Deaf Education, 3(1)*, 4–14.

Bell, A. G. (1883). *Memoir upon the formation of a deaf variety of the human race.* New Haven, CT: National Academy of Science.

Bellugi, U., Marks, S., Bihrle, A., & Sabo, H. (1994). Dissociation between language and cognitive functions in Williams Syndrome. In D. Bishop & K. Mogford (Eds.), *Language development in exceptional children* (pp. 177–189). Mahwah, NJ: Erlbaum Associates

Bellugi, U., O'Grady, L., Lillo-Martin, D., O'Grady, M., van Hoek, K., & Corina, D. (1990). Enhancement of spatial cognition in deaf children. In V. Volterra & C. Erting (Eds.), *From gesture to language in hearing and deaf children* (pp. 278–298). New York: Springer-Verlag.

Bernstein, M., & Morrison, M. (1992). Are we ready for PL 99–457? *American Annals of the Deaf, 137(1)*, 7–13.

Bialystok, E., & Hakuta, K. (1994). *In other words: The psychology of second language acquisition.* New York: Basic Books.

Biesold, H. (1999). *Crying hands: Eugenics and deaf people in Nazi Germany.* Washington, DC: Gallaudet University Press.

Blanchfield, B., Feldman, J., Dunbar, J., & Gardner, E. (2001). The severely to profoundly hearing-impaired population in the United States: Prevalence estimates and demographics. *Journal of the American Academy of Audiology, 12*, 183–189.

Blatt, S., Auerbach, J., & Levy, K. (1997). Mental representations in personality development, psychopathology, and the therapeutic process. *Review of General Psychology, 1*, 351–374.

Blennerhassett, L. (2000). Psychological assessments. In P. Hindley & N. Kitson (Eds.), *Mental health and deafness* (pp. 185–205). London: Whurr Publishers.

Bloch, N. (2001, April/May). Executive view. *NADmag, 1*, 13.

Blotzer, M., & Ruth, R. (1995). *Sometimes you just want to feel like a human being.* Baltimore: Paul H. Brookes.

Bodner-Johnson, B., & Sass-Lehrer, M. (1999). *Family-school relationships: Concepts and premises.* Washington, DC: Gallaudet University Pre-College National Mission Programs.

Bornstein, H. (1982). Toward a theory of use of signed English: From birth through adulthood. *American Annals of the Deaf, 127*, 69–72.

Bowe, F. (1991). *Approaching equality: Education of the deaf.* Silver Spring, MD: T. J. Publishers.

Bowen, S. (1999). *Building bridges: Case studies in literacy and deafness.* Unpublished doctoral dissertation, The University of Arizona.

Bowlby, J. (1958). The nature of the child's tie to his mother. *International Journal of Psycho-Analysis, 39*, 350–373.

Brackett, D., & Henniges, M. (1976). Communicative interaction of preschool hearing impaired children in an integrated setting. *The Volta Review, 78*, 276–285.

Braden, J. (1994). *Deafness, deprivation, and IQ.* New York: Plenum.

Braden, J. P. (2001). The clinical assessment of deaf people's cognitive abilities. In M. Clark, M. Marschark, & M. Karchmer (Eds.), *Context, cognition, and deafness* (pp. 14–37). Washington, DC: Gallaudet University Press.

Bradley-Johnson, S., & Evans, L. (1991). *Psychoeducational assessment of hearing-impaired students: Infancy through high school.* Austin, TX: Pro-Ed.

Bragg, B., & Bergman, E. (1989). *Lessons in laughter: The autobiography of a deaf actor.* Washington, DC: Gallaudet University Press.

Branson, J., & Miller, D. (2002). *Damned for their difference: The cultural construction of deaf people as disabled.* Washington, DC: Gallaudet University Press.

Brauer, B. (1980). The dimensions of perceived interview relationship as influenced by deaf person's self-concepts and interviewer attributes as deaf or non-deaf. Doctoral dissertation, New York University, 1979. *Dissertation Abstracts International, 40*, 1352B.

Brauer, B. (1993). Adequacy of a translation of the MMPI into American Sign Language for use with deaf individuals: Linguistic equivalency issues. *Rehabilitation Psychology, 38*, 247–260.

Brauer, B., Braden, J., Pollard, R., & Hardy-Braz, S. (1998). Deaf and hard of hearing people. In J. Sandoval, C. Frisby, K. Geisinger, J. Scheuneman, & J. Grenier (Eds.), *Test interpretation and diversity* (pp. 297–315). Washington, DC: American Psychological Association.

Brelje, H. W. (Ed.). (1999). *Global perspectives on the education of the deaf in selected countries.* Hillsboro, OR: Butte Publications.

British Broadcast Company (BBC). March 2, 2000. London, England.

Brougham v. Town of Yarmouth (1993). 20 IDELR 12. *Individuals with Disabilities Education law report, 20(1),* 12–18.

Brown, P. M., Rickards, F., & Bortoli, A. (2001). Structures underpinning pretend play and word production in young hearing children and children with hearing loss. *Journal of Deaf Studies and Deaf Education, 6,* 15–31.

Brueggemann, B. (1999). *Lend me your ear: Rhetorical constructions of deafness.* Washington, DC: Gallaudet University Press.

Buchanan, R. (1994). Building a silent colony: Life and work in the deaf community of Akron, Ohio from 1910 through 1950. In C. J. Erting, R. C. Johnson, D. L. Smith, & B. D. Snider (Eds.), *The Deaf way* (pp. 250–259). Washington, DC: Gallaudet University Press.

Buchanan, R. (1999). *Illusions of equality: Deaf Americans in school and factory 1850–1950.* Washington, DC: Gallaudet University Press.

Buck, D. (2000). *Deaf peddler: Confessions of an inside man.* Washington, DC: Gallaudet University Press.

Burke, F., Gutman, V., & Dobosh, P. (1999). Treatment of deaf survivors of sexual abuse: A process of healing. In I. W. Leigh (Ed.), *Psychotherapy with deaf clients from diverse groups* (pp. 279–305). Washington, DC: Gallaudet University Press.

Busby, H. (2001). *Working with Deaf American Indians and Alaskan Natives.* Paper Presented at the National Symposium on Childhood Deafness: Families, Children, and Literacy in the 21st Century. Sept. 29 – October 2, 2001, Sioux Falls, SD.

Butler, K., & Prinz, P. (1998). ASL proficiency and English literacy acquisition: New perspectives. *Topics in Language Disorders, 18(4),* 1–88.

Calderon, R., & Greenberg, M. (1997). The effectiveness of early intervention for deaf and hard of hearing children. In M. J. Guralnick (Ed.), *The effectiveness of early intervention: Directions for second generation research* (pp. 455–482). Baltimore: Paul Brookes.

Callaway, A. (2000). *Deaf children in China.* Washington, DC: Gallaudet University Press.

Camilleri, C., & Malewska-Peyre, H. (1997). Socialization and identity strategies. In J. W. Berry, P. R. Dasen, & T. S. Saraswathi (Eds.), *Handbook of cross-cultural psychology, Volume 2: Basic processes and human development* (2nd ed., pp. 41–67). Boston: Allyn and Bacon.

Cantor, D. W., & Spragins, A. (1977). Delivery of service to the hearing impaired child in the elementary school. *American Annals of the Deaf, 122(5),* 330–336.

Capirici, O., Iverson, J., Pizzuto, E., & Volterra, V. (1996). Gestures and words during the transition to two-word speech. *Journal of Child Language, 23,* 645–673.

Capirci, O., Cattani, A., Rossini, P., & Volterra, V. (1998). Teaching sign language to hearing children as a possible factor in cognitive enhancement. *Journal of Deaf Studies and Deaf Education, 3(2),* 135–142.

Carroll, C., & Fischer, C. H. (2001). *Orchid of the bayou: A deaf woman faces blindness.* Washington, DC: Gallaudet University Press.

Case, L., & Smith, T. (2000). Ethnic representation in a sample of the literature of applied psychology. *Journal of Consulting and Clinical Psychology, 68,* 1107–1110.

Census. (2000). *Resident population and apportionment counts.* Retrieved December 15, 2001, from http://www.census.gov/main/www/cen2000.html.

Chamberlain, C., Morford, J., & Mayberry, R. (2000). *Language acquisition by eye.* Mahwah, NJ: Erlbaum.

Chase, P., Hall, J., & Werkhaven, J. (1996). Sensorineural hearing loss in children: Etiology and pathology. In F. Martin & J. Clark (Eds.), *Hearing care for children* (pp. 73–91). Boston: Allyn and Bacon.

Cheng, L. (2000). Deafness: An Asian/Pacific perspective. In K. Christensen (Ed.), *Deaf plus: A multicultural perspective* (pp. 59–92). San Diego, CA: DawnSignPress.

Chess, S., & Fernandez, P. (1980). Neurologic damage and behavior disorders in rubella children. *American Annals of the Deaf, 125,* 998–1001.

Christensen, K. (1993). A multicultural approach to education of children who are deaf. In K. M. Christensen & G. L. Delgado (Eds.), *Multicultural issues in deafness* (pp. 17–27). White Plains, NY: Longman Publishing Group.

Christensen, K. (Ed.). (2000). *Deaf plus: A multicultural perspective.* San Diego, CA: DawnSign Press.

Christiansen, J. (1994). Deaf people and the world of work: A case study of deaf printers in Washington, DC. In C. J. Erting, R. C. Johnson, D. L. Smith, & B. D. Snider (Eds.), *The Deaf way* (pp. 260–267). Washington, DC: Gallaudet University Press.

Christiansen, J., & Barnartt, S. (1995). *Deaf president now! The 1988 revolution at Gallaudet University.* Washington, DC: Gallaudet University Press.

Christiansen, J. B., & Leigh, I. W. (2002). *Cochlear implants in children: Ethics and choices.* Washington, DC: Gallaudet University Press.

Church, M. W., Eldis, F., Blakley, B. W., & Bawle, E. V. (1997). Hearing, language, speech, vestibular, and dentofacial disorders in fetal alcohol syndrome. *Alcoholism, Clinical and Experimental Research, 21,* 227–237.

Clarcq, J., & Walter, G. (1997–98). Supplemental Security Income payments made to young adults who are deaf and hard of hearing. *Journal of the American Deafness and Rehabilitation Association, 31,* 1–9.

Clark, J. (1994). Reading the Silver Screen. *Technology Review.* Massachusetts Institute of Technology Alumni Association, Boston.

Clark, M., Marschark, M., & Karchmer, M. (2001). *Context, cognition, and Deafness.* Washington, DC: Gallaudet University Press.

Clark, M., Schwanenflugel, P., Everhart, V., & Bartini, M. (1996). Theory of mind in deaf adults and the organization of verbs of knowing. *Journal of Deaf Studies and Deaf Education, 1,* 179–189.

Cochlear Implant Association, Inc. (2001, January 19). *A brief history of the Cochlear Implant Association, Inc.* Retrieved September 27, 2001, from http://www.cici.org/historyciai.html.

Cohen, H., & Jones, E. (1990). Interpreting for cross-cultural research: Changing written English to American Sign Language. *Journal of the American Deafness and Rehabilitation Association, 24,* 41–48.

Cohen, N., & Gordon, M. (1994, February). Cochlear implants: Basics, history, and future possibilities. *SHHH Journal,* pp. 8–10.

Cohen, O. P. (1991). At-risk deaf adolescents. *The Volta Review, 93,* 57–72.

Cohn, J. (1999). *Sign mind: Studies in American Sign Language poetics.* Boulder, CO: Museum of American Poetics Publications.

Collins, F. (2001, July). *The human genome project: Healthcare implications.* Presentation at the Human Genome Project and Hearing Loss Conference, Bethesda, MD.

Collins, W. A., & Gunnar, M. (1990). Social and personality development. *Annual Review of Psychology, 41,* 387–416.

Commission on Education of the Deaf (COED). (1988). *Toward equality: Education of the deaf.* Washington, DC: USGPO.

Conrad, R. (1979). *The deaf school child.* London: Harper & Row Ltd.

Corbett, C. (1999). Mental health issues for African-American deaf people. In I. W. Leigh (Ed.), *Psychotherapy with deaf clients from diverse groups* (pp. 151–176). Washington, DC: Gallaudet University Press.

Corina, D. (1998). Studies of neural processing in deaf signers: Toward a neurocognitive model of language processing in the deaf. *Journal of Deaf Studies and Deaf Education, 3(1),* 35–48.

Corker, M. (1994). *Counselling: The deaf challenge.* London: Jessica Kingsley Publishers.

Corker, M. (1996). *Deaf transitions.* London: Jessica Kingsley Publishers.

Corker, M. (1998). *Deaf and disabled, or deafness disabled?* Buckingham, England: Open University Press.

Cornett, O. (1967). Cued speech. *American Annals of the Deaf, 112,* 3–13.

Coster, W. J., Gersten, M. S., Beeghly, M., & Cicchetti, D. (1989). Communicative functioning in maltreated toddlers. *Developmental Psychology, 25,* 1020–1029.

Courtin, C. (2000). The impact of sign language on the cognitive development of deaf children: The case of theories of mind. *Journal of Deaf Studies and Deaf Education, 5(3),* 266–276.

Crocker, J., & Major, B. (1989). Social stigma and self-esteem: The self-protective properties of stigma. *Psychological Review, 96,* 608–630.

Crouch, R. (1997). Letting the deaf be deaf: Reconsidering the use of cochlear implants in prelingually deaf children. *Hastings Center Report, 27(4),* 14–21.

Crowe, T. (2002). Translation of the Rosenberg Self-Esteem Scale into American Sign Language: A principal components analysis. *Social Work Research, 26 (1),* 57–63.

Crowley, M., Keane, K., & Needham, C. (1982). Fathers: The forgotten parents. *American Annals of the Deaf, 127,* 38–40.

Crystal, D. (1997). *The Cambridge encyclopedia of language* (2nd ed.). New York: Cambridge University Press.

Cumming, C., & Rodda, M. (1989). Advocacy, prejudice, and role modeling in the deaf community. *The Journal of Social Psychology, 129,* 5–12.

Cummins, J. (2000). *Language, power and pedagogy: Bilingual children in the crossfire.* Cleveton, England: Multilingual Matters.

Curtiss, S. (1977). *Genie: A psycholinguistic study of a modern day "wild child."* New York: Academic Press.

Daigle, B. V. (1994) *An analysis of a deaf psychotic inpatient population.* Unpublished master's thesis, Western Maryland College, Westminster, MD.

Daniels, M. (2001). *Dancing with words: Signing for hearing children's literacy.* Westport, CT: Bergin & Harvey.

Davis, H., & Silverman, R. (1964). *Hearing and deafness.* New York: Holt, Rinehart and Winston.

Davis, J. (Ed.). (2002). *Our forgotten children: Hard of hearing children in the public schools* (3rd ed.). SHHH Publications.

Davis, L. (1995). *Enforcing normalcy: Disability, deafness, and the body.* London: Versace.

Davis, L. (Ed.). (1997). *The disability studies reader.* New York: Routledge.

Deaf American. (1969). Deaf post office clerks being trained in Ohio. *The Deaf American, 22,* 29.

Deaf American. (1970). New Orleans post office employs deaf workers. *The Deaf American, 22,* 34.

Deaf Aztlan: Deaf Latino/a Network. Retrieved September 27, 2001, from http://www.deafvision.net/aztlan/welcome.html.

Deaf Churches. (2001). Retrieved September 27, 2001, from http://members.aol.com/deaflist/deafch.htm.

Deaf Latino Organizations. (2001). *Deaf Aztlan: Deaf Latino/a network.* Retrieved September 27, 2001, http://www.deafvision.net/aztlan/resources/index.html.

Deaf Seniors of America. (2001). *Deaf seniors of America: An organization created for seniors by seniors.* Brochure.

Deaf Women United. (2000, January 7). *About DWU.* Retrieved September 27, 2001, from http://dwu.org.

Dean, R., & Pollard, R. (2001). Application of demand-control theory to sign language interpreting: Implications for stress and interpreter training. *Journal of Deaf Studies and Deaf Education, 6,* 1–14.

Delgado, G. (Ed.). (1984). *The Hispanic deaf: Issues and challenges for special bilingual education.* Washington, DC: Gallaudet University Press.

Denmark, J. (1973). The education of deaf children. *Hearing, 70,* 3–12.

Denmark, J. C., & Warren, F. (1972). A psychiatric unit for the deaf. *British Journal of Psychiatry, 120,* 423–428.

Denoyelle, F., Weil, D., Maw, M., Wilcox, S., Lench, N., Allen-Powell, D., Osborn, A., Dahl, H., Middleton, A., Houseman, M., Dode, C., Marlin, S., Boulila-ElGaied, A., Grati, M., Ayadi, H., BenArab, S., Bitoun, P., Lina-Granade, G., Godet, J., Mustapha, M., Loiselet, J., El-Zir, E., Aubois, A., Joannard, A., McKinlay Gardner, R., & Petit, C. (1997). Prelingual deafness: High prevalence of a 30delG mutation in the connexin 26 gene. *Human Molecular Genetics, 6,* 2173–2177.

Desselle, D., & Pearlmutter, L. (1997). Navigating two cultures: Deaf children, self-esteem, and parents' communication patterns. *Social Work in Education, 19,* 23–30.

DeVilliers, P. (1991). English literacy development in deaf children: Directions for research and intervention. In J. Miller (Ed.), *Research on child language disorders: A decade of progress* (pp. 349–378). Austin, TX: Pro-Ed.

Dew, D. (Ed.). (1999). *Serving individuals who are low-functioning deaf: Report from the study group, 25th Institute on Rehabilitation Issues.* Washington, DC: George Washington University, Regional Rehabilitation Continuing Education Program.

Diefendorf, A. (1996). Hearing loss and its effects. In F. Martin & J. Clark (Eds.), *Hearing care for children* (pp. 3–19). Boston: Allyn and Bacon.

Diefendorf, A. (1999). Screening for hearing loss in infants. *The Volta Review, 99,* 43–61.

Drasgow, E., & Paul, P. (1995). A critical analysis of the use of MCE systems with deaf students: A review of the literature. *ACEHI/ACEDA, 21(3),* 80–93.

Drolsbaugh, M. (2000, November). You deaf people. *Silent News, 32,* 12.

Duncan, E., Prickett, H., Finkelstein, D., Vernon, M., & Hollingsworth, T. (1988). *Usher's Syndrome: What it is, how to cope, and how to help.* Springfield, IL: Charles C. Thomas.

Eastabrooks, W. (2000). Auditory-verbal practice. In S. Waltzman & N. Cohen (Eds.), *Cochlear implants* (pp. 225–246). New York: Thieme.

Eckenrode, J., Laird, M., & Doris, J. (1993). School performance and disciplinary problems among abused and neglected children. *Developmental Psychology, 29,* 53–62.

Eckhardt, E., Goldstein, M., Montoya, L., Steinberg, A. (under review). *Psychiatric diagnosis in a deaf sample using an American Sign Language version of the Diagnostic Interview Schedule-IV.*

Eckhardt, E., Steinberg, A., Lipton, D., Montoya, L., & Goldstein, M. (1999). Innovative directions in mental health assessment Part III: Use of interactive video technology in assessment: A research project. *Journal of the American Deafness and Rehabilitation Association, 33,* 20–30.

Egeland, B., Jacobvitz, D., & Stroufe, L. A. (1988). Breaking the cycle of abuse. *Child Development, 59,* 1080–1088.

Einhorn, K. (1999, February). Noise-induced hearing loss in the performing arts: An otolaryngologic perspective. *The Hearing Review,* pp. 28–30.

Eldredge, N. (1999). Culturally responsive psychotherapy with American Indians who are deaf. In I. W. Leigh (Ed.), *Psychotherapy with deaf clients from diverse groups* (pp. 177–201). Washington, DC: Gallaudet University Press.

Elliot, L., Stinson, M., McKee, B., Everhart, V., & Francis, P. (2001). College students' perceptions of the C-Print Speech-to-text transcription system. *Journal of Deaf Studies and Deaf Education, 6(4),* 285–298.

Emerson, R. (1870). Society and solitude. In L. Frank (Ed.), *Quotationary* (p. 362). New York: Random House.

Emmorey, K. (1998). The impact of sign language use on visuospatial cognition. In M. Marschark (Ed.), *Psychological perspectives on deafness* (Vol. 2, pp. 19–52). Mahwah, NJ: Erlbaum.

Emmorey, K. (2002). *Language, cognition, and the brain.* Mahwah, NJ: Erlbaum.

Emmorey, K., Kosslyn, S. M., & Bellugi, U. (1993). Visual imagery and visual-spatial language: Enhanced imagery abilities in deaf and hearing ASL signers. *Cognition, 46,* 139–181.

Emmorey, K., & Lane, H. (2000). *The sign of language revisited: An anthology to honor Ursula Bellugi and Edward Klima.* Mahwah, NJ: Erlbaum.

Epstein, S. (1999). Introduction–An evaluation of the diagnosis and management of hearing loss during the past 50 years. *The Volta Review, 99,* v–vii.

Erikson, E. H. (1972). Eight ages of man. In C. S. Lavatelli & F. Stendler (Eds.), *Readings in child behavior and child development.* San Diego, CA: Harcourt Brace Jovanovich.

Erting, C. J. (1982). *Deafness, communication, and social identity.* Unpublished doctoral dissertation, American University, Washington, DC.

Erting, C. J., Johnson, R. C., Smith, D., & Snider, B. (Eds.). (1994). *The Deaf way: Perspectives from the international conference on Deaf culture.* Washington, DC: Gallaudet University Press.

Erting, C. J., Prezioso, C., & Hynes, M. O. (1990). The interactional context of deaf mother-infant communication. In V. Volterra & C. Erting (Eds.),

From gesture to language in hearing and deaf children. Berlin, Germany: Springer.

Ervin-Tripp, S. (1966). Language development. In M. L. Hoffman & L. W. Hoffman (Eds.), *Review of child development research, Vol. 11* (pp. 55–105). New York: Russell Sage.

Essex, E., Seltzer, M., & Krauss, M. (2002). Fathers as caregivers for adult children with mental retardation. In B. Kramer & E. Thompson (Eds.), *Men as caregivers: Theory, research, and service implications* (pp. 250–268). New York: Springer.

European Deaf Sport Organization. (2001). *EDSO history.* Retrieved September 27, 2001, from http://www.edso.net/histo.htm.

Evans, R. B. (1999, December). Psychology continues to redefine itself. *APA Monitor, 30(11),* 20.

Ewoldt, C. (1981). A psycholinguistic description of selected deaf children reading in sign language. *Reading Research Quarterly, XVII,* 58–89.

Feuerstein, R. (1980). *Instrumental enrichment: An intervention program for cognitive modifiability.* Baltimore, MD: University Park Press.

Fischel-Ghodsian, N., Prezant, T., Chaltraw, W., Wendt, K., Nelson, R., Arnos, K., & Falk, R. (1997). Mitochondrial gene mutation is a significant predisposing factor in aminoglycoside ototoxicity. *American Journal of Otolaryngology, 18,* 173–178.

Fischer, L. C. (2000). *Cultural identity development and self concept of adults who are deaf: A comparative analysis.* Doctoral dissertation, Arizona State University, Tempe. Dissertation Abstracts International, 61–10B, 5609.

Fischgrund, J. E., & Akamatsu, C. T. (1993) Rethinking the education of ethnic/multicultural deaf people: Stretching the boundaries. In K. M. Christensen & G. L. Delgado (Eds.), *Multicultural issues in deafness.* White Plains, NY: Longman Publishing Group.

Foster, S. (1989). Social alienation and peer identification: A study of the social construction of deafness. *Human Organization, 48(3),* 226–235.

Fowler, K., Dahle, A., Boppana, S., & Pass, R. (1999). Newborn hearing screening: Will children with hearing loss caused by congenital cytomegalovirus infection be missed? *Journal of Pediatrics, 135,* 60–64.

Freeman, R. (1977). Psychiatric aspects of sensory disorders and interpretation. In P. Graham (Ed.), *Epidemiological approaches in child psychiatry* (pp. 275–304). New York: Academic Press.

Freeman, R. D., Malkin, S. F., & Hastings, J. O. (1975). Psychosocial problems of deaf children and their families: A comparative study. *American Annals of the Deaf, 120,* 391–403.

Freeman, S. T. (1989). Cultural and linguistic bias in mental health evaluations of deaf people. *Rehabilitation Psychology, 34,* 51–63.

French, M. (1999). *Starting with assessment: A developmental approach to deaf children's literacy.* Pre-College National Mission Programs. Washington, DC: Gallaudet University.

Fried, J. (1997, November 18). Woman pleads guilty in case of deaf Mexican peddlers. *The New York Times,* p. B13.

Friedburg, I. (2000). *Reference group orientation and self-esteem of deaf and hard-of-hearing college students.* Unpublished doctoral dissertation, Gallaudet University, Washington, DC.

Friedlander, H. (1999). Introduction. In H. Biesold. *Crying hands: Eugenics and deaf people in Nazi Germany* (pp. 1–12). Washington, DC: Gallaudet University Press.

Friere, P. (1970). *Pedagogy of the oppressed.* New York: Continuum.

Fujikawa, S. (2001). Healthy People 2010. *Audiology Today, 13(2),* 38.

Galenson, E., Miller, R., Kaplan, E., & Rothstein, A. (1979). Assessment of development in the deaf child. *Journal of the American Academy of Child Psychiatry, 18,* 128–142.

Gallaudet Research Institute, Gallaudet University. (2002, January). *Race/ethnic background of deaf children in U.S. regional and national summary report of data from 1973 to 2001.* Annual surveys of deaf and hard of hearing children & youth. Washington, DC: GRI, Gallaudet University.

Gallimore, L. (1999). *Teachers' stories: Teaching American Sign Language and English literacy.* Unpublished doctoral dissertation, The University of Arizona.

Gannon, C. L. (1998). The deaf community and sexuality education. *Sexuality and Disability, 16,* 283–293.

Gannon, J. (1981). *Deaf heritage: A narrative history of Deaf America.* Silver Spring, MD: National Association of the Deaf.

Gannon, J. (1989). *The week the world heard Gallaudet.* Washington, DC: Gallaudet University Press.

Garbarino, J., Guttmann, E., & Wilson Seeley, J. (1986). *The psychologically battered child.* San Francisco: Jossey-Bass.

Garber, C., Garne, G., & Testut, E. (1984). A survey of certification requirements for teachers of the hearing impaired. *Volta Review, 86(4),* 342–346.

Geers, A., & Moog, J. (1992). Speech perception and production skills of students with impaired hearing from oral and total communication settings. *Journal of Speech and Hearing Research, 35,* 1384–1393.

Geers, A., & Moog, J. (Eds.). (1994). Effectiveness of cochlear implants and tactile aids for deaf children: The sensory aids study at Central Institute for the Deaf. *Volta Review, 96,* 12–31.

Gentry, M. (1999). *Deaf readers: Transfer of factual information using multimedia and multimedia presentation options.* Unpublished doctoral dissertation, Lamar University, Beaumont, TX.

Gerber, S. (2001). *The handbook of genetic communicative disorders.* New York: Academic Press.

Gerber, S. E., Epstein, L., & Mencher, L. S. (1995). Recent changes in the etiology of hearing disorders: Perinatal drug exposure. *Journal of the American Academy of Audiology, 6,* 371–377.

Gianelli, D. (1999). Protect doctors from "undue burdens" of ADA. *American Medical News, 42(2),* 5.

Girocelli, L. (1982). *The comprehension of some aspects of figurative language by deaf and hearing subjects.* Unpublished doctoral dissertation, University of Illinois, Urbana-Champaign.

Glickman, N. (1996a). The development of culturally deaf identities. In N. Glickman & M. Harvey (Eds.), *Culturally affirmative psychotherapy with Deaf persons* (pp. 115–153). Mahwah, NJ: Erlbaum.

Glickman, N. (1996b). What is culturally affirmative psychotherapy. In N. Glickman & M. Harvey (Eds.), *Culturally affirmative psychotherapy with Deaf persons* (pp. 1–55). Mahwah, NJ: Erlbaum.

Glickman, N. S., & Carey, J. C. (1993). Measuring deaf cultural identities: A preliminary investigation. *Rehabilitation Psychology, 38,* 275–283.

Goldberg, D. (1996). Early intervention. In F. Martin & J. Martin (Eds.), *Hearing care for children* (pp. 287–302). Boston: Allyn and Bacon.

Goldberg, D., & Flexer, C. (2001). Auditory-verbal graduates: Outcome survey of clinical efficacy. *Journal of the American Academy of Audiology, 12(8),* 406–414.

Goldin-Meadow, S., & Mylander, C. (1990). Beyond the input given: The child's role in the acquisition of language. *Language, 66(2),* 323–355.

Goldsmith, H., & Harman, C. (1994). Temperament and attachment: Individuals and relationships. *Current Directions in Psychological Science, 3,* 53–61.

Gorlin, R. J., Toriello, H. V., & Cohen, M. M. (1995). *Hereditary hearing loss and its syndromes.* New York: Oxford University Press.

Gould, S. (1981). *The mismeasure of man.* New York: W. W. Norton.

Gonsoulin, T. (2001). Cochlear implant/Deaf World dispute: Different bottom elephants. *Otolaryngology-Head and Neck Surgery, 125,* 552–556.

Gray, C., & Hosie, J. (1996). Deafness, story understanding, and theory of mind. *Journal of Deaf Studies and Deaf Education, 1(4),* 217–233.

Green, G., Scott, D., McDonald, J., Woodworth, G., Sheffield, V., & Smith, R. (1999). Carrier rates in the Midwestern United States for GJB2 mutations causing inherited deafness. *The Journal of the American Medical Association, 281,* 2211–2216.

Greenberg, M. T. (2000). Educational interventions: Prevention and promotion of competence. In P. Hindley & N. Kitson (Eds.), *Mental health and deafness.* London: Whurr Publishers.

Greenberg, M. T., Calderon, R., & Kusche, C. (1984). Early intervention using simultaneous communication with deaf infants: The effect on communication development. *Child Development, 55,* 607–616.

Greenberg, M. T., & Kusche, C. (1998, Winter). Preventive intervention for school-age deaf children: The PATHS curriculum. *Journal of Deaf Studies and Deaf Education, 3(1),* 49–63.

Greenberg, M. T., & Marvin, R. S. (1979). Attachment patterns in profoundly deaf preschool children. *Merrill-Palmer Quarterly, 25,* 265–279.

Greenberg, J., Vernon, M., DuBois, J., & McKnight, J. (1982). *The language arts handbook.* Baltimore, MD: University Park Press.

Grinker, R. R. (Ed.). (1969). *Psychiatric diagnosis, therapy, and research on the psychotic deaf.* Final Report, Grant # RD 2407 S. Social and Rehabilitation Service, Department of Health, Education and Welfare, Chicago.

Grosjean, F. (1998). Living with two languages and two cultures. In I. Parasnis (Ed.), *Cultural and language diversity and the deaf experience.* New York: Cambridge University Press.

Groth-Marnat, G. (1999). *Handbook of psychological assessment* (3rd ed.). New York: John Wiley & Sons.

Groth-Marnat, G. (2000). Introduction to neuropsychological assessment. In G. Groth-Marnat (Ed.), *Neuropsychological assessment in clinical practice* (pp. 3–25). New York: John Wiley & Sons.

Grundfast, K., Siparsky, N., & Chuong, D. (2001, June). Genetics and molecular biology: Update. *Otolaryngology Clinical North America, 34(6),* 1367–1394.

Grushkin, D. (1998). Why shouldn't Sam read? Toward a new paradigm for literacy and the deaf. *Journal of Deaf Studies and Deaf Education, 3(3),* 179–198.

Gustason, G., Pfetzing, D., & Zawolkow, E. (1978). *Signing exact English: Supplement 1 & 2.* Los Angeles: Modern Signs Press.

Guthman, D. (1996). An analysis of variables that impact treatment outcomes of chemically dependent deaf and hard of hearing individuals. (Doctoral dissertation, University of Minnesota, 1996). *Dissertation Abstracts International, 56(7A),* 2638.

Guthman, D., Lybarger, R., & Sandberg, K. (1993). Providing chemical dependency treatment to the deaf or hard of hearing mentally ill client. *Journal of the American Deafness and Rehabilitation Association, 27,* 1–15.

Guthman, D., Sandberg, K., & Dickinson, J. (1999). Chemical dependency: An application of a treatment model for deaf people. In I. W. Leigh (Ed.), *Psychotherapy with deaf clients from diverse groups* (pp. 349–371). Washington, DC: Gallaudet University Press.

Gutman, V. (1999). Therapy issues with deaf lesbians, gay men, and bisexual men and women. In I. W. Leigh (Ed.), *Psychotherapy with deaf clients from diverse groups* (pp. 97–120). Washington, DC: Gallaudet University Press.

Hairston, E., & Smith, L. (1983). *Black and deaf in America: Are we that different?* Silver Spring, MD: TJ Publishers.

Hall, S. (1994). Silent club: An ethnographic study of folklore among the deaf. In C. J. Erting, R. C. Johnson, D. L. Smith, & B. D. Snider (Eds.), *The Deaf way* (pp. 522–527). Washington, DC: Gallaudet University Press.

Handler, L. (1996). The clinical use of figure drawings. In C. Newmark (Ed.), *Major psychological assessment instruments* (2nd ed., pp. 206–293). Boston: Allyn and Bacon.

Hansen, V. C. (1929). *Beretning om sindslidelse blaudt Danmarks d ovstumme.* Copenhagen, Denmark: Johansens Bogtrykkei.

Hardy, M. P. (1970). Speechreading. In H. Davis & S. Silverman (Eds.), *Hearing and deafness* (pp. 335–345). New York: Holt, Rinehart and Winston.

Hardy, M. P., Haskins, H. L., Hardy, W. G., & Shimizi, H. (1973). Rubella: Audiologic evaluation and follow up. *Archives of Otolaryngology, 98,* 237–245.

Hardy, S. T., & Kachman, W. (1995). Inclusion and students who are deaf or hard of hearing: School psychology's perspective. In B. D. Snider (Ed.), *Inclusion? Defining quality education for deaf and hard of hearing students* (pp. 103–114). Washington, DC: Gallaudet University.

Harmer, L. (1999). Health care delivery and deaf people: Practice, problems, and recommendations for change. *Journal of Deaf Studies and Deaf Education, 4*, 73–110.

Harris, R. I. (1978). Impulse control in deaf children: Research and clinical issues. In L. Liben (Ed.), *Deaf children: Developmental perspectives* (pp. 137–156). New York: Academic Press.

Harrison, J. (1998). Schools for the deaf make accommodations to support children with implants. *NECCI News: Network of Educators of Children with Cochlear Implants, 9(2)*, 1, 4.

Harter, S. (1997). The personal self in social context. In R. D. Ashmore & L. Jussim (Eds.), *Self and identity* (pp. 81–105). New York: Oxford University Press.

Harty-Golder, B. (1998). Meet ADA regs for treating hearing-impaired. *American Medical News, 41(25)*, 26.

Harvey, M. (1989). *Psychotherapy with deaf and hard of hearing persons: A systemic model.* Hillsdale, NJ: Erlbaum.

Harvey, M. (1993). Cross cultural psychotherapy with deaf persons: A hearing, white, middle class, middle aged, non-gay, Jewish, male, therapist's perspective. *Journal of the American Deafness and Rehabilitation Association, 26*, 43–55.

Hauser, P., Maxwell-McCaw, D., Leigh, I. W., & Gutman, V. (2000). Internship accessibility issues for deaf and hard-of-hearing applicants: No cause for complacency. *Professional Psychology: Research and Practice, 31*, 569–574.

Heath, S. B. (1983). *Way with words.* Cambridge: Cambridge University Press.

Hernandez, M. (1999). The role of therapeutic groups in working with Latino deaf adolescent immigrants. In I. W. Leigh (Ed.), *Psychotherapy with deaf clients from diverse groups* (pp. 227–249). Washington, DC: Gallaudet University Press.

Hickok, G., Bellugi, U., & Klima, E. (2001). Sign language in the brain. *Scientific American, 285(6)*, 58–65.

Hickok, G., Poeppel, D., Clark, K., Buxton, R., Rowley, H., & Roberts, T. (1997). Sensory mapping in a congenitally deaf subject: MEG and MRI studies of cross-modal non-plasticity. *Human Brain Mapping, 5*, 437–444.

Higginbotham, D. J., & Baker, B. M. (1981). Social participation and cognitive play differences in hearing-impaired and normally hearing preschoolers. *The Volta Review, 83*, 135–149.

Hintermair, M. (2000). Hearing impairment, social networks, and coping: The need for families with hearing-impaired children to relate to other parents and to hearing-impaired adults. *American Annals of the Deaf, 145*, 41–53.

Hirshoren, A., & Schnittjer, D. J. (1979). Dimensions of problem behavior in deaf children. *Journal of Abnormal Child Psychology, 7*, 221–228.

Hoffmeister, R. (2000). A piece of the puzzle: ASL and reading comprehension in deaf children. In C. Chamberlain, J. Morford, & R. Mayberry (Eds.), *Language acquisition by eye* (pp. 143–163). Mahwah, NJ: Erlbaum.

Hoffmeister, R. & Harvey, M. (1996). Is there a psychology of the hearing? In N. Glickman & M. Harvey (Eds.), *Culturally affirmative psychotherapy with deaf persons* (pp. 73–97). Mahwah, NJ: Erlbaum.

Holcomb, M., & Wood, S. (1989). *Deaf women: A parade through the decades.* Berkeley, CA: DawnSign Press.

Holcomb, T. K., Coryell, J., & Rosenfield, E. (1992, March/April). Designing a supportive mainstream environment. In *A folio of mainstream articles from Perspectives in Education and Deafness.* Washington, DC: Pre-College Programs of Gallaudet University.

Holden-Pitt, L. (1997a). A look at residential school placement patterns for students from deaf- and hearing-parented families: A ten year perspective. *American Annals of the Deaf, 142(2)*, 108–114.

Holden-Pitt, L. (1997b). Annual survey. *American Annals of the Deaf, 142(2)*, 68–74.

Holden-Pitt, L., & Diaz, J. A. (1998). Thirty years of the Annual Survey of Deaf and Hard-of-Hearing Children and Youth: A glance over the decades. *American Annals of the Deaf, 142*, 72–76.

Holzrichter, A., & Meier, R. (2000). Child-directed signing in American Sign Language. In C. Chamberlain, J. Morford, & R. Mayberry (Eds.), *Language acquisition by eye* (pp. 25–40). Mahwah, NJ: Erlbaum.

Hotto, S. (2001). *Gallaudet Research Institute. Regional and national summary report of data from 1999–2000. Annual survey of deaf and hard of hearing youth.* Washington, DC: Graduate Research Institute, Gallaudet University.

Howell, R. (1985). Maternal reports of vocabulary development in four-year-old deaf children. *American Annals of the Deaf, 129*, 459–465.

Hu, D., Qiu, W., Wu, B., Fang, L., Zhou, F., Gu, Y., Zhang, Q., Yan, J., Ding, Y., & Wong, H. (1991). Genetic aspects of antibiotic induced deafness: Mitochondrial inheritance. *Journal of Medical Genetics, 28*, 79–83.

Hui, C. H., & Triandis, H. C. (1985). Measurement in cross-cultural psychology: A review and comparison of strategies. *Journal of Cross-Cultural Psychology, 16,* 131–152.

Humphries, T. (1993). Deaf culture and cultures. In K. Christensen & G. Delgado (Eds.), *Multicultural issues in deafness.* White Plains, NY: Longman.

Humphries, T. (1996). Of Deaf-mutes, the strange, and the modern deaf self. In N. Glickman & M. Harvey (Eds.), *Culturally affirmative psychotherapy with deaf persons* (pp. 99–114). Mahwah, NJ: Erlbaum.

Intertribal Deaf Council. (1999). Retrieved September 27, 2001 from http://www.bigriver.net/~rasmith/idc/idc.html.

Jacobs, L. (1981). *A deaf adult speaks out.* Silver Spring, MD: National Association of the Deaf.

Jacobs, R. (1987). Use of the Sixteen Personality Factor Questionnaire, Form A, with deaf university students. *Journal of Rehabilitation of the Deaf, 21,* 19–26.

Jankowski, K. (1997). *Deaf empowerment: Emergence, struggle, and rhetoric.* Washington, DC: Gallaudet University Press.

Jensema, C., McCann, R., & Ramsey, S. (1996). Close-captioned television presentation speech and vocabulary. *American Annals of the Deaf, 14(4),* 284–292.

Jensema, C., Sharkawy, S., Danturthi, R., Burch, R., & Hsu, D. (2000). Eye movement patterns of captioned television viewers. *American Annals of the Deaf, 145(3),* 275–285.

Johnson, R. C. (2001, Spring/Summer). High stakes testing and deaf students: Some research perspectives. *Research at Gallaudet,* pp. 1–6.

Johnston, E. (1997). Residential schools offer students deaf culture. *Perspectives in Education and Deafness, 16(2),* 4–5, 24.

Joint Committee on Infant Hearing. (2000). Year 2000 position statement: principles and guidelines for early hearing detection and intervention programs. *American Journal of Audiology, 9,* 9–29.

Jones, B. E. (1999, February). Providing access: "New roles" for educational interpreters. *Views, 16(2),* 15.

Jordan, J. (1991). Preface. In D. Stewart (Ed.), *Deaf sport: The impact of sports within the deaf community* (pp. vii–viii). Washington, DC: Gallaudet University Press.

Kagan, J. (1998). Is there a self in infancy? In M. Ferrari & R. J. Sternberg (Eds.), *Self-awareness: Its nature and development* (pp. 137–147). New York: Guilford Press.

Kampfe, C. (1989). Parental reaction to a child's hearing impairment. *American Annals of the Deaf, 134,* 255–259.

Karchmer, M. A., & Allen, T. E. (1999, April). The functional assessment of deaf and hard of hearing students. *American Annals of the Deaf, 144(2),* 68–77.

Katz, C. (1994). *VisMa and the child: Its myth and history.* Unpublished manuscript, Ohlone College, Fremont, CA.

Katz, C. (1996). *A history of the Deaf community in Beaumont, Texas.* Unpublished paper, Lamar University, Beaumont, TX.

Katz, C. (1999). *The establishment of bachelor degree programs in deaf studies.* Unpublished doctoral dissertation, Lamar University, Beaumont, TX.

Katz, D., Vernon, M., Penn, A., & Gillece, J. (1992). The consent decree: A means of obtaining mental health services for people who are deaf. *Journal of the American Deafness and Rehabilitation Association, 26(2),* 22–28.

Kauffman, J. M. (2001). *Characteristics of emotional and behavioral disorders of children and youth* (7th ed.). Columbus OH: Merrill Prentice Hall.

Kaufman, J., & Zigler, E. (1987). Do abused children become abusive parents? *American Journal of Orthopsychiatry, 57, (2),* 186–192.

Keane, K., & Kretschmer, R. (1987). Effect of mediated learning intervention on cognitive task performance with a deaf population. *Journal of Education Psychology, 79(1),* 49–53.

Keane, K., Tannenbaum, A., & Krapf, G. (1992). Cognitive competence: Reality and potential in the deaf. In C. Haywood & T. Tzuriel (Eds.), *Interactive assessment.* New York. Springer-Verlag.

Keats, B. (2001). *Introduction to genes and hearing loss.* Presentation at the Human Genome Project and Hearing Loss Conference, Bethesda, MD.

Keats, B., & Corey, D. (1999). The Usher syndromes. *American Journal of Medical Genetics, 89,* 158–166.

Kelly, R. (1996). The interaction of syntactic competence and vocabulary during reading by deaf students. *Journal of Deaf Studies and Deaf Education, 1(1),* 75–90.

Kenny, V. (1962). A better way to teach deaf children. *Harpers Magazine,* pp. 61–65.

Kersting, S. (1997). Balancing between deaf and hearing worlds: Reflections of mainstreamed college students on relationships and social interactions. *Journal of Deaf Studies and Deaf Education, 2,* 252–263.

Kestenbaum, R., Farber, E. A., & Sroufe, L. A. (1989). Individual differences in empathy among preschoolers: Relation to attachment history. In N. Eisenberg (Ed.), *Empathy and related emotional responses* (New Directions for Child development, No. 33, pp. 51–64). San Francisco: Jossey-Bass.

Koester, L. S., & Meadow-Orlans, K. P. (1990). Parenting a deaf child: Stress, strength, and support. In D. F. Moores & K. P. Meadow-Orlans (Eds.), *Educational and developmental aspects of deafness.* Washington, DC: Gallaudet University Press.

Koester, L. S., Papousek, H., & Smith-Gray, S. (2000). Intuitive parenting, communication, and interaction with deaf infants. In P. E. Spencer, C. J. Erting, & M. Marschark (Eds.), *The deaf child in the family and at school* (pp. 55–71). Mahwah, NJ: Erlbaum.

Koppe, J. G., & Kloosterman, G. J. (1982). Congenital toxoplasmosis: Long-term follow-up. *Padiatrie und Padologie, 17,* 171–179.

Krashen, S., Long, M., & Scarcella, R. (1982). Age, rate, and eventual attainment in second language acquisition. In S. Krashen, R. Scarcella, & M. Long (Eds.), *Child-adult differences in second language acquisition* (pp. 161–172). Rowley, MA: Newbury House.

Kricos, P. (1993). The counseling process: Children and parents. In J. Alpiner & P. McCarthy (Eds.), *Rehabilitative audiology: Children and adults* (pp. 211–233). Philadelphia: Lippincott Williams & Wilkens.

Kroger, J. (1993). Ego identity: An overview. In J. Kroger (Ed.), *Discussions on ego identity.* Hillsdale, NJ: Erlbaum.

Kusche, C. A., & Greenberg, M. T. (1994). *The PATHS curriculum.* Seattle, WA: Developmental Research And Programs.

LaBarre, A. (1998). Treatment of sexually abused children who are deaf. *Sexuality & Disability, 16,* 321–324.

LaFromboise, T., Coleman, H., & Gerton, J. (1993). Psychological impact of biculturalism: Evidence and theory. *Psychological Bulletin, 114,* 395–412.

Lane, H. (1993). Mask of irreverence (Letter to the editor). *American Annals of the Deaf, 138(4),* 316–319.

Lane, H. (1996). Cultural self-awareness in hearing people. In N. Glickman & M. Harvey (Eds.), *Culturally affirmative psychotherapy with deaf people* (pp. 57–72). Mahwah, NJ: Erlbaum.

Lane, H. (1997). Constructions of deafness. In L. Davis (Ed.), *The disability studies reader* (pp. 153–171). New York: Routledge.

Lane, H. (1999). *The mask of benevolence: Disabling the Deaf community.* San Diego, CA: DawnSign Press.

Lane, H., & Bahan, B. (1998). Ethics of cochlear implantation in young children: A review and reply from a Deaf-world perspective. *Otolaryngology—Head and Neck Surgery, 119,* 297–307.

Lane, H., Hoffmeister, R., & Bahan, B. (1996). *A journey into the Deaf-world.* San Diego, CA: Dawn Sign Press.

Lane, H., Pillard, R., & French, H. (2000). Origins of the American Deaf-world: Assimilating and differentiating societies and their relation to genetic patterning. *Sign Language Studies, 1,* 17–44.

Lang, H. (2000). *A phone of our own: The deaf insurrection against Ma Bell.* Washington, DC: Gallaudet University Press.

Lang, H., & Meath-Lang, B. (1995). *Deaf persons in the arts and sciences.* Westport, CT: Greenwood Press.

Langholtz, D., & Ruth, R. (1999). Deaf people with HIV/AIDS: Notes on the psychotherapeutic journey. In I. W. Leigh (Ed.), *Psychotherapy with deaf clients from diverse groups* (pp. 253–277). Washington, DC: Gallaudet University Press.

LaSasso, C. (1999). Test-taking skills: A missing component of deaf students' curriculum. *American Annals of the Deaf, 144,* 35–43.

LaSasso, C., & Metzger, M. (1998). An alternate route for preparing deaf children for BiBi programs: The home language L1 and Cued Speech for conveying traditionally spoken languages. *Journal of Deaf Studies and Deaf Education, 3(4),* 265–289.

LaSasso, C., & Wilson, A. (2000). Results of two national surveys of leadership personnel needs in deaf education. *American Annals of the Deaf, 145(5),* 429–435.

Lederberg, A. R. (1993). The impact of deafness on mother-child and peer relationships. In M. Marschark & M. D. Clark (Eds.), *Psychological perspectives on deafness* (pp. 93–119). Hillsdale, NJ: Erlbaum.

Lederberg, A. R., (1998, August). *Maternal stress and social support: Hearing impaired versus hearing toddlers.* Poster displayed at the meeting of the American Psychological Association, Atlanta, GA.

Lederberg, A. R., & Mobley, C. E. (1990). The effect of hearing impairment on the quality of attachment and mother-toddler interaction. *Child Development, 61,* 1596–1604.

Lederberg, A. R., & Prezbindowski, A. K. (2000). Impact of child deafness on mother-toddler interaction: Strengths and weakness. In P. E. Spencer, C. J. Erting, & M. Marschark (Eds.), *The deaf child in the family and at school* (pp. 73–92). Mahwah, NJ: Erlbaum.

Lederberg, A. R., Rosenblatt, V., Vandell, D. L., & Chapin, S. L. (1987). Temporary and long term friendships in hearing and deaf preschoolers. *Merrill-Palmer Quarterly, 33,* 515–533.

Lederberg, A. R., & Spencer, P. (2001). Vocabulary development of deaf and hard of hearing children. In M. Clark, M. Marschark, & M. Karchmer (Eds.), *Context, cognition, and deafness* (pp. 88–112). Washington, DC: Gallaudet University Press.

Leigh, I. W. (1987). Parenting and the hearing impaired: Attachment and coping. *The Volta Review, 89,* 11–21.

Leigh, I. W. (1994). Psychosocial implications of full inclusion for deaf children and adolescents. In R. C. Johnson & O. P. Cohen (Eds.), *Implications and complications for deaf students of the full inclusion movement* (pp. 73–77). Washington, DC: Gallaudet University Press.

Leigh, I. W. (1999a, March/April). Book review: We can hear and speak. *Perspectives in Education and Deafness,* 18–19.

Leigh, I. W. (1999b). Inclusive education and personal development. *Journal of Deaf Studies and Deaf Education, 4,* 236–245.

Leigh, I. W. (Ed.). (1999c). *Psychotherapy with deaf clients from diverse groups.* Washington, DC: Gallaudet University Press.

Leigh, I. W. (2000). *Mental health access for deaf and hard-of-hearing consumers.* Presentation, Access Is the Issue: Access to Mental Health for Deaf and Hard-of-Hearing Persons, Training Conference, New York City.

Leigh, I. W., & Anthony, S. (1999). Parent bonding in clinically depressed deaf and hard-of-hearing adults. *Journal of Deaf Studies and Deaf Education, 4,* 28–36.

Leigh, I. W., & Anthony-Tolbert, S. (2001). Reliability of the BDI-II with deaf persons. *Rehabilitation Psychology, 46,* 195–202.

Leigh, I. W., Corbett, C., Gutman, V., & Morere, D. (1996). Providing psychological services to deaf individuals: A response to new perceptions of diversity. *Professional Psychology: Research and Practice, 27,* 364–371.

Leigh, I. W., & Lewis, J. (1999). Deaf therapists and the deaf community: How the twain meet. In I. W. Leigh (Ed.), *Psychotherapy with deaf clients from diverse groups* (pp. 45–65). Washington, DC: Gallaudet University Press.

Leigh, I. W., Marcus, A., Dobosh, P., & Allen, T. (1998). Deaf/hearing identity paradigms: Modification of the Deaf Identity Development Scale. *Journal of Deaf Studies and Deaf Education, 3,* 329–338.

Leigh, I. W., Robins, C., & Welkowitz, J. (1988). Modification of the Beck Depression Inventory for use with a deaf population. *Journal of Clinical Psychology, 44,* 728–732.

Leigh, I. W., & Sommer, J. P. (1998). *Politics of deafness.* Presentation at the A.G. Bell Association Convention, Little Rock, AR.

Leigh, I. W., & Stinson, M. (1991). Social environment, self-perceptions, and identity of hearing-impaired adolescents. *The Volta Review, 93,* 7–22.

LeNard, J. M. (2001). *How public input shapes the Clerc Center's priorities: Identifying critical needs in transition from school to postsecondary education and employment.* Washington, DC: Gallaudet University, Laurent Clerc National Deaf Education Center.

Lenneberg, E. (1967). *Biological foundations of language.* New York: Wiley.

Levanen, S., Jourmaki, V., & Hari, R. (1998). Vibration-induced auditory cortex activation in a congenitally deaf adult. *Current Biology, 8,* 869–872.

Levanen, S., Uutela, K., Salenius, S., & Hari, R. (2001). Cortical representation of sign language comparison of deaf signers and hearing non-signers. *Cerebral Cortex, 11,* 506–512.

Levine, E. S. (1951). Psycho-educational characteristics of children following maternal rubella. *American Journal of Disabilities of Children,* 627–632.

Levine, E. S. (1956). *Youth in a silent world.* New York: New York University Press.

Levine, E. S. (1960). *Psychology of deafness.* New York: Columbia University Press.

Levine, E. S. (1977). The preparation of psychological service providers to the deaf. Report of the Spartanburg Conference. Monograph #4. *Journal of Rehabilitation of the Deaf.*

Levine, E. S. (1981). *The ecology of early deafness: Guides to fashioning environments and psychological assessments.* New York: Columbia University Press.

Levine, E. S., & Wagner, E. E. (1974). Personality patterns of deaf persons: An interpretation based on research with the hand test. *Perceptual and Motor Skills Monograph Supplement, 39,* 23–44.

Lezak, M. (1995). *Neuropsychological assessment* (3rd ed.). New York: Oxford University Press.

Liben, L. S. (1978). Developmental perspectives on experiential deficiencies of deaf children. In L. Liben (Ed.), *Deaf children: Developmental perspectives* (pp. 195–215). New York: Academic Press.

Ling, D. (1976). *Speech and the hearing impaired child: Theory and practice. Washington, DC:* Alexander Graham Bell Association for the Deaf.

Linton, S. (1998). *Claiming disability: Knowledge and identity.* New York: New York University Press.

Lipton, D., & Goldstein, M. (1997). Measuring substance abuse among the Deaf. *Journal of Drug Issues, Inc.,* 733–754.

Litchenstein, E. (1998). The relationships between reading processes and English skills of deaf college students. *Journal of Deaf Studies and Deaf Education, 3(2),* 80–134.

Livingston, S. (1997). *Rethinking the education of deaf students: Theory and practice from a teacher's perspective.* Portsmouth, NH: Heinemann.

Lopez, J. (2001). Hispanic from a Latino perspective. Unpublished manuscript.

Lucas, C., & Valli, C. (1992). *Language contact in the American deaf community.* San Diego, CA: Academic Press.

Lucker, J. (2002). Cochlear implants: A technological overview. In J. Christiansen & I. W. Leigh, *Cochlear implants in children: Ethics and choices* (pp. 45–64). Washington, DC: Gallaudet University Press.

Luterman, D. (1999). Emotional aspects of hearing loss. *The Volta Review, 99,* 75–83.

Luterman, D., & Kurtzer-White, E. (1999). Identifying hearing loss: Parents' needs. *American Journal of Audiology, 8,* 13–18.

Lyons, C., & Pinnell, G. (2001). *Systems for change in literacy education: A guide to professional development.* Portsmouth, NH: Heinemann.

Lytle, L. (1987). Identify formation and developmental antecedents in deaf college women (Doctoral dissertation, The Catholic University, 1987). *Dissertation Abstracts International, 48(3–A),* 606–607.

Lytle, R., & Rovins, M. R. (1997). Reforming deaf education: A paradigm shift from how to teach to what to teach. *American Annals of the Deaf, 142(1),* 7–15.

MacCollin, M. (1998). Neurofibromatosis 2. *GeneClinics: Clinical Genetics Information Resource.* Retrieved October 12, 2001, from University of Washington, Seattle website: http://www.geneclinics.org/profiles/nf2/index.html.

Mackelprang, R., & Salsgiver, R. (1999). *Disability: A diversity model approach in human service practice.* Pacific Grove, CA: Brooks Cole.

Madriz, J. J., & Herrera, G. (1995). Human immunodeficiency virus and acquired immune deficiency syndrome AIDS-related hearing disorders. *Journal of the American Academy of Audiology, 6,* 358–364.

Maher, J. (1996). *Seeing language in sign: The work of William C. Stokoe.* Washington, DC: Gallaudet University Press.

Maller, S., Singleton, J., Supalla, S., & Wix, T. (1999). The development and psychometric properties of the American Sign Language Proficiency Assessment (ASL-PA). *Journal of Deaf Studies and Deaf Education, 4,* 249–269.

Malzkuhn, M. (1994). The human rights of the deaf. In C. J. Erting, R.C. Johnson, D. L. Smith, & B. D. Snider (Eds.), *The Deaf way* (pp. 780–785). Washington, DC: Gallaudet University Press.

Marazita, M., Ploughman, L., Rawlings, B., Remington, E., Arnos, K., & Nance, W. (1993). Genetic epidemiological studies of early-onset deafness in the U.S. school-age population. *American Journal of Medical Genetics, 46,* 486–491.

Marcia, J. E. (1993). The relational roots of identity. In J. Kroger (Ed.), *Discussions on ego identity.* Hillsdale, NJ: Erlbaum.

Marschark, M. (1993). *Psychological development of deaf children.* New York: Oxford University Press.

Marschark, M. (1997). *Raising and educating a deaf child: A comprehensive guide to the choices, controversies, and decisions faced by parents and educators.* New York York: Oxford University Press.

Marschark, M. (2000a). Education and development of deaf children or is it development and education? In P. E. Spencer, C. J. Erting, & M. Marschark (Eds.), *The deaf child in the family and at school* (pp. 275–301). Mahwah, NJ: Erlbaum.

Marschark, M. (2000b). *Language development in children who are deaf: A research synthesis.* National Association of State Directors of Special Education (NASDSE), 1800 Diagonal Road, Suite 320, Alexandria, VA 22314.

Marschark, M. (2001). Language development in children who are deaf: A research synthesis. *Project Forum.* Alexandria, VA: National Association of State Directors of Special Educators (NASDSE).

Marshark, M., & Clark, M. (Eds.). (1993). *Psychological perspectives on deafness.* Hillsdale, NJ: Erlbaum.

Marschark, M., & Everhart, V. (1999). Problem-solving by deaf and hearing children: Twenty questions. *Deafness and Education International, 1,* 63–79.

Marschark, M., & Lukomski, J. (2001). Understanding language and learning in deaf children. In M. Clark, M. Marschark, & M. Karchmer (Eds.), *Context, cognition, and deafness* (pp. 71–87). Washington, DC: Gallaudet University Press.

Martin, D., Craft, A., & Zhang, Z. (2001). The impact of cognitive strategy instruction on deaf learners: An international comparative study. *American Annals of the Deaf, 146(4)*, 366–378.

Martin, F., & Clark, J. (2000). *Introduction to audiology* (7th ed.). Boston: Allyn and Bacon.

Mather, S. (1997). Initiation in visually constructed dialogue: Reading books with three to eight year old students who are deaf and hard of hearing. In C. Lucas (Ed.), *Multicultural aspects of sociolinguistics in deaf communities* (pp. 109–131). Washington, DC: Gallaudet University Press.

Mauk, G. W., & Mauk, P. P. (1992). Somewhere, out there: Preschool children with hearing impairment and learning disabilities. *Topics in Early Childhood Special Education: Hearing Impaired Preschoolers, 12*, 174–195.

Maxon, A., & Brackett, D. (1992). *The hearing impaired child: Infancy through high school years.* Boston: Andover Medical Publishers.

Maxwell, M., & Doyle, J. (1996). Language codes and sense-making among deaf schoolchildren. *Journal of Deaf Studies and Deaf Education, 1(2)*, 122–136.

Maxwell-McCaw, D. L. (2001). *Acculturation and psychological well-being in deaf and hard-of-hearing people.* (Doctoral dissertation, George Washington University). *Dissertation Abstracts International, 61(11–B)*, 6141.

Mayberry, R., & Eichen, E. B. (1991). The long-lasting advantage of learning sign language in childhood: Another look at the critical period for language acquisition. *Journal of Memory, 30(4)*, 486–512.

Mayer, C., & Akamatsu, T. (1999). Bilingual-bicultural models of literacy education for deaf students: Considering the claims. *Journal of Deaf Studies and Deaf Education, 4(1)*, 1–8.

McCartney, B. (1986). An investigation of the factors contributing to the ability of hearing-impaired children to communicate orally as perceived by oral deaf adults and parents and teachers of the hearing impaired. *The Volta Review, 88*, 133–143.

Mayer, C., & Wells, G. (1996). Can the linguistic interdependence theory support a bilingual-bicultural model of literacy education for deaf students? *Journal of Deaf Studies and Deaf Education, 1*, 93–107.

McCracken, G. (1986). Aminoglycoside toxicity in infants and children. *American Journal of Medicine, 80*, 172–178.

McCullough, C., & Emmorey, K. (1997). Face processing by deaf ASL signers: Evidence for expertise in distinguishing local features. *Journal of Deaf Studies and Deaf Education, 2*, 212–222.

McGhee, H. (1996). An evaluation of modified written and American Sign Language versions of the Beck Depression Inventory with the prelingually deaf. (Doctoral dissertation, The California School of Professional Psychology, Alameda, 1995). *Dissertation Abstracts International, Section B: The Sciences & Engineering, 56 (11–B)*, 6456.

McIntosh, R., Sulzen, L., Reeder, L., & Kidd, D. (1994). Making science accessible to deaf students. *American Annals of the Deaf, 139(5)*, 480–484.

Meadow, K. P. (1980). *Deafness and child development.* Berkeley: University of California Press.

Meadow-Orlans, K. P. (1996). Socialization of deaf children and youth. In P. Higgins & J. Nash (Eds.), *Understanding deafness socially: Continuities in research and theory* (2nd ed., pp. 71–95). Springfield, IL: Charles C. Thomas.

Meadow-Orlans, K. P. (1997). Effects of mother and infant hearing status on interactions at twelve and eighteen months. *Journal of Deaf Studies and Deaf Education, 2(1)*, 27–36.

Meadow-Orlans, K., Mertens, D., Sass-Lehrer, M., & Scott-Olson, K. (1997). Support services for parents and their children who are deaf and hard of hearing. *American Annals of the Deaf, 142*, 278–293.

Mertens, D., Sass-Lehrer, M., & Scott-Olson, K. (2000). Sensitivity in the family-professional relationship: Parental experiences in families with young deaf and hard of hearing children. In P. Spencer, C. Erting, & M. Marschark (Eds.), *The deaf child in the family and at school* (pp. 133–150). Mahwah, NJ: Erlbaum.

Metzger, M. (1999). *Sign language interpreting: Deconstructing the myth of neutrality.* Washington, DC: Gallaudet University Press.

Metzger, M. (2000). *Bilingualism and identity in deaf communities.* Washington, DC: Gallaudet University Press.

Meyer, G., Finn, S., Eyde, L., Kay, G., Moreland, K., Dies, R., Eisman, E., Kubiszyn, T., & Reed, G. (2001). Psychological testing and psychological assessment. *American Psychologist, 56*, 128–165.

Meyerhof, W., Cass, S., Schwaber, M., Sculerati, N., & Slattery, W. (1994). Progressive sensorineural hearing loss in children. *Otolaryngology—Head and Neck Surgery, 110*, 560–570.

Middleton, A., Hewison, J., & Mueller, R. (2001). Prenatal diagnosis for inherited deafness—What is the potential demand? *Journal of Genetic Counseling, 10*, 121–131.

Miles, B. (2000, January). Literacy for persons who are deaf-blind. Monmouth, OR: *DB-LINK*. The National Clearinghouse on Children Who Are Deaf-Blind.

Miller, K. (2000). Welcome to the real world: Reflections on teaching and administration. *American Annuals of the Deaf, 145(5),* 404–410.

Miller, K. (2001). Access to sign language interpreters in the criminal justice system. *American Annals of the Deaf, 146,* 328–330.

Miller, K., & Vernon, M. (2001, June). Deaf rights card. *Silent News,* 4.

Miller, M. S., & Moores, D. F. (2000). Bilingual/bicultural education for deaf students. In M. A. Winzer & K. Mazurek (Eds.), *Special education in the 21st century: Issues of inclusion and reform* (pp. 221–237). Washington, DC: Gallaudet University Press.

Mills v. Board of Education of the District of Columbia, 348. (1972). F. Supp. 866, 868, 875, D.D.C.

Mindel, E. D., & Vernon, M. (1971). *They grow in silence: The deaf child and his family.* Silver Spring, MD: National Association of the Deaf.

Miner, I. (1999). Psychotherapy for people with Usher Syndrome. In I. W. Leigh (Ed.), *Psychotherapy with deaf clients from diverse groups* (pp. 307–327). Washington, DC: Gallaudet University Press.

Mitrushina, M., Boone, K., & D'Elia, L. (1999). *Handbook of normative data for neuropsychological assessment.* New York: Oxford University Press.

Moeller, M., & Condon, M. (1998). Family matters: Making sense of complex choices. In F. Bess (Ed.), *Children with hearing impairment: Contemporary trends* (pp. 305–310). Nashville, TN: Vanderbilt-Bill Wilkerson Center Press.

Mogford, K. (1994). Oral language acquisition in the prelinguistically deaf. In D. Bishop & K. Mogford (Eds.), *Language development in exceptional children* (pp. 110–131). Mahwah, NJ: Erlbaum.

Mohay, H. (2000). Language in sight: Mothers' strategies for making language visually accessible to deaf children. In P. Spencer, C. Erting, & M. Marschark (Eds.), *The deaf child in the family and at school* (pp. 151–166). Mahwah, NJ: Erlbaum.

Moll, L. (1990). *Vygotsky and education.* Cambridge: Cambridge University Press.

Montanini Manfredi, M. (1993). The emotional development of deaf children. In M. Marschark & M. D. Clark (Eds.), *Psychological perspectives on deafness* (pp. 49–63). Hillsdale NJ: Erlbaum.

Moores, D. F. (1973). Families and deafness. In A. Norris (Ed.), *Deafness annual* (pp. 115–130). Silver Spring, MD: Professional Rehabilitation Workers with the Adult Deaf.

Moores, D. F. (1990, January). An open letter to the campus community: Old w(h)ine in new bottles. Unpublished paper. Gallaudet University, Washington, D.C.

Moores, D. F. (1993a). Mask of confusion. *American Annals of the Deaf, 138(4),* 319–321.

Moores, D. F. (1993b). Book reviews: The mask of benevolence: Disabling the deaf community. *American Annals of the Deaf, 138,* 4–9.

Moores, D. F. (2001a). *Educating the Deaf: Psychology, principles, and practices* (5th ed.). Boston: Houghton Mifflin.

Moores, D. F. (2001b). Testing revisited. *American Annals of the Deaf, 146(4),* 307–308.

Moores, D. F., Jatho, J., & Creech, C. (2001). Families with deaf members: American Annals of the Deaf, 1996–2000. *American Annals of the Deaf, 146,* 245–250.

Moose, M. (1999, February). Educational interpreting: Raising the standards. *VIEWS, 16,* 2, 10.

Morton, D. (2000). Beyond parent education: The impact of extended family dynamics in deaf education. *American Annals of the Deaf, 145,* 359–365.

Morton, D., & Christensen, J. N. (2000). *Mental health services for deaf people: A resource directory.* Washington, DC: Department of Counseling, Gallaudet University.

Moulton, R., Andrews, J. F., & Smith, M. (1996). The deaf world. In R. Brown, D. Baine, & A. Newfeldt (Eds.), *Beyond basic care: Special education and community rehabilitation in low income countries* (pp. 168–182). North York, Ontario, Canada: Captus Press.

Mounty, J. (1986). *Nativization and input in the language development of two deaf children of hearing parents.* Unpublished doctoral dissertation, Boston University.

Muller, C. (2001). *Sudden sensorineural hearing loss.* Paper presented at Grand Rounds in the Department of Otolaryngology Head/Neck Surgery. University of Texas Medical Branch, Galveston, TX.

Munro-Ludders, B. (1992). Deaf and dying: Deaf people and the process of dying. *Journal of the American Deafness and Rehabilitation Association, 26,* 31–41.

Murphy, K., & Davidshofer, C. (1998). *Psychological testing: Principles and applications* (4th ed.). Upper Saddle River, NJ: Prentice Hall.

Musselman, C., & Churchill, A. (1991). Conversational control in mother-child dyads. *American Annals of the Deaf, 136,* 99–117.

Musselman, C., & Kircaali-Iftar, G. (1998). The development of spoken language in deaf children.

Explaining the unexplained variance. *Journal of Deaf Studies and Deaf Education, 1(2)*, 108–121.

Myers, R. (Ed.). (1995). *Standards of care for the delivery of mental health services to deaf and hard-of-hearing persons.* Retrieved October 13, 2001, from http://www.deafhoh-health.org/html/professionals/standards_guidelines.html.

Myklebust, H. R. (1954). *Auditory disorders in children: A manual for differential diagnosis.* New York: Grune & Stratton.

Myklebust, H. R. (1960). *The psychology of deafness.* New York: Grune & Stratton.

Naito, Y., Hirano, S., Honjo, I., Okazawa, H., Ishizu, K., Takahashi, H., Fujiki, N., Shiomi, Y., Yonekura, Y., & Konishi, J. (1997). Sound-induced activation of auditory cortices in cochlear implant users with post- and prelingual deafness demonstrated by positron emission tomography. *Acta Otolaryngol, 117*, 490–496.

Napier, J. (2002). The D/deaf-H/hearing debate. *Sign Language Studies, 2*, 141–149.

National Asian Deaf Congress. (2001). *About National Asian Deaf Congress.* Retrieved September 27, 2001, from http://www.nadc-usa.org/about.html.

National Association of the Deaf. (2000a). *Legal rights: The guide for deaf and hard of hearing people* (5th ed.). Washington, DC: Gallaudet University Press.

National Association of the Deaf. (2000b, November). NAD position statements. *The NAD Broadcaster*, p. 5.

National Association of the Deaf. (2001, March) The NAD's position on the statewide assessment of deaf and hard of hearing students. *The NAD Broadcaster*, pp. 9–10.

National Association of the Deaf (2002, January). NAD position statement on inclusion. Silver Spring, MD: NAD Education Policy and Program Development Center.

National Deaf Children's Society (NDCS). (1999). *PATHS: The way towards personal and social empowerment for deaf children: A report on the NDCS deaf children in mind project-personal and social initiative.* London: National Deaf Children's Society.

National Information Center on Deafness (NICD). (1991). *Mainstreaming D/HH students: Q and A research, reading, resources.* Washington, DC: Gallaudet University.

National Organization for Rare Disorders. (2000). *Neurofibromatosis Type 2 (NF-2).* Retrieved September 7, 2000, from http://www.stepstn.com/cgi-win/nord.exe?proc=GetDocument&rectype=0&recnum=792.

National Research Council (NRC). (1993). *Understanding child abuse and neglect.* Washington, DC: National Academy Press.

Neville, H., Bavelier, D., Corina, D., Rauschecker, J., Karni, A., Laiwani, A., Braun, A., Clark, V., Jezzard, P., & Turner, R. (1998). Cerebral organization for language in deaf and hearing subjects: Biological constraints and effects of experience. *Proceedings of the National Academy of Science, USA, 95*, 922–929.

Newport, E. (1990). Maturational constraints on language learning. *Cognitive Science, 14*, 11–28.

Newport, E., & Meier, R. (1985). Acquisition of American Sign Language. In D. Slobin (Ed.), *The cross-linguistic study of language acquisition: Volume 1. The Data* (pp. 881–938). Hillsdale, NJ: Erlbaum.

Ng, M., Niparko, J., & Nager, G. (1999). Inner ear pathology in severe to profound sensorineural hearing loss. In J. Niparko, K. I. Kirk, N. Mellon, A. M. Robbins, D. Tucci, & B. Wilson (Eds.), *Cochlear implants: Principles and practices* (pp. 57–92). Philadelphia: Lippincott Williams & Wilkins.

Nishimura, H., Hashikawa, K., Doi, K., Iwaki, T., Watanabe, Y., Kusuoka, H., Nishimura, T., & Kubo, T. (1999). Sign language heard in the auditory cortex. *Nature, 397*, 116.

Nover, S. (1995a). Full inclusion for deaf students: An ethnographic perspective. In B. Snider (Ed.), *Inclusion? Defining quality education for deaf and hard of hearing students* (pp. 33–50). Washington, DC: Gallaudet University, College of Continuing Education.

Nover, S. (1995b). Politics and language: American Sign Language and English in deaf education. In C. Lucas (Ed.), *Sociolinguistics in deaf communities* (pp. 109–163). Washington, DC: Gallaudet University Press.

Nover, S., & Andrews, J. (2000). *Critical pedagogy in deaf education: Teachers' reflections on creating a bilingual classroom for deaf learners.* Year 1, year 2, year 3 and year 4 reports. Star Schools Project. Santa Fe: New Mexico School for the Deaf. www.starschools.org/nmsd.

Nover, S., Christensen, K., & Cheng, L. (1998). Development of ASL and English competencies for learners who are deaf. In K. Butler & P. Prinz (Eds.), ASL proficiency and English language acquisition: New Perspectives. *Topics in Language Disorders, 18(4)*, 61–72.

Nover, S., & Moll, L. (1997). Cultural mediation of deaf cognition. In M. P. Moeller & B. Schick (Eds.), *Deafness and diversity: Sociolinguistic issues* (pp. 39–50). Omaha, NE: Boys Town Research Hospital.

Nover, S., & Ruiz, R. (1994). The politics of American Sign Language in deaf education. In B. Schick & M. Moeller (Eds.), *The use of sign language in instructional settings: Current concepts and controversies* (pp. 73–84). Omaha, NE: Boys Town National Research Hospital.

Nowak, C. B. (1998). Genetics and hearing loss: A review of Stickler Syndrome. *Journal of Communication Disorders, 31,* 437–454.

Oberkotter, M. (Ed.). (1990). *The possible dream.* Washington, DC: Alexander Graham Bell Association for the Deaf.

Ogden, P. (1996). *The silent garden: Raising your deaf child.* Washington, DC: Gallaudet University Press.

Olkin, R. (1999). *What psychotherapists should know about disability.* New York: Guilford Press.

Ouellette, S. (1988). The use of projective drawing techniques in the personality assessment of prelingually deafened young adults: A pilot study. *American Annals of the Deaf, 133,* 212–218.

Padden, C. (1980). The deaf community and the culture of deaf people. In C. Baker & R. Battison (Eds.), *Sign language and the deaf community* (pp. 89–102). Silver Spring, MD: National Association of the Deaf.

Padden, C. (1998). From the cultural to the bicultural: The modern deaf community. In I. Parasnis (Ed.), *Cultural and language diversity and the deaf experience* (pp. 79–98). New York: Cambridge University Press.

Padden, C., & Humphries, T. (1988). *Deaf in America: Voices from a culture.* Cambridge, MA: Harvard University Press.

Padden, C., & Ramsey, C. (2000). American Sign Language and reading ability in deaf children. In C. Chamberlain, J. Morford, & R. Mayberry (Eds.), *Language acquisition by eye* (pp. 165–189). Mahwah, NJ: Erlbaum.

Padden, C., & Rayman, J. (2002). The future of American Sign Language. In D. Armstrong, M. Karchmer, & J. Van Cleve (Eds.), *The study of signed languages: Essays in honor of William Stokoe* (pp. 247–261). Washington, DC: Gallaudet University Press.

Pal Kapur, Y. (1996). Epidemiology of childhood hearing loss. In S. Gerber (Ed.), *The handbook of pediatric audiology* (pp. 3–14). Washington, DC: Gallaudet University Press.

Pappas, D., & Pappas, D. (1999). Medications and characteristics of drugs causing ototoxicity. *The Volta Review, 99,* 195–203.

Paradise, J. L. (1999). Universal newborn hearing screening: Should we leap before we look? *Pediatrics, 103(3),* 670–672.

Parasnis, I. (1996). On interpreting the deaf experience within the context of cultural and language diversity. In I. Parasnis (Ed.), *Cultural and language diversity and the deaf experience* (pp. 3–19). New York: Cambridge University Press.

Parasnis, I., Samar, V., Bettger, J., & Sathe, K. (1996). Does deafness lead to enhancement of visual spatial cognition in children? Negative evidence from deaf nonsigners. *Journal of Deaf Studies and Deaf Education, 1(2),* 145–152.

Parents and Families of Natural Communication, Inc. (1998). *We can hear and speak.* Washington, DC: Alexander Graham Bell Association of the Deaf.

Payne, J. A., & Quigley, S. (1987). Hearing-impaired children's comprehension of verb particle combinations. *Volta Review, 89,* 133–143.

Pennsylvania Association for Retarded Children (PARC) v. Pennsylvania, 334 F. Supp. 1257 (E.D. Pa. 1971) modified, 33 F. Supp. 279 (E.D. Pa. 1972).

Peters, C. (2000). *Deaf American literature: From carnival to cannon.* Washington, DC: Gallaudet University Press.

Peterson, C., & Siegel, M. (1995). Deafness, conversation and theory of mind. *Journal of Child Psychology and Psychiatry and Allied Disciplines, 36(3),* 459–474.

Peterson, C., & Siegel, M. (1998). Changing focus on the representational mind: Deaf, autistic, and normal children's concepts of false photos. *Journal of Developmental Psychology, 16(3),* 301–320.

Petitto, L. (2000). The acquisition of natural signed languages: Lessons in the nature of human language and its biological foundations. In C. Chamberlain, J. Morford, & R. Mayberry (Eds.), *Language acquisition by eye* (pp. 41–59). Mahwah, NJ: Erlbaum.

Petitto, L., & Holowka, S. (2002). Evaluating attributions of delay and confusion in young bilinguals: Special insights from infants acquiring a signed and a spoken language. *Sign Language Studies, 3(1),* 4–33.

Pettito, L., Zatorre, R., Gauna, K., Nikelski, E., Dostie, D., & Evans, A. (2000, December). Speech-like cerebral activity in profoundly deaf people processing signed languages: Implications for the neural basis of human language. *tPNAS, 97(25),* 13961–13966.

Piaget, J. (1929). *The child's conception of the world.* New York: Harcourt, Brace.

Pinker, S. (1994). *The language instinct: How the mind creates language.* New York: Harper.

Pipp-Siegel, S., Sedey, A., & Yoshinaga-Itano, C. (2002). Predictors of parental stress in mothers of young children with hearing loss. *Journal of Deaf Studies and Deaf Education*, 7, 1–17.

Poizner, H., Klima, E., & Bellugi, U. (1987). *What the hands reveal about the brain*. Cambridge, MA: MIT Press.

Pollard, E. (2002). The president's corner. *NADmag*, 1, p. 9.

Pollard, R. (1992–93). 100 years in psychology and deafness: A centennial retrospective. *Journal of the American Deafness and Rehabilitation Association*, 26, 32–46.

Pollard, R. (1994). Public mental health service and diagnostic trends regarding individuals who are deaf or hard of hearing. *Rehabilitation Psychology*, 39, 147–160.

Pollard, R. (1996). Professional psychology and deaf people: The emergence of a discipline. *American Psychologist*, 51, 389–396.

Pollard, R. (1998). Psychopathology. In M. Marschark & M. D. Clark (Eds.), *Psychological perspectives on deafness* (pp. 171–197). Mahwah, NJ: Erlbaum.

Powers, S., Gregory, S., & Thortehhoofd, E. (1998). *The educational achievements of deaf children: A literature review, research report 65*. London: Department of Education and Employment.

Preston, P. (1994). *Mother father deaf: Living between sound and silence*. Cambridge, MA: Harvard University Press.

Price, J. M. (1996). Friendships of maltreated children and adolescents: Contexts for expressing and modifying relationship history. In W. M. Bukowski, A. F. Newcomb, & W. W. Hartup (Eds.), *The company they keep: Friendship in childhood and adolescence* (pp. 262–285). New York: Cambridge University Press.

Psychological Corporation. (1997). *WAIS III – WMS III technical manual*. San Antonio, TX: The Psychological Corporation, Harcourt Brace & Co.

Quigley, S., & Kretchmer, R. (1982). *The education of deaf children: Issues, theory and practice*. Baltimore: University Park Press.

Quigley, S., Montanelli, D., & Wilbur, R. (1976). Some aspects of the verb system in the language of deaf students. *Journal of Speech and Hearing Research*, 19, 536–550.

Quigley, S., Power, D., & Steinkemp, M. (1977). The language structure of deaf children. *Volta Review*, 79, 73–84.

Raifman, L., & Vernon, M. (1996a). Important implications for psychologists of the Americans with Disabilities Act: Case in point, the patient who is deaf. *Professional Psychology: Research and Practice*, 27, 372–377.

Raifman, L., & Vernon, M. (1996b). New rights for deaf patients: New responsibilities for mental hospitals. *Psychiatric Quarterly*, 67, 209–219.

Rainbow Alliance of the Deaf. (2000, 9 November). *RAD: Fact sheet*. Retrieved September 27, 2001, from http://www.rad.org.

Rainer, J. D., & Altshuler, K. Z. (1966). *Comprehensive mental health services for the deaf*. New York: Columbia University Press.

Rainer, J. D., Altshuler, K. Z., Kallman, F. J., & Deming, W. E. (Eds.). (1963). *Family and mental health populations in a deaf population*. New York: New York State Psychiatric Institute.

Ralston, E., Zazove, P., & Gorenflo, D. (1995). Communicating with deaf patients. *Journal of the American Medical Association*, 274, 794.

Ramsey, C. L. (1997). *Deaf children in public schools: Placement, context and consequences*. Washington, DC: Gallaudet University Press.

Ramsey, C. L. (2001). Beneath the surface: Theoretical frameworks shed light on educational interpreting. *Odyssey*, 2(2), 19–24.

Ramsey, C. L., & Noriega, J. (2001). Ninos Milagrizados: Language attitudes, deaf education, and miracle cures in Mexico. *Sign Language Studies*, 1(3), 254–280.

Randall, K., McAnally, P., Rittenhouse, B., Russell, D., & Sorensen, G. (2000). High stakes testing: What is at stake? *American Annals of the Deaf*, 145(5), 390–393.

Registry of Interpreters for the Deaf, Inc. (2000). Code of Ethics of the Registry of Interpreters for the Deaf, Inc. *Educational interpreting: A collection of articles from views*. Silver Spring, MD: RID Publications.

Rehkemper, G. (1996). *Executive functioning and psychosocial adjustment in deaf subjects with nonhereditary and hereditary etiologies*. Unpublished doctoral dissertation, Gallaudet University, Washington, DC.

Reich, E. (1996a). *Treacher Collins syndrome: An overview*. Norwich, VT: Treacher Collins Foundation.

Reich, E. (1996b). *Frequency of Treacher Collins syndrome*. Retrieved October 13, 1999, from Treacher Collins Foundation Newsletter website: http://www.teachercollinsfnd.org/news 96/freqtcs.htm.

Reichman, A. (2000, November). What's happening with VR services to deaf and hard of hearing individuals? *The NAD Broadcaster*, p. 8.

Remvig, J. (1969). Deaf-mutism and psychiatry. *Acta Scandinavieu, Supplementum*, 210, Copenhagen, Munksgaard.

Remvig, J. (1972). Psychic deviations of the prelingual deaf. *Scandinavian Audiology*, 1, 35–42.

Reschly, D. J. (2000). Assessment and eligibility determination in Individuals with Disabilities Education Act of 1997. In C. F. Telzrow & M. Tankersley (Eds.), *IDEA admendments of 1997: Practice guidelines for school-based teams* (pp. 65–104). Bethesda, MD: National Association of School Psychologists.

Ridgeway, J. (1969). Dumb children. *New Republic*, pp. 19–22.

Rittenhouse, R., Johnson, C., Overton, B., Freeman, S., & Jaussi, K. (1991). The black and deaf movements in America since 1960: Parallelism and an agenda for the future. *American Annals of the Deaf, 136,* 392–400.

Robbins, A. (1994). Guidelines for developing oral communication skills in children with cochlear implants. *The Volta Review, 96(5),* 75–82.

Robbins, A. (1998). Two paths of auditory development for children with cochlear implants. *Loud and Clear: A Cochlear Implant Rehabilitation Newsletter, 1(1),* 1–4.

Robinson, L. (1978). *Sound minds in a soundless world.* Washington, DC: U.S. Department of Health, Education and Welfare.

Rodriguez, Y. (2001). *Toddlerese: Conversations between hearing parents and their deaf toddlers in Puerto Rico.* Unpublished doctoral dissertation. Lamar University, Beaumont, TX.

Rogers, C. (1951). *Client-centered therapy.* Boston: Houghton Mifflin.

Romig, L. (1985). *The cognitive processing and cuing systems used by young hearing impaired children when spelling.* Unpublished doctoral dissertation, University of Missouri, Columbia.

Rosen, S., & Virnig, S. (1997). *A synopsis of the Bill of Rights for deaf and hard of hearing children.* Retrieved February 8, 2002, from the National Association of the Deaf website: http://www.nad.org.

Roy, C. (Ed.). (2000). *Innovative practices for teaching sign language interpreters.* Washington, DC: Gallaudet University Press.

Rutherford, S. (1989). Funny in deaf—Not in hearing. In S. Wilcox (Ed.), *American Deaf culture: An anthology.* Burtonsville, MD: Linstok Press.

Samar, V. J. (1999, Winter). Identifying learning disabilities in the deaf population: The leap from Gibraltar. *NTID Research Bulletin, 4(1),* 1–5.

Samar, V. J., Parasnis, I., & Berent, G. P. (1998). Learning disabilities, attention deficit disorders and deafness. In M. Marschark & M. D. Clark (Eds.), *Psychological perspectives on deafness: Volume 2* (pp. 199–242). Mahwah, NJ: Erlbaum.

Sandoval, J., Frisby, C., Geisinger, K., Scheuneman, J., & Grenier, J. (Eds.). (1998). *Test interpretation and diversity.* Washington, DC: American Psychological Association.

Schein, J. (1981). *A rose for tomorrow: Biography of Frederick C. Schreiber.* Silver Spring, MD: National Association of the Deaf.

Schein, J. (1986). Some demographics aspects of religion and deafness. In J. Schein & L. Waldman (Eds.), *The deaf Jew in the modern world* (pp. 76–87). New York: Ktav Publishing House.

Schein, J. (1989). *At home among strangers.* Washington, DC: Gallaudet University Press.

Schein, J. (1996). The demography of deafness. In P. C. Higgins & J. E. Nash (Eds), *Understanding deafness socially: Continuities in research and theory* (2nd ed., pp. 21–43). Springfield, IL: Charles C. Thomas.

Schein, J., & Delk, M. (1974). *The deaf population of the United States.* Silver Spring, MD: National Association of the Deaf.

Schick, B. (2001). Interpreting for children: How it is different. *Odyssey, 2(2),* 8–11.

Schildroth, A. (1994, July). Congenital cytomegalovirus and deafness. *American Journal of Audiology,* pp. 27–38.

Schleper, D. (1997). *Reading to deaf children: Learning from deaf adults.* Washington, DC: Gallaudet University Press.

Schlesinger, H. S. (1985). Deafness, mental health, and language. In F. Powell, T. Finitzo-Hieber, S. Friel-Patti, & D. Henderson (Eds.), *Education of the hearing impaired child* (pp. 103–116). San Diego, CA: College-Hill Press.

Schlesinger, H. S. (2000). A developmental model applied to problems of deafness. *Journal of Deaf Studies and Deaf Education, 5(4),* 349–361.

Schlesinger, H. S., & Meadow, K. P. (1972). Development of maturity in deaf children. *Exceptional Children, 38,* 461–467.

Schmidt, T., & Stipe, M. (1991, March/April). A clouded map for itinerant teachers: More questions than answers. In *A folio of mainstream articles from Perspectives in Education and Deafness.* Washington, DC: Pre-college Programs of Gallaudet University.

Schonbeck, J. (2000). The unit in Westborough. *Hearing Health, 39,* 41–42.

Schott, L. A. (2002, January). Sexual abuse at deaf schools in America. *The FAED Eagle* (pp. 5–6). Gastonia, NC: The FAED Eagle Newsletter.

Schrader, S. (1995). *Silent alarm: On the edge with a deaf EMT.* Washington, DC: Gallaudet University Press.

Schreiber, F. (1981). Priority needs of deaf people. In J. D. Schein (Ed.), *A rose for tomorrow* (pp. 74–77).

Silver Spring, MD: National Association of the Deaf.

Schroedel, J., & Geyer, P. (2000). Long-term career attainments of deaf and hard of hearing college graduates: Results from a 15–year follow-up survey. *American Annals of the Deaf, 145,* 303–314.

Schuchman, J. (1988). *Hollywood speaks: Deafness and the film entertainment history.* Urbana: University of Illinois Press.

Schwartz, N. S., Mebane, D. L., & Malony, H. N. (1990). Effects of alternate modes of administration on Rorschach performance of deaf adults. *Journal of Personality Assessment, 54,* 671–683.

Schwartz, S. (1996). *Choices in deafness: A parents' guide to communication options.* Bethesda, MD: Woodbine House.

Seeman, J. (1989). Toward a model of positive health. *American Psychologist, 44,* 1099–1109.

Self Help for Hard of Hearing People. (2001, August). *About SHHH.* Retrieved September 27, 2001, from www.shhh.org.

Seligman, M., & Csikszentmihalyi, M. (2000). Positive psychology: An introduction. *American Psychologist, 55,* 5–14.

Shapiro, J. (1993). *No pity: People with disabilities forging a new civil rights movement.* New York: Times Books.

Sheldon, K., & King, L. (2001). Why positive psychology is necessary. *American Psychologist, 56,* 216–217.

Sheridan, M. (2001). *Inner lives of deaf children: Interviews and analysis.* Washington, DC: Gallaudet University Press.

Sheridan, S. M., Cowan, R. J., & Eagle, J. W. (2000). Partnering with parents in educational programming for students with special needs. In C. F. Telzrow & M. Tankersley (Eds.), *IDEA amendments of 1997: Practice guidelines for school-based teams.* Bethesda, MD: National Association of School Psychologists.

Shore, K. (1994). *The parents' public school handbook: How to make the most of your child's education, from kindergarten through middle school.* New York: Fireside.

Siedlecki, T. (1999). Intelligent use of the Rorschach Inkblot Technique with deaf persons. *Journal of the American Deafness and Rehabilitation Association, 33,* 31–46.

Siegel, L. (2000). The educational and communication needs of deaf and hard of hearing children: A statement of principle regarding fundamental systemic educational changes. *National Deaf Education Project.* Greenbrae, CA: National Deaf Education Project.

SignFont Handbook. (1989). Bellevue, WA: Edmark Corp.

Silverman, F., & Moulton, R. (2002). *The impact of a unique cooperative American university USAID funded speech-language pathologist, audiologist, and deaf educator B.S. degree program in the Gaza Strip.* Lewiston, NY: Edwin Mellen Press.

Singleton, J., Supalla, S., Litchfield, S., & Schley, S. (1998). From sign to word: Considering modality constraints in ASL/English bilingual education. In K. Butler & P. Prinz (Eds.), *ASL proficiency and English literacy acquisition: New perspectives. Topics in Language Disorders, 18(4),* 16–29.

Singleton, J., & Tittle, M. (2000). Deaf parents and their hearing children. *Journal of Deaf Studies and Deaf Education, 5(3),* 221–236.

Smith, M. D. (1997). *The art of itinerant teaching for teachers of the deaf and hard of hearing.* Hillsboro, OR: Butte Publication.

Smith, R., & Schwartz, C. (1998). Branchio-oto-renal syndrome. *Journal of Communication Disorders, 31,* 411–421.

Smith, R., Green, G., & Van Camp, G. (1999, February). *Hereditary hearing loss and deafness overview.* Retrieved March 13, 1999, from GeneClinics: Clinical Genetic Information Resource University of Washington, Seattle website: http://www.geneclinics.org.

Smith, S., & Harker, L. (1998). Single gene influences on radiologically-detectable malformations of the inner ear. *Journal of Communication Disorders, 31,* 391–410.

Smith, S., Kolodziej, P., & Olney, A. H. (n.d.). Waardenburg Syndrome. *ENT Syndrome Clinic.* University of Nebraska Medical Center, Omaha: Munroe-Meyer Institute for Genetics and Rehabilitation.

Smith, S., Schafer, G., Horton, M., & Tinley, S. (1998). Medical genetic evaluation for the etiology of hearing loss in children. *Journal of Communication Disorders, 31,* 371–389.

Smith, Z. (1999). *A study of four African American families reading to the young deaf children.* Unpublished doctoral dissertation, Lamar University, Beaumont, TX.

Sonnenstrahl, D. (2002). *Deaf artists in America: Colonial to contemporary.* San Diego: DawnSign Press.

Spencer, P. (2002). Language development of children with cochlear implants. In J. B. Christiansen & I. W. Leigh, *Cochlear implants in children: Ethics and choices* (pp. 222–249). Washington, DC: Gallaudet University Press.

Spencer, P. E., & Deyo, D. A. (1993). Cognitive and social aspects of deaf children's play. In M. Marschark & M. D. Clark (Eds.), *Psychological perspectives on deafness* (pp. 65–91). Hillsdale, NJ: Erlbaum.

Sroufe, L. A. (1983). Infant-caregiver attachment and patterns of adaptations in preschool: The roots of maladaptation and competence. In M. Perlmutter (Ed.), Development and policy concerning children with special needs. *Minnesota Symposium on Child Psychology, 16*, 41–83. Hillsdale, NJ: Erlbaum.

Sroufe, L. A. (1995, September). Quoted in Beth Azar, The bond between mother and child. *APA Monitor, 26(9)*, 28.

Stansfield, M., & Veltri, D. (1987). Assessment from the perspective of the sign language interpreter. In H. Elliott, L. Glass, & J. Evans (Eds.), *Mental health assessment of deaf clients* (pp. 153–163). Boston: Little, Brown.

Stedt, J., & Moores, D. (1990). Manual Codes on English and American Sign Language. In H. Bornstein (Ed.), *Manual communication: Implications for education* (pp. 1–20). Washington, DC: Gallaudet University Press.

Stein, L., & Boyer, K. (1994). Progress in the prevention of hearing loss in infants. *Ear & Hearing, 15*, 116–125.

Steinberg, A. G., Davila, R., Collazo, J., Loew, R., & Fischgrund, J. (1997). "A little sign and a lot of love . . . ": Attitudes, perceptions, and beliefs of Hispanic families with deaf children. *Qualitative Health Research, 7*, 202–222.

Steinberg, A. G., Loew, R., & Sullivan, V. J. (1999). The diversity of consumer knowledge, attitudes, beliefs, and experiences: Recent findings. In I. W. Leigh (Ed.), *Psychotherapy with deaf clients from diverse groups* (pp. 23–43). Washington, DC: Gallaudet University Press.

Stewart, D. (1991). *Deaf sport: The impact of sports within the deaf community*. Washington, DC: Gallaudet University Press.

Stewart, D., & Kluwin, T. (2001). *Teaching deaf and hard of hearing students: Content, strategies, and curriculum*. Boston: Allyn and Bacon.

Stewart, L. (1972). A truly silent minority. *Deafness Annual, V. II*. Silver Spring, MD: Professional Rehabilitation Workers with the Adult Deaf.

Stewart, L. (1992). Debunking the bilingual/bicultural snow job in the American deaf community. In M. Garretson (Ed.), *Viewpoints on deafness: A deaf American monograph* (pp. 129–142). Silver Spring, MD: National Association of the Deaf.

Stinson, M., & Antia, S. D. (1999). Considerations in educating deaf and hard-of-hearing students in inclusive settings. *Journal of Deaf Studies and Deaf Education, 4(3)*, 163–175.

Stinson, M., Chase, K., & Kluwin, T. (1990, April). *Self-perceptions of social relationships in hearing impaired adolescents*. Paper presented at the American Educational Research Association Convention, Boston.

Stinson, M., & Foster, S. (2000). Socialization of deaf children and youths in schools. In P. E. Spencer, C. J. Erting, & M. Marschark (Eds.), *The deaf child in the family and at school* (pp. 191–210). Mahwah, NJ: Erlbaum.

Stinson, M., & Kluwin, T. (1996). Social orientations toward deaf and hearing peers among deaf adolescents in local public high schools. In P. C. Higgins & J. E. Nash (Eds.), *Understanding deafness socially: Continuities in research and theory* (2nd ed., pp. 113–134). Springfield, IL: Charles C. Thomas.

Stinson, M., & Leigh, I. W. (1995). Inclusion and the psychosocial development of deaf children and youths. In B. D. Snider (Ed.), *Inclusion? Defining quality education for deaf and hard of hearing students* (pp. 153–161). Washington, DC: Gallaudet University.

Stinson, M., & Whitmire, K. (1992). Students' views of their social relationships. In T. Kluwin, D. Moores, & M. Gonter Gaustad (Eds.), *Toward effective public school programs for deaf students: Context, process, and outcomes* (pp. 149–174). New York: Teachers College Press.

Stokoe, W. (1960). *Sign language structure: A outline of visual communication systems of the American deaf*. Studies in Linguistics, Occasional Paper, Buffalo, NY.

Stokoe, W. (1975). The use of sign language in teaching English. *American Annals of the Deaf, 120(4)*, 417–421.

Stokoe, W. (Ed.). (1980). *Sign and culture: A reader for students of American Sign Language*. Silver Spring, MD: Linstok Press.

Stokoe, W. (1989). Dimensions of difference: ASL and English based cultures. In S. Wilcox (Ed.), *American deaf culture: An anthology* (pp. 49–59). Burtonsville, MD: Linstok Press.

Stokoe, W. (1990). An historical perspective on sign language research: A personal view. In C. Lucas (Ed.), *Sign language research: Theoretical issues*. Washington, DC: Gallaudet University Press.

Stokoe, W. (2001a). Deafness, cognition, and language. In M. Clark, M. Marschark, & M. Karchmer (Eds.), *Context, cognition, and deafness* (pp. 6–13). Washington, DC: Gallaudet University Press.

Stokoe, W. (2001b). *Language in hand: Why sign came before speech*. Washington, DC: Gallaudet University Press.

Stokoe, W., Casterline, D. C., & Croneberg, C. G. (1965). *A dictionary of American Sign Language on linguistic principles*. Washington, DC: Gallaudet University Press.

Strand, V. C. (1991). Victim of sexual abuse: Case of Rosa, age 6. In N. B. Webb (Ed.), *Play therapy with children in crisis: A casebook for practitioners* (pp. 69–91). New York: Guildford Press.

Strauss, M. (1999). Hearing loss and cytomegalovirus. *The Volta Review, 99*, 71–74.

Strong, M., & Prinz, P. (2000). Is American Sign Language skill related to English literacy? In C. Chamberlain, J. Morford, & R. Mayberry (Eds.), *Language acquisition by eye* (pp. 131–141). Mahwah, NJ: Erlbaum.

Stuckless, E. R., & Birch, J. W. (1966). The influence of early manual communication on linguistic development in deaf children. *American Annals of the Deaf, 111*, 452–460.

Sue, D. W., & Sue, D. (1999). *Counseling the culturally different: Theory and practice* (3rd ed.). New York: John Wiley & Sons.

Suggs, T. (2001a, July). NFSD celebrates 100 years of fraternalism. *Silent News, 33*, p. 1.

Suggs, T. (2001b, December). Threat of anthrax real for these postal workers. *Silent News, 33(12)*, 1, 18.

Sullivan, P., Brookhouser, P., & Scanlan, J. (2000). Maltreatment of deaf and hard of hearing children. In P. Hindley & N. Kitson (Eds.), *Mental health and deafness* (pp. 149–184). London: Whurr Publishers.

Sullivan, P., & Knutson, J. (1998). Maltreatment and behavioral characteristics of youth who are deaf and hard of hearing. *Sexuality and Disability, 16*, 295–319.

Sullivan, P. M., & Vernon, M. (1979). Psychological assessment of hearing-impaired children. *School Psychology Digest, 8*, 271–290.

Supalla, S. (1991). Manually-coded English: The modality question in signed language language development. In P. Siple & S. Fischer (Eds.), *Theoretical issues in sign language research, Vol. 2: Acquisition* (pp. 85–109). Chicago: University of Chicago Press.

Supalla, S. (1992). *The book of name signs: Naming in American Sign Language*. San Diego, CA: Dawn Sign Press.

Supalla, S., Wix, T., & McKee, C. (2001). Print as a primary source of English for deaf learners. In J. Nicol & T. Langendoen (Eds.), *One mind, two languages: Studies in bilingual language processing* (pp. 177–190). Oxford: Blackwell.

Sussman, A. (1974). An investigation into the relationship between self concepts of deaf adults and their perceived attitudes toward deafness (Doctoral dissertation, New York University, 1973). *Dissertation Abstracts International, 34*, 2914B.

Sussman, A., & Brauer, B. (1999). On being a psychotherapist with deaf clients. In I. W. Leigh (Ed.), *Psychotherapy with deaf clients from diverse groups* (pp. 3–22). Washington, DC: Gallaudet University Press.

Sussman, K., & Lopez-Holzman, G. (2001). Bilingualism: Addressing cultural needs in the classroom. *Volta Voices, 8(4)*, 11, 13–16.

Swisher, V. (2000). Learning to converse: How deaf mothers support the development of attention and conversation skills in their young deaf children. In P. Spencer, C. Erting, & M. Marschark (Eds.), *The deaf child in the family and at school* (pp. 21–39). Mahwah, NJ: Erlbaum.

Tajfel, H. (1981). *Human groups and social categories*. Cambridge: Cambridge University Press.

Terwilliger, L., Kamman, T., & Koester, L. S. (1997, April). *Self-regulation by deaf and hearing infants at 9 months*. Poster session presented at the annual meeting of the Rocky Mountain Psychological Association, Reno, NV.

Thompson, D., McPhilips, H., Davis, R., Lieu, T., Homer, C., & Helfand, M. (2001). Universal newborn hearing screening: Summary of the evidence. *Journal of the American Medical Association, 286*, 2000–2010.

Traxler, C. (2000). The Stanford Achievement Test, 9th Edition: National norming and performance standards for deaf and hard of hearing students. *Journal of Deaf Studies and Deaf Education, 5(4)*, 337–348.

Trumbetta, S., Bonvillian, J., Siedlecki, T., & Haskins, B. (2001). Language-related symptoms in persons with schizophrenia and how deaf persons may manifest these symptoms. *Sign Language Studies, 1*, 228–253.

Trybus, R. (1983). Hearing-impaired patients in public psychiatric hospitals throughout the United States. In D. Watson & B. Heller (Eds.), *Mental health and deafness: Strategic perspectives* (pp. 1–19). Silver Spring, MD: American Deafness and Rehabilitation Association.

Trybus, R., Karchmer, M., & Kerstetter, P. (1980). The demographics of deafness resulting from maternal rubella. *American Annals of the Deaf, 125*, 977–984.

Trzepacz, P., & Baker, R. (1993). *The psychiatric mental status examination*. New York: Oxford University Press.

Tucker, B. (1998a). *Cochlear implants: A handbook*. Jefferson, NC: McFarland & Company.

Tucker, B. (1998b). Deaf culture, cochlear implants, and elective disability. *Hastings Center Report, 28*, 6–14.

Tucker, J. (2000, Spring/Summer). The home plate. *MDAD News, 40 (No. 2/3)*, 26–27.

Tucker, S., & Bhattacharya, J. (1992). Screening of hearing impairment in the newborn using the auditory response cradle. *Archives of Disease in Childhood, 67*, 911–919.

Turner, E. (2001). Roles in educational interpreting. *Odyssey, 2(2)*, 40–41.

Turner, J., Klein, H., & Kitson, N. (2000). Interpreters in mental health settings. In P. Hindley & N. Kitson (Eds.), *Mental health and deafness* (pp. 297–310). London: Whurr.

U.S. Department of Health and Human Services (USDHHS). (1999). *Blending perspectives and building common ground: A report to Congress on substance abuse and child protection*. Washington, DC: U.S. Government Printing Office.

USA Deaf Sports Federation. (2001). *What is USADSF?* Retrieved September 27, 2001, from http://www.usadsf.org/About_Us/What_is_USADSF/what_is_usadsf.html.

Usami, S., Abe, S., & Shinkawa, H. (1998). Sensorineural hearing loss caused by mitochondrial DNA mutations: Special reference to the A1555G mutation. *Journal of Communication Disorders, 31*, 423–435.

Valli, C., & Lucas, C. (2000). *Linguistics of American Sign Language: An introduction* (3rd ed.). Washington, DC: Gallaudet University Press.

Van Camp, G., & Smith, R. (2001). *Hereditary hearing loss homepage*. Retrieved October 14, 2001, from http://dnalab-www.uia.ac.be/dnalab/hhh/.

Van Cleve, J. (Ed.). (1993). *Deaf history unveiled: Interpretations from the new scholarship*. Washington, DC: Gallaudet University Press.

Van Cleve, J., & Crouch, B. (1989). *A place of their own: Creating the deaf community in America*. Washington, DC: Gallaudet University Press.

Vandell, D. L., & George, L. B. (1981). Social interaction in hearing and deaf preschoolers: Successes and failures in initiations. *Child Development, 53*, 1354–1363.

Van Gurp, S. (2001). Self-concept of deaf secondary school students in different educational settings. *Journal of Deaf Studies and Deaf Education, 6(1)*, 54–69.

Van Naarden, K., Decoufle, P., & Caldwell, K. (1999). Prevalence and characteristics of children with serious hearing impairment in metropolitan Atlanta, 1991–1993. *Pediatrics, 103*, 570–575.

Vernon, M. (1967). Meningitis and deafness: The problem, its physical, audiological, psychological, and educational manifestations in deaf children. *The Laryngoscope, 10*, 1856–1974.

Vernon, M. (1968). Fifty years of research on the intelligence of deaf and hard of hearing children: A review of literature and discussion of implications. *Journal of Rehabilitation of the Deaf, 1*, 1–12.

Vernon, M. (1969a). *Multiply handicapped deaf children: Medical, educational, and psychological considerations*. Reston, VA: Council of Exceptional Children.

Vernon, M. (1969b). Sociological and psychological factors associated with profound hearing loss. *Speech and Hearing Research, 12*, 541–563.

Vernon, M. (1970). The role of deaf teachers in the education of deaf children. *Deaf American, 23*, 17–20.

Vernon, M. (1983). Deafness and mental health: Emerging responses. In E. Petersen (Ed.), *Mental health and deafness: Emerging responses* (pp. 1–15). Silver Spring, MD: American Deafness and Rehabilitation Association.

Vernon, M. (1991). At the crossroads: The future workplace and implications for rehabilitation. In D. Watson & M. Taff-Watson (Eds.), *At the crossroads: A celebration of diversity, Monograph No. 15* (pp. 3–10). Little Rock, AR: American Deafness and Rehabilitation Association.

Vernon, M. (2001). Assessment of individuals who are deaf or hard of hearing. In B. Bolton (Ed.), *Handbook of measurement and evaluation in rehabilitation* (pp. 385–395). Gaithersburg, MD: Aspen Publishers.

Vernon, M., & Andrews, J. (1990). *The psychology of deafness: Understanding deaf and hard-of-hearing people*. New York: Longman.

Vernon, M., & Daigle-King, B. (1999). Historical overview of inpatient care of mental patients who are deaf. *American Annals of the Deaf, 144*, 51–61.

Vernon, M., & Koh, S. D. (1971). Effects of oral preschool compared to early manual communication in deaf children. *American Annals of the Deaf, 116*, 569–574.

Vernon, M., & Makowsky, B. (1969). Deafness and minority group dynamics. *Deaf American, 21(11)*, 3–6.

Vernon, M., Raifman, L., & Greenberg, S. (1996). The Miranda warnings and the deaf suspect. *Behavioral Sciences and the Law, 14*, 121–135.

Vernon, M., Raifman, L., Greenberg, S., & Monteiro,

B. (2001). Forensic pre-trial police interviews of deaf suspects: Avoiding legal pitfalls. *International Journal of Law and Psychiatry, 24,* 43–59.

Vernon, M., & Rich, S. (1997). Pedophilia and deafness. *American Annals of the Deaf, 142,* 300–311.

Volterra, V., & Erting, C. (1994). *From gesture to language in hearing and deaf children.* Washington, DC: Gallaudet University Press.

Vygotsky, L. S. (1978). *Mind in society: The development of higher psychological processes.* Cambridge, MA: Harvard University Press.

Walker, L. A. (1986). *A loss for words: The story of deafness in a family.* New York: Harper & Row.

Waltzman, S., & Cohen, N. (Eds). (2000). *Cochlear implants.* New York: Thieme.

Wampler, D. (1971). *Linguistics of visible English.* Santa Rosa, CA: Early Childhood Education Department, Aurally Handicapped Program, Santa Rosa City Schools.

Waterman, A. S. (1992). Identity as an aspect of optimal psychological functioning. In G. R. Adams, T. P. Gullotta, & R. Montemayor (Eds.), *Adolescent identity formation* (pp. 50–72). Newbury Park, CA: Sage Publications.

Watkin, P., Beckman, A., & Baldwin, M. (1995). The views of parents of hearing impaired children on the need for neonatal hearing screening. *British Journal of Audiology, 29,* 259–262.

Watt, J. D., & Davis, F. E. (1991). The prevalence of boredom proneness and depression among profoundly deaf residential school adolescents. *American Annals of the Deaf, 136,* 409–413.

Wax, T. (1999). The evolution of psychotherapy for deaf women. In I. W. Leigh (Ed.), *Psychotherapy with deaf clients from diverse groups* (pp. 69–95). Washington, DC: Gallaudet University Press.

Wax, T., Haskins, B., Mason, T., Ramirez, W., & Savoy-McAdory, M. (2001). Inpatient psychiatric services for deaf and hard-of-hearing people: Where are we now? *JADARA, 35,* 8–14.

Weinberg, N., & Sterritt, M. (1986). Disability and identity: A study of identity patterns in adolescents with hearing impairments. *Rehabilitation Psychology, 31,* 95–102.

Welch, O. M. (2000). Building a multicultural curriculum: Issues and dilemmas. In K. Christensen (Ed.), *Deaf plus: A multicultural perspective* (pp. 1–28). San Diego, CA: DawnSign Press.

White, B. (1999). *The effect of perceptions of social support and perceptions of entitlement on family functioning in deaf-parented adoptive families.* Unpublished doctoral dissertation, Washington, DC: Catholic University of America.

Wilbur, R. (2000). The use of ASL to support the development of English and literacy. *Journal of Deaf Studies and Deaf Education, 5(1),* 81–104.

Willems, P. (2000). Genetic causes of hearing loss. *The New England Journal of Medicine, 342(15),* 1101–1109.

Willis, R. (1999). *Diagnosis and treatment characteristics of deaf children and adolescents in psychiatric residential treatment.* A paper given at the World Congress on Mental Health and Deafness, Gallaudet University, Washington, DC.

Willis, R., & Vernon, M. (2002). Residential psychiatric treatment of emotional disturbed deaf youth. *American Annals of the Deaf, 147(1),* 31–37.

Wilson, T., & Hyde, M. (1997). The use of signed English pictures to facilitate reading comprehension by deaf students. *American Annals of the Deaf, 142,* 333–341.

Winefield, R. (1987). *Never the twain shall meet: Bell, Gallaudet, and the communications debate.* Washington, DC: Gallaudet University Press.

Winston, E. A. (2001). Visual inaccessibility: The elephant (blocking the view) in interpreted education. *Odyssey, 2(2),* 5–7.

Witte, T., & Kuzel, A. (2000). Elderly deaf patients' health care experiences. *Journal of the American Board of Family Practice, 13,* 17–22.

Wolff, A., & Thatcher, R. (1990). Cortical reorganization in deaf children. *Journal of Clinical and Experimental Neuropsychology, 12,* 209–211.

Woodroffe, T., Gorenflo, D., Meador, H., & Zazove, P. (1998). Knowledge and attitudes about AIDS among deaf and hard of hearing persons. *AIDS Care, 103,* 377–386.

Woodward, J. (1989). How you gonna get to heaven if you can't talk with Jesus? The educational establishment vs. the deaf community. In S. Wilcox (Ed.), *American Deaf culture: An anthology* (pp. 163–172). Burtonsville, MD: Linstok Press.

Wright, M. H. (1999). *Sounds like home: Growing up black and deaf in the South.* Washington, DC: Gallaudet University Press.

Wu, C., & Grant, N. (1999). Asian American and Deaf. In I. W. Leigh (Ed.), *Psychotherapy with deaf clients from diverse groups* (pp. 203–226). Washington, DC: Gallaudet University Press.

www.urmc.rochester.edu/strongconnections/. StrongConnections: *Telehealth sign language solutions.* Retrieved 20 November.

www.whitehouse.gov. *Fact sheet: No Child Left Behind Act.* http://www.whitehouse.gov/news/releases/2002/01/20020108.html

Wynne, M., Diefendorf, A., & Fritsch, M. (2001, December 26). Sudden hearing loss. *The ASHA Leader, 6(23),* 6–8.

Yarger, C. C., & Luckner, J. L. (1999). Itinerant teaching: The inside story. *American Annuals, 144(4)*, 309–314.

Yoshinaga-Itano, C. (2000). Development of audition and speech: Implications for early intervention with infants who are deaf and hard of hearing. *Volta Review, 100*, 213–234.

Yoshinaga-Itano, C., Sedley, A., Coulter, D. K., & Mehl, A. L. (1998). Language of early and late identified children with hearing loss. *Pediatrics, 102(5)*, 1161–1171.

Yoshinaga-Itano, C., & Snyder, L. (1985). Form and meaning in the written language of hearing impaired children. *Volta Review, 87*, 75–90.

Zwiebel, A. (1994). Judaism and deafness: A humanistic heritage. In C. J. Erting, R.C. Johnson, D. L. Smith, & B. D. Snider (Eds.), *The Deaf way* (pp. 231–238). Washington, DC: Gallaudet University Press.

Abbe, S., 44
Achtzehn, J., 176
Acredolo, L., 68, 69
Afrin, J., 243
Ainsworth, M. D. S., 159
Akamatsu, T., 99, 127, 150
Al Muhaimeed, H., 41
Allen, T., 174, 186
Altshuler, K. Z., 8, 9, 197
Anderson, G., 210
Anderson, J., 174
Andersson, Y., 24
Andrews, J., 2, 6, 10, 28, 29, 40, 41,
    42, 43, 45, 46, 47, 51, 53, 55, 68,
    72, 79, 80, 91, 92, 93, 94, 97, 98,
    101, 103, 106, 107, 129, 131,
    132, 141, 142, 145, 146, 148,
    149, 150, 153, 160, 183, 187,
    190, 192, 195, 196, 213, 215,
    229, 232, 233
Anthony, D., 146,147
Anthony, S., 193
Anthony-Tolbert, S., 193
Antia, S. D., 117, 118, 120, 169, 170
Aramburo, A., 210, 237
Arnos, K., 44, 45, 46, 47, 49, 50, 51,
    52, 249, 250

Bahan, B., 11, 19, 52, 56, 111, 113,
    115, 116, 130, 172, 177, 192,
    211, 215, 232, 237, 245
Bailes, C., 99, 100, 245
Baker, C., 70, 81, 82, 83, 138, 152,
    153
Baker, R., 195
Baker-Shenk, C., 6
Baldwin, D., 26
Baldwin, M., 53
Baldwin, R., 194
Baldwin, S., 31
Bangs, D., 32
Barnartt, S., 12, 27, 184, 202, 204,
    214, 223, 225, 238
Barry, D., 216
Bartini, M., 87
Basilier, T., 8

Bat-Chava, Y., 58, 169, 171, 172,
    185, 187, 188
Bateman, G., 204, 205, 206
Battison, R., 6
Bavelier, D., 194
Bawle, E. V., 43
Baynton, D., 31, 224, 229
Bebko, J., 82
Beckman, A., 53
Beeghly, M., 176
Bell, A. G., 12
Bellugi, U., 6, 69, 70, 72, 76, 79, 81,
    82, 194, 244
Berent, G. P., 175
Bernstein, M., 163, 164
Bettger, J., 82
Bhattacharya, J., 53
Bialystok, E., 152, 155
Biesold, H., 52, 249
Bihrle, A., 81
Blakley, B. W., 43
Blanchfield, B., 17, 21, 215
Blehar, M. C., 159
Blennerhassett, L., 177, 178
Bloch, N., 207
Blotzer, M., 226
Bodner-Johnson, B., 115
Bonvillian, J., 9, 196
Boone, K., 190
Boppana, S., 41
Bornstein, H., 146, 147
Bortoli, A., 166, 167
Bowe, F., 109
Bowlby, J., 159
Boyer, K., 41, 42
Brackett, D., 57, 162, 166
Braden, J., 5, 82, 178, 183, 184, 188,
    190, 191, 192, 193
Bradley-Johnson, S., 146, 191
Branson, J., 225
Brauer, B., 7, 181, 183, 184, 191, 192,
    193, 198, 226
Brelje, H. W., 131, 132
Brookhouser, P., 176
Brown, P. M., 166, 167
Brueggemann, B., 38, 222

Buchanan, R., 213, 214, 215
Buck, D., 24, 216
Burch, R., 92
Burke, F., 175, 176, 196, 197
Busby, H., 18
Butler, K., 79, 98, 153, 155, 245

Calderon, R., 113, 114, 163, 165,
    167, 169
Caldwell, K., 17, 53
Callaway, A.,127, 150
Camilleri, C., 184
Cantor, D. W., 5
Capirci, O., 69
Carroll, C., 30
Case, L., 187
Cass, S., 39
Casterline, D. C., 6, 95
Cattani, A., 69
Chamberlain, C., 79, 98, 153, 155,
    245
Chase, P., 39, 41, 42, 43, 185
Cheng, L., 54, 153
Chess, S., 174
Chomsky, N., 6, 69
Christensen, J. N., 195, 197
Christensen, K., 17, 30, 126, 127,
    128, 153, 206
Christiansen, J. B., 12, 23, 27, 53, 57,
    58, 60, 125, 142, 143, 144, 158,
    160, 164, 184, 202, 204, 208,
    213, 214, 223, 224, 238, 251
Chuong, D., 249
Church, M. W., 43
Churchill, A., 167
Cicchetti, D., 176
Clarcq, J., 215
Clark, J., 39, 42, 60, 61, 104
Clark, M., 82, 87
Cohen, H., 191, 192
Cohen, M. M., 43, 44, 48, 49, 50, 242
Cohen, N., 139, 142, 143, 144
Cohen, O. P., 210
Cohn, J., 31
Coleman, H., 187
Collazo, J., 54

Collins, F., 41
Collins, W. A., 159
Condon, M., 55
Conrad, R., 6, 93
Corbett, C., 127, 173, 183, 184, 187, 191, 192, 196, 198, 210, 237
Corey, D., 49, 50
Corina, D., 23, 82, 194
Corker, M., 20, 185, 187, 221, 225, 228, 230, 231
Cornett, O., 139, 145, 148
Coster, W. J., 176
Courtin, C., 82, 87
Craft, A., 83, 86
Creech, C., 131
Critchfield, B., 243
Croneberg, C. G., 6, 95
Crouch, B., 16, 20, 25, 114, 144, 202, 206, 210, 214, 238
Crowe, T., 192
Crowley, M., 165
Crystal, D., 93
Csikszentmihalyi, M., 182
Cummins, C., 99, 102, 138, 152, 153, 227
Curtiss, S., 78

D'Elia, L., 190
Dahle, A., 41
Daigle-King, B., 8, 9, 10
Daniels, M., 107
Danturthi, R., 92
Davila, R., 54
Davis, F. E, 193
Davis, J., 183, 184
Davis, L., 223, 224, 225
Davis, R., 4
Dean, R., 234, 235, 236
Decoufle, P., 17, 53
Deignan, E., 58, 169
Delgado, G., 206
Delk, M., 56
Deming, W. E., 8
Denmark, J., 8, 9
Denoyelle, F., 46
Desselle, D., 188
DeVilliers, P., 92, 96, 97
Devlin, L., 44, 51
Dew, D., 195
Deyo, D. A., 166
Diaz, J. A., 206
Dickinson, J., 196
Diefendorf, A., 39, 52, 57, 63

Dobosh, P., 175, 176, 186, 196, 197
Doris, J., 176
Doyle, J., 138
Drasgow, E., 95, 150
Drolsbaugh, M., 227
DuBois, J., 107
Dunbar, J., 17, 215
Duncan, E., 30, 107
Dunn, C., 55

Eastabrooks, W., 138
Eckenrode, J., 176
Eckhardt, E., 194
Egeland, B., 176
Eichen, E. B., 23
Einhorn, K., 43
Eldis, F., 43
Eldredge, N., 54, 199, 237
Elliot, L., 104
Emerson, R. W., 1
Emmorey, K., 70, 71, 76, 77, 78, 190, 194, 245
Epstein, L., 42, 43
Epstein, S., 41
Erikson, E., 167, 170, 171
Erting, C. J., 24, 26, 30, 32, 34, 68, 69, 76, 161, 226, 237
Essex, E., 165
Evans, L., 149, 191
Everhart, V., 87, 97, 104
Ewoldt, C., 92, 98, 101

Farber, E. A., 159
Feldman, J., 17, 215
Fernandez, P., 174
Feuerstein, R., 83, 84, 86
Finkelstein, D., 30, 107
Fischel-Ghodsian, N., 42, 48
Fischer, C. H., 30, 186
Fischgrund, J., 54, 127
Flexer, C., 144
Foster, S., 169
Fowler, K., 41
Francis, P., 104
Franklin, T., 10
Freeman, R. D., 174, 191
French, H., 25
French, M., 149
Fried, J., 216
Friedburg, I., 186
Friedlander, H., 52
Friere, P., 135
Frisby, C., 190

Fujikawa, S., 17, 29

Galenson, E., 161
Gallimore, L., 97, 99, 100, 245
Gannon, C. L., 31
Gannon, J., 33, 176, 204, 207, 211, 213, 214, 216
Garbarino, J., 175
Gardner, E., 17, 215
Geers, A., 142
Geisinger, K., 190
Gentry, M., 106
Gerber, S. E., 42, 43, 249, 250
Gersten, M. S., 176
Gerton, J., 187
Geyer, P., 24, 184, 214, 215
Gianelli, D., 212, 236
Gillece, J., 9
Glickman, N., 185, 186, 198, 227
Goldberg, D., 144, 162
Goldin-Meadow, S., 78
Goldsmith, H., 159
Goldstein, M., 194
Gonsoulin, T., 21, 22, 23
Goodwyn, S., 68, 69
Gorenflo, D., 212
Gorlin, R. J., 43, 44, 48, 49, 50, 242
Gould, S., 3
Grant, N., 187, 199, 210
Gray, C., 87, 98
Green, G., 46, 48
Greenberg, J., 107
Greenberg, M., 113, 114, 160, 163, 165, 167, 169, 170
Greenberg, S., 217
Grenier, J., 190
Grinker, R. R., 8
Grosjean, F., 22, 35, 136, 151, 227
Groth-Marnat, G., 189, 190, 193, 194
Grundfast, K., 249
Grushkin, D., 28, 70, 96, 98, 137
Gunnar, M., 159
Gustason, G., 146
Guthman, D., 9, 196, 243
Gutman, V., 30, 173, 175, 176, 183, 184, 191, 192, 196, 197, 209, 223, 237
Guttmann, E., 175

Hairston, E., 17, 206, 210
Hakuta, K., 152, 155
Hall, J., 39

Hall, S., 211
Handler, L., 193
Hansen, V. C., 8
Hardy, M. P., 40, 141
Hardy, S. T., 118
Hardy, W. G., 40
Hardy-Braz, S., 183, 192, 193
Hari, R., 194
Harker, L., 49, 50
Harman, C., 159
Harmer, L., 205, 212, 236
Harter, S., 184, 187
Harvey, M., 158, 198, 227, 229, 231
Haskins, B., 9, 196, 197
Haskins, H. L., 40
Hastings, J. O., 174
Hauser, P., 223, 236
Heath, S. B., 101
Helfand, M., 4
Hernandez, M., 54, 198
Herrera, G., 41
Hewison, J., 51
Hickok, G., 79, 244
Hintermair, M., 54, 58
Hoffmeister, R., 11, 19, 56, 111, 113,
    115, 116, 130, 153, 172, 177,
    192, 211, 215, 229, 227, 231,
    232, 237, 245
Holcomb, M., 213, 214, 237
Holden-Pitt, L., 124, 169, 206
Hollingsworth, T., 30, 107
Holowka, S., 80, 245
Holzrichter, A., 75
Homer, C., 4
Horton, M., 48
Hosie, J., 87, 98
Howell, R., 92
Hsu, D., 92
Hui, C. H., 191
Humphries, T., 11, 15, 19, 22, 26,
    30, 127, 201, 226
Hyde, M., 95
Hynes, M. O., 161

Israel, J., 44, 51

Jacobs, R., 24, 193
Jacobvitz, D., 176
Jankowski, K., 22, 25, 30, 204, 206,
    210, 229, 230, 237
Jatho, J., 55, 131
Jensema, C., 92, 106
Johnson, B., 6

Johnson, R. C., 24, 34, 126, 130, 191,
    226
Jones, B. E., 121, 122
Jones, E., 191, 192
Jordan, D., 131, 215
Jordan, I. K., 12, 109, 247
Jordan, J., 212
Jourmaki, V., 194

Kachman, W., 118
Kagan, J., 187
Kallman, K. J., 8
Kallmann, F., 8
Kamman, T., 162
Kampfe, C., 54
Kaplan, E., 161
Karchmer, M., 39, 82,
    174
Katz, C., 31, 33, 34
Katz, D., 9
Kauffman, J. M., 111
Kaufman, J., 176
Keane, K., 83, 84, 85, 165
Keats, B., 49, 50, 51
Kelly, R., 96
Kerstetter, P., 39
Kersting, S., 223
Kestenbaum, R., 159
Kidd, D., 100
King, L., 182
Kirtzer-White, 54
Kitson, N., 198
Klein, H., 198
Klima, E., 69, 70, 72, 76, 79, 244
Kluwin, T., 56, 110, 118, 120, 123,
    185
Knutson, J., 177
Koester, L. S., 158, 161, 162, 165,
    166
Koh, S., 6
Kosslyn, S. M., 194
Krapf, G., 84
Krashen, S., 78
Krauss, M., 165
Kretchmer, R., 136
Kricos, P., 53
Kroger, J., 173
Kurtzer-White, E., 53
Kusche, C., 167, 170
Kuzel, A., 212

LaBarre, A., 176
LaFromboise, T., 187

Laird, M., 176
Lane, H., 10, 11, 19, 23, 25, 27, 30,
    52, 56, 70, 111, 113, 115, 116,
    130, 168, 172, 173, 177, 183,
    192, 202, 203, 210, 211, 214,
    215, 222, 228, 232, 237, 245
Lang, H., 23, 33, 204, 209, 213
Langholtz, D., 212, 237
LaSasso, C., 72, 93, 94, 95, 97, 131,
    145
Lederberg, A. R., 96, 160, 161, 165,
    169
Leigh, I. W., 7, 9, 20, 23, 30, 53, 55,
    56, 57, 58, 60, 112, 125, 142,
    143, 144, 158, 160, 164, 169,
    172, 173, 183, 184, 185, 186,
    191, 192, 193, 196, 197, 206,
    208, 223, 224, 237, 251, 252
LeNard, J. M., 130, 216
Lenneberg, E., 6, 78
Levanen, S., 194
Levine, E., 2, 3–4, 192
Lewis, J., 206, 237
Lichtenstein, E., 70, 94
Lieu, T., 4
Lillo-Martin, D., 82
Linton, S., 225
Lipton, D., 194
Litchenstein, E., 93
Livingston, S., 89
Loew, R., 54, 195, 198
Long, M., 78
Lopez, J., 215
Lopez-Holzman, G., 128
Lucas, C., 22, 71, 72, 73, 138, 145,
    150
Luckner, J. L., 119
Lukomski, J., 93
Luterman, D., 53, 54, 55
Lybarger, R., 9
Lyons, C., 99
Lytle, R., 129, 172

MacCollin, M., 48
Mackelprang, R., 203
Madriz, J. J., 41
Makowsky, B., 10, 26
Malewska-Peyre, H., 184
Malkin, S. F., 174
Maller, S., 154
Malony, H. N., 193
Malzkuhn, M., 202
Marazita, M., 39, 43, 44, 45, 47

Marcia, J. E., 172, 173
Marcus, A., 186
Marks, S., 81
Marschark, M., 3, 23, 58, 82, 83, 92, 93, 97, 98, 111, 113, 115, 136, 137, 141, 160, 163, 166, 168, 169, 170, 172, 183, 191
Martin, D., 83, 86
Martin, F., 39, 42, 60, 61
Marvin, R. S., 160
Mason, J., 101
Mather, S., 102
Mauk, G. W., 175
Mauk, P. P., 175
Maxon, A., 57, 162, 166
Maxwell, M., 138
Maxwell-McCaw, D. L., 172, 186, 188, 223
Mayberry, R., 23, 98, 153, 245
Mayer, C., 99, 150
McAnally, P., 126
McCann, R., 106
McCracken, G., 42
McGhee, H., 192
McIntosh, R., 100
McKee, B., 104
McKee, C., 95, 151
McKnight, J., 107
McPhilips, H., 4
Meador, H., 212
Meadow, K., 6, 10
Meadow-Orlans, K. P., 30, 56, 146, 158, 161, 163, 165, 166, 184
Meath-Lang, B., 33, 213
Mebane, D. L., 193
Meier, R., 70, 75, 76, 77
Mencher, L. S., 42, 43
Mertens, D., 53, 55, 57, 146
Metzger, M., 72, 93, 94, 95, 145, 150, 235
Meyberry, R., 79
Meyer, G., 190
Meyerhof, W., 39, 40
Middleton, A., 51
Miles, B., 108
Miller, D., 225
Miller, K., 129, 217, 247
Miller, R., 161
Mindel, E., 6, 8, 10, 23, 141
Miner, I., 208, 237
Miner, L., 49
Mitrushina, M., 190
Mobley, C. E., 160

Moeller, M., 55
Mogford, K., 72, 80
Mohay, H., 146, 165, 166, 184
Moll, L., 23, 24, 138, 151
Monteiro, B., 217
Montgomery, G., 6
Montoya, L., 194
Moog, J., 142
Moores, D. F., 5, 6, 11, 23, 39, 43, 55, 111, 112, 113, 116, 124, 129, 130, 131, 145, 158, 163, 164, 175, 193, 228, 229
Morere, D., 173, 183, 184, 191, 192, 196
Morford, J., 79, 98, 153, 245
Morrison, M., 163, 164
Morton, D., 54, 195, 197
Moulton, R., 131
Mounty, J., 137, 152
Mueller, R., 51
Muller, C., 242
Munro-Ludders, B., 212–213
Musselman, C., 166–167
Myers, R., 197
Myklebust, H., 3
Mylander, C., 78

Nager, G., 41, 49
Needham, C., 165
Neville, H., 194
Newport, E., 70, 76, 77, 152
Ng, M., 41, 49
Niparko, J., 41, 48, 49
Nishimura, H., 194
Nover, S., 23, 24, 99, 103, 122, 123, 129, 149, 150, 151, 153, 154, 229, 232, 235
Nowak, C. B., 49

O'Grady, L., 82
O'Grady, M., 82
Oberkotter, M., 203
Ogden, P., 37
Olkin, R., 203
Olson, K., 146
Ouellette, S., 193

Padden, C., 11, 19, 22, 26, 27, 30, 95, 96, 153, 186, 201, 211, 226, 245, 248
Pal Kapur, Y., 39, 40, 41, 42, 43
Papousek, H., 161, 162
Pappas, D., 42

Parasnis, I., 82, 175, 187
Pass, R., 41
Paul, P., 95, 150
Payne, J. A., 98
Pearlmutter, L., 188
Penn, A., 9
Peters, C., 26, 31
Peterson, C., 87
Petitto, L., 27, 75, 76, 80, 92, 245
Pfetzing, D., 146, 148
Pillard, R., 25
Pinker, S., 69, 70, 152
Pinnell, G., 99
Pipp-Siegel, S., 55, 161
Poizner, H., 69, 70, 72, 76, 79, 244
Pollard, E., 234
Pollard, R., 3, 9, 183, 192, 193, 195, 196, 197, 198, 229, 233, 234, 235, 236
Power, D., 74, 92
Preston, P., 56, 184
Prezbindowski, A. K., 161, 165
Prezioso, C., 161
Price, J. M., 176,
Prickett, H., 30, 107
Prinz, P., 79, 98, 153, 155, 245

Quigley, S., 74, 92, 97, 98, 136

Raifman, L., 5, 205, 217, 226
Rainer, J., 8, 9
Ralston, E., 212
Ramirez, W., 197
Ramsey, C. L., 95, 96, 111, 112, 153, 245
Ramsey, S., 106
Randall, K., 126
Rayman, J., 211
Reeder, L., 100
Rehkemper, G., 174
Reich, E., 49
Reichman, A., 215
Remvig, J., 8
Reschly, D. J., 115
Rich, S., 176
Rickards, F., 166, 167
Rittenhouse, B., 126, 210
Robins, C., 191, 193
Robinson, L., 8, 195
Rodda, M., 227
Rodriguez, Y., 27, 75, 102
Romig, L., 96
Rossini, P., 69

Rothstein, A., 161
Rovins, M. R., 129
Roy, C., 235
Ruiz, R., 229
Russell, D., 126
Ruth, R., 212, 226, 237
Rutherford, S., 82

Sabo, H., 81
Salenius, S., 194
Salsgiver, R., 203
Samar, V., 82, 175
Sandberg, K., 9, 196
Sandoval, J., 190
Sass-Lehrer, M., 53, 55, 57, 115, 146
Sathe, K., 82
Savoy-McAdory, M., 197
Scanlan, J., 176
Scarcella, R., 78
Schafer, G., 48
Schein, J., 17, 18, 25, 56, 204, 206,
     207, 210, 211, 213, 233, 241
Scheuneman, J., 190
Schick, B., 121, 123
Schildroth, A., 40
Schleper, D., 99
Schlesinger, H., 10, 167, 168, 172
Schonbeck, J., 7, 196, 197
Schott, L. A., 176
Schreiber, F., 33
Schroedel, J., 24, 184, 214, 215
Schuchman, J., 32, 213, 224
Schwaber, M., 39
Schwanenflugel, P., 87
Schwartz, C., 48
Schwartz, N. S., 193
Scotch, R., 204, 225
Scott-Olson, K., 53, 55, 57
Sculerati, N., 39
Sedey, A., 55, 161
Seeman, J., 182
Seligman, M., 182
Seltzer, M., 165
Shapiro, J., 203, 204, 225
Sharkawy, S., 92
Sheldon, K., 182
Sheridan, M., 157, 159
Shimizi, H., 40
Shinkawa, H., 44
Siedlecki, T., 9, 193, 196
Siegel, L., 111, 112, 117, 124, 125,
     217, 252
Siegel, M., 87

Singleton, J., 16, 27, 28, 154
Siparsky, N., 249
Slattery, W., 39
Smith, D., 24, 34, 226
Smith, L., 17, 206, 210
Smith, M., 131, 132
Smith, M. D., 119
Smith, R., 46, 47, 48
Smith, S., 48, 49, 50
Smith, T., 187
Smith, Z., 97, 102
Smith-Gray, S., 161, 162
Snider, B., 24, 34, 226
Snyder, L., 97
Sonnenstrahl, A., 33, 205
Sorensen, G., 126
Spencer, P., 96, 137, 140, 143, 166
Spragins, A., 5
Stansfield, M., 198
Stedt, J., 145
Stein, L., 41, 42
Steinberg, A., 8, 54, 194, 195, 198
Steinkemp, M., 74, 92
Sterritt, M., 185
Stewart, D., 18, 19, 20, 21, 22, 24, 27,
     28, 29, 30, 31, 56, 110, 118, 120,
     123, 211
Stewart, L., 10, 230, 231
Stinson, M., 104, 112, 117, 118, 169,
     170, 172, 185, 252
Stokie, W., 67
Stokoe, W., 6, 26, 69, 71, 95,
     151
Strand, V. C., 176
Strauss, M., 40
Strong, M., 153
Stroufe, L. A., 159, 176
Stuckless, R., 6
Sue, D., 185
Sue, D. W., 185
Suggs, T., 207, 228
Sullivan, P., 176–177
Sullivan, V. J., 195, 198
Sulzen, L., 100
Supalla, S., 26, 71, 95, 138, 151, 154
Sussman, A., 7, 181, 183, 184, 188,
     198, 246
Sussman, K., 128
Swisher, V., 162, 184

Tajfel, H., 171
Tannenbaum, A., 84
Terwilliger, L., 162

Thompson, D., 4, 250
Tinley, S., 48
Tittle, M., 16, 27, 28
Toriello, H. V., 43, 44, 48, 49, 50, 242
Traxler, C., 108, 247
Triandis, H. C., 191
Trumbetta, S., 9, 196
Trybus, R., 39, 198
Trzepacz, P., 195
Tucker, B., 205
Tucker, S., 53
Turner, J., 198
Turrentine-Jenkins, 5

Usami, S., 44
Uutela, K., 194

Valli, C., 22, 71, 72, 73, 138, 145, 150
Van Camp, G., 46, 47, 48
Van Cleve, J., 16, 20, 25, 31, 114,
     144, 202, 206, 210, 213–214,
     238
van Hoek, K., 82
Van Naarden, K., 17, 53
Veltri, D., 198
Vernon, M., 1, 2, 3, 5, 6, 7, 8, 9, 10,
     23, 26, 28, 29, 30, 40, 41, 42, 43,
     45, 46, 47, 51, 53, 55, 68, 72, 79,
     80, 82, 98, 106, 107, 141, 142,
     145, 146, 148, 153, 160, 176,
     183, 187, 190, 192, 195, 196,
     205, 216, 217, 226, 229
Volterra, V., 68, 69, 76
Vygotsky, L. S., 70, 84, 91, 166, 252

Wagner, E. E., 4
Wall, S., 159
Walter, G., 215
Waltzman, S., 139, 142, 143, 144
Wampler, D., 146, 149
Warren, F., 8
Waterman, A. S., 185
Waters, E., 159
Watkin, P., 53
Watt, J. D., 193
Wax, T., 7, 197, 209
Weinberg, N., 185
Welch, O. M., 128
Welkowitz, J., 191, 193
Wells, G., 99, 150
Werkhaven, J., 39
Werry, J. S., 174
White, B., 29

Wilbur, R., 21, 23, 70, 96, 98, 103, 153, 155
Willems, P., 39, 43, 44, 45
Willis, R., 7
Wilson Seeley, J., 175
Wilson, A., 131
Wilson, H., 213
Wilson, M. P., 44, 51
Wilson, T., 95
Winefield, R., 10, 141
Winston, 122, 123, 124

Witte, T., 212
Wix, T., 95, 151, 154
Wood, S., 213, 214, 237
Woodroffe, T., 212
Woodward, J., 226
Wright, M. H., 30, 206
Wu, C., 187, 199, 210

Yarger, C. C., 119
Yoshinaga-Itano, C., 55, 97, 137, 138, 161

Zakzouk, S., 41
Zawolkow, E., 146
Zazove, P., 212
Zhang, Z., 83, 86
Zigler, E., 176
Zmijewski, G., 92
Zwalkow, E., 148
Zwiebel, A., 210

SUBJECT INDEX

Abusive situations with deaf children, 175–177
Academic learning, 83–87
Adaptive devices, 25
Alcoholism in deaf people, 9
Alerting devices, 65
American Association of the Deaf-Blind (AADB), 208
American Sign Language (ASL), 6, 11
  competency and higher reading scores, 98
  grammar vs. English grammar, 70–75
  graphemes, 93–94
  growing recognition and acceptance of, 244–246
  and spoken language acquisition, 77
Americans with Disabilities Act (ADA), 4, 9, 204
Amplification systems/tools, 57–58, 64–65
Analog hearing aids, 65
Artists in deaf community, 33
ASL (see American Sign Language)
Assistive listening devices (ALDs), 65
Association of Late-Deafened Adults (ALDA), 208
Attachment theory, 159–163
Attitudes within deaf community, 237–238
Audiogram sample form, 62
Audiology, basics of, 60–65
Auditory aids, 20, 57–58
Auditory technologies, 103
Auditory-oral programs, 138–139, 140
Auditory-verbal programs, 138, 140
Auditory-vocal paths of language, 75–77
Autosomal dominant inheritance, 44–45

Autosomal recessive inheritance, 45–47
Auxiliary aids, 25

Babbling by deaf babies, 75–76, 92
Bilingualism, 22, 80
  and intelligence, 81–82
  and reading English as a second language, 102–103
  as teaching approach, 150–155
Bill of Rights for deaf and hard-of-hearing children, 132
Brain-environment relationship, 79–81
Branchial-oto-renal syndrome, 48

C-Print system, 104
Charter schools, 116–117
Child abuse, 175–177
Child development and deafness, 165–173
Childhood bilingualism, 80
Childhood psychological issues, 157–179
  abuse, 175–177
  attachment, 159–163
  deafness and childhood development, 165–173
  early intervention programs, 163–165
  parent/child relationship, 158–163
  psychological evaluation, 177–178
  psychopathology, 173–175
Closed-captioned TV, 104
Cochlear Implant Association, Inc. (CIAI), 208
Cochlear implantation, 57–58, 65, 139, 142–144
  advances in, 249, 250–251
Cognitive development and play, 166–167
Cognitive functioning of deaf people, 81–87

Cognitive skills assessment in deaf children, 178
Collaboration between classroom teacher and special education teacher, 120
Communication Access Real-Time Translation (CART), 104
Communication:
  evolving to language, 68–75, 90–92
  technologies, 103
Communities of deaf people, 33–34
Computer-assisted note-taking (CAN) systems, 104
Computer-assisted psychological assessment, 194
Congenital toxoplasmosis, 42
Connexin 26 gene, 46–47
Consultation services by itinerant teachers, 119
Contact Signing, 22
Court decisions and legislation regarding deafness, 4
Critical period hypothesis, 78–79
Cued speech, 95, 145
  definition of, 72
Customs and values of Deaf culture, 26
Cytomegalovirus (CMV), 40–41

Day schools, 116
Deaf adoptive and foster children, 28–29
Deaf adults, psychological issues, 181–199
  identity, 184–187
  "normalcy," 183–184
  positive psychology, 182
  psychological assessment, 188–195
  psychologically healthy, 184
  psychopathology, 195–199
  self-concept, 187–188
Deaf adults, sociological issues, 201–218

deaf clubs/organizations, 206–212
ethnic deaf groups, 210
health care, 212–213
legal issues, 216–217
religious groups, 210–211
sociopolitical implications, 203–206
specialized organizations, 208–209
sports, 211–212
work world, 213–216
Deaf children:
with deaf parents, 161, 167
with disabilities, 107–108
with hearing parents, 23, 27, 80, 159–163
Deaf clubs, 211
Deaf community, 15–35
anthropological view, 25
belief system, 23–25
changes in, 246–248
demographics, 17–18, 19
medical/disability model, 20–22, 202–203
membership, 27–30
sociolinguistic/cultural model, 22
terminology, 18–20
transmission of Deaf culture, 30–33
values and customs, 26
Deaf culture, 10–12
Deaf and Hard of Hearing Section (DHHS), 207
Deaf identity, 184–187
Deaf Latino organizations, 210, 256
Deaf organizations, 206–212, 255–256
Deaf parents:
of deaf children, 167
during diagnosis of children, 56
Deaf President Now movement, 203–206
Deaf Pride movement, 12
Deaf professionals:
opportunities for, 7–8, 11–12, 213
role of, 173
Deaf Seniors of America (DSA), 209
Deaf studies programs, 33

Deaf teachers, training, 130
Deaf Women United (DWU), 209
Deaf-blindness, 29–30, 49–50, 107, 237
Deaf-hearing relationships, 221–239
how deaf see hearing, 226–227
how hearing see deaf, 225–226
interpreter issues, 233–237
oppression, 228, 230–231
perceptions, influence of, 224
professional attitudes, 227–230
relating in healthy ways, 231–233
Deafness as a disability, 12
distinguished from disability, 225–226
Decoding words, 95
Diagnosis of deafness, 38, 52–58, 158–159
Differences among the Deaf, 30
Digital hearing aids, 65
Diversity within deaf community, 237, 248
Drama groups and actors in deaf community, 31–32
Dual diagnoses, 9

Early conversation skills, 90–92
Early intervention programs, 113–114, 163–165
Education for All Handicapped Children Act, 4
Education of deaf children, 109–133
charter schools, 116–117
day schools, 116
early intervention programs, 113
future goals, 251–253
Individuals with Disabilities Education Act, 111–113
international deaf education, 131–132
multicultural issues, 126–128
placement issues, 110–111, 124–125
public schools, 117–124
residential schools, 114–116
school placement issues, 113–125
teacher-training issues, 128–131
testing issues, 125–126

Educational interpreting, 120–124
Electronic devices for communication and signaling, 25
Emotional and behavioral disorders, 174
English vs. ASL, 70–75
Environment and development of deaf child, 4
Error analysis in reading, 101
Erythroblastosis fetalis, 42
Ethnic deaf groups, 210, 255–256
Etiology (see Hearing loss, causes of)
Eye gaze and eye contact during interaction, 162
Eye movements of captioned deaf viewers, 101

Fetal alcohol syndrome (FAS), 42–43
Finger-babbling, 75–76, 92
Finger-spelling, 6, 92
for children with disabilities, 107
early attempts, 93–94

Genetic causes of deafness, 43–44
Genetic counseling, 50–52
Genetic research, 249–250
Genetic syndromes involving deafness, 48–50
Genetic transmission of deafness, 44–50
German measles, 39–40
Gestural behaviors, 68–70
of infants, 74–75
Grammar of English, difficulties in, 97–98
Grief after diagnosis, 53–54

Hard-of-hearing people of deaf or hearing parents, 28
Health care issues of deaf adults, 212–213
Hearing:
measurement of, 61–64
mechanics of, 60
Hearing aids, 57–58, 64–65, 142–143
Hearing-deaf relationships (see Deaf-hearing relationships)
Hearing loss, causes of, 38–52
genetic, 43–50

nongenetic, 39–43
Hearing loss, types of, 61
Hearing parents of deaf children, 158, 167
Hearing people in deaf families, 27–28
Herpes simplex virus infection, 41
High school drop-outs, 215
High-stakes testing, 126
Historical perspectives, 1–13
Human immunodeficiency virus (HIV), 41

Iconicity, definition of, 72
Identity of deaf adults, 184–187
achievement of, 172–173
Inclusion:
vs. mainstreaming, 112, 117–118
philosophy of, 118
Individuals with Disabilities Education Act (IDEA), 111–113
Infections as cause of deafness, 39–42
Instrumental Enrichment (IE), 84–85
Intellectual abilities of deaf people, 81–87
Interactive multimedia, 104–105
Interlanguage grammar, 102–103
International deaf education, 131–132
Interpreted education, 120–124
Intuitive parenting, definition of, 162
IQ tests, 2
Itinerant teachers, 119–120

Jervell and Lange-Nielsen syndrome, 48

Labels of different perspectives, 18–20
Language acquisition by deaf children, 70–81 (*see also* Language to literacy)
Language acquisition device (LAD), 69
Language development of deaf children, 69–70
foundations for, 165–166
Language learning and language teaching, 135–156
bilingual approaches, 150–155

communication competence, 136–138
language-mixing, 144–150
monolingual approaches, 138–144
Language to literacy, 89–108
early conversation skills, 90–92
reading process, 92–101
sociocultural processes, 101–108
Language-mixing, 137–138, 144–150
definition of, 145
Language paths, 75–77
Language-teaching approaches, 98–100
Late-deafened people, 29
Late-onset hearing loss, 41
Learning disabilities and deaf children, 175
Learning Potential Assessment Device (LPAD), 83–84
Legislation and court decisions regarding deafness, 4, 216–217
Linguistic Interdependence model, 99
Lip-reading, 6, 10
Literacy:
and content subjects, 100–101
and language teaching, 98–100
and reading, 92–101
Literature of Deaf people, 31
Low reading levels, 23–24

Mainstreaming:
vs. inclusion, 112, 117–118
philosophy of, 118
Maternal stress, 161
Mediated learning experiences, definition of, 84–85
Medical/disability model, 20–22, 203
Meningitis, 41–42
Mental health services for deaf people, 195–198
advances in, 242–244
Mental illness and deaf people, 2–3, 8–10
Mental status examinations, 195
Metacognitive abilities, 83–87
Metalinguistic awareness, definition of, 81
Minority teachers, training, 131

Miscue (error) analysis, 101
Mitrochondial inheritance, 47–48
Molecular genetics, advances in, 249–250
Monolingual approaches in teaching, 138–144
Morphology, definition of, 72
Multicultural issues, 126–128, 187, 198–199

National Asian Deaf Congress, 210, 256
National Association of the Deaf (NAD), 21, 132, 206–207
National Black Deaf Advocates, 210
National Fraternal Society for the Deaf (NFSD), 207
National Theater for the Deaf, 31–32
Neurofibromatosis Type 2 (NF-2), 48, 65
Neuropsychology, 194–195
Newborn hearing screening, 52–53, 137, 158–159, 250
Newborn Infant Hearing Screening and Intervention Act, 4
No Child Left Behind Act, 125
Noise-induced hearing loss, 43
Nongenetic causes of deafness, 39–43
"Normalcy" of deafness, 183–184

Oppression, 228, 230–231
Oral-manual controversy, 141
Oral-only education, 6
Organizations for Deaf culture, 31
Ototoxic drugs, 42

Parent-child relationship, 158–163
Parents using sign language, 23
Peer socialization, 30
Pendred syndrome, 49
Perceptions of deaf people, influence of, 224
Phonological coding, 94
Phonology of words, 71–72
Play and early cognitive development, 166–167
Political involvement of deaf people, historically, 204
Positive psychology, 182

Prematurity as cause of deafness, 43
Professionals:
    attitudes of, 227–230
    opportunities for deaf, 7–8, 11–12
    training of, 7
Promoting Alternative Thinking Strategies (PATH), 170–171
Psychiatry and mental health, 8–10
Psychological assessment of deaf adults, 188–195
Psychological considerations after diagnosis, 56–58
Psychological evaluation of deaf children, 177–178
Psychological impact of deafness, 3
Psychological issues during childhood (*see* Childhood psychological issues)
Psychological maladjustment problems among deaf children, 174
Psychologically healthy deaf adults, 184
Psychologists and educational policy, 6–7
Psychopathology:
    in childhood, 173–175
    of deaf adults, 195–199
Psychosocial development of child, 167–173
Public school settings for deaf children, 5, 21
    placement alternatives, 117–124

Rainbow Alliance of the Deaf (RAD), 209
Reading by eye/reading by ear, 92–93
Reading process, 92–101
    comprehension, 97–98
    language-teaching approaches, 98–100
    progression development, 96–97
    readiness, 91
    word recognition, 93–96
Registry of Interpreters for the Deaf (RID), 120–121
Rehabilitation Act of 1973, 4
Religious groups for deaf people, 210–211

Residential schools, 114–116
Resource room classes, 118
RH factor, 42
Rubella, 39–40

Screening for hearing loss, 52–53
Second language acquisition, 78–79, 152
Second language learners, 102
Self-concept/Self-esteem:
    of deaf adults, 187–188
    of deaf children, 168–173
Self Help for Hard of Hearing People, Inc., 209
Sex-linked recessive conditions of deafness, 47
Sign language, 6–7, 9–10, 69
    for deaf children with disabilities, 107
    historical change in, 72
    interpreter issues, 233–237
Sign-meaning-print connection, 94–95
Signing avatars, 105–106
Social competency, 168–169
Socialization and residential schools, 115
Sociocultural processes via language and literacy learning, 101–108
Socioemotional assessment of deaf adults, 192–193
Sociolinguistic/cultural model, 22, 203
Speaking-signing bilinguals, 80
Special education teachers, 119–120
Special populations using sign language, 107–108
Speech-reading, 141–142
Speech-to-text transcription systems, 104
Spelling skills, 96–97
Sports organizations for deaf people, 211–212
Standardized tests, 125–126
Stickler syndrome, 49
Substance abuse diagnoses, 196
Surgical auditory brainstem implants, 65
Surgically implanted hearing devices, 65

Teacher-training issues, 128–131
    programs for deaf, 11–12
Teaching reading to deaf students (graphic), 100
Team teaching classroom, 120
Technology:
    changes in, 253–254
    in the classroom, 103–106
Telecommunications for the Deaf, Inc., 209
Terminology, 18–20
Testing in education, 125–126
Theory of mind, 86–87
Total communication, definition of, 145
Transmission of Deaf culture, 30–33
Treacher-Collins syndrome, 49
Tympanometry, definition of, 63

Usher syndrome, 49–50

Values and customs of Deaf culture, 26
Videoconferencing, 105
Vision, loss of, 50
Visual alerts, 25
Visual communication strategies, 165
Visual teaching techniques, 98–99
Visual technologies, 20
Vocabulary difficulties, 97–98

Waardenburg syndrome, 50
Web-based courses with video-streaming, 105
Websites of organizations, 219, 255–258
Williams syndrome, 79, 80–81
Word processing by eye or ear, 92–93
Word recognition, 93–96
Work world of deaf adults, 213–216
World Federation of the Deaf (WFD), 207
Writing sample, 96

X-linked recessive inheritance, 47

Zone of proximal development, 91